Recent Advances in Ophthalmology—11

Recent Advances in Ophthalmology—11

Editors

HV Nema MS
Former Professor and Head
Department of Ophthalmology
Banaras Hindu University
Varanasi, Uttar Pradesh, India

Nitin Nema MS DNB
Associate Professor
Department of Ophthalmology
Sri Aurobindo Institute of Medical Sciences
Indore, Madhya Pradesh, India

Editorial Board

JAYPEE BROTHERS MEDICAL PUBLISHERS (P) LTD

New Delhi • London • Philadelphia • Panama

Jaypee Brothers Medical Publishers (P) Ltd

Headquarters

Jaypee Brothers Medical Publishers (P) Ltd
4838/24, Ansari Road, Daryaganj
New Delhi 110 002, India
Phone: +91-11-43574357
Fax: +91-11-43574314
Email: jaypee@jaypeebrothers.com

Overseas Offices

J.P. Medical Ltd.,
83, Victoria Street, London
SW1H 0HW (UK)
Phone: +44-2031708910
Fax: +02-03-0086180
Email: info@jpmedpub.com

Jaypee-Highlights Medical Publishers Inc.
City of Knowledge, Bld. 237, Clayton
Panama City, Panama
Phone: +507-301-0496
Fax: +507-301-0499
Email: cservice@jphmedical.com

Jaypee Brothers Medical Publishers Ltd
The Bourse
111 South Independence Mall East
Suite 835, Philadelphia, PA 19106, USA
Phone: + 267-519-9789
Email: joe.rusko@jaypeebrothers.com

Jaypee Brothers Medical Publishers (P) Ltd
17/1-B Babar Road, Block-B, Shaymali
Mohammadpur, Dhaka-1207
Bangladesh
Mobile: +08801912003485
Email: jaypeedhaka@gmail.com

Jaypee Brothers Medical Publishers (P) Ltd
Shorakhute, Kathmandu
Nepal
Phone: +00977-9841528578
Email: jaypee.nepal@gmail.com

Website: www.jaypeebrothers.com
Website: www.jaypeedigital.com

Inquiries for bulk sales may be solicited at: jaypee@jaypeebrothers.com

Recent Advances in Ophthalmology—11

First Edition: **2013**

ISBN: 978-93-5090-435-0

Printed at: S. Narayan & Sons

Dedicated to

The Loving Memory of
Pratibha

Contributors

A Ramanan MS
Medical Vision Research Foundation
Sankara Nethralaya
Chennai, Tamil Nadu, India

Aditi Gupta MS
Shri Mahavir Vitrcorctinal Service
Medical Research Foundation
Sankara Nethralaya
Chennai, Tamil Nadu, India

Ajit Majji MS
Consultant, LV Prasad Eye Institute
Hyderabad, Andhra Pradesh, India

AK Grover MD (AIIMS)
MNAMS FRCS (Glasgow) FIMSA FICO
Chairman
Department of Ophthalmology
Sir Ganga Ram Hospital
Chairman, Vision Eye Center
New Delhi, India

Alay Banker MS
Banker's Retina Clinic and Retina Centre
Ahmedabad, Gujarat, India

Amol D Kulkarni MS
Department of Ophthalmology and Visual Sciences
University of Wisconsin School of Medicine and Public Health
Madison, WI, USA

Arjit Mithara MS
Glaucoma Service
Aravind Eye Hospital
Tirunelveli, Tamil Nadu, India

Arup Chakrabarty MS
Founder Director
Chakrabarti Eye Care Center
Thiruvananthapuram, Kerala, India

Ashwin Mohan MS
Resident Ophthalmologist
Sankara Nethralaya
Chennai, Tamil Nadu, India

Chandra Sekhar Garudadri MD FRCS
Director
Kallam Anji Reddy Campus
LV Prasad Eye Institute
Hyderabad, Andhra Pradesh, India

C Veerajayalakshmi MS
Aravind Eye Hospital
Madurai, Tamil Nadu, India

Deependra Vikram Singh MD
Consultant Vitreoretinal Surgeon
DRS Northex Eye Institute
New Delhi, India
Sheetla Hospital and Eye Institute Pvt Ltd
Gurgaon, Haryana, India

Dananjay Shukla MS MAMS
Professor of Ophthalmology and Consultant
Retina Vitreous Service, Aravind Eye Hospital and Postgraduate Institute
Madurai, Tamil Nadu, India

Deepa Banker MD
Associate Professor of Pediatrics
NHL Municipal Medical College
VS Hospital
Ahmedabad, Gujarat, India

Frank Joseph Goes MD
Director
Oagchirurgie-Oagheelkunde
Antwerp, Belgium

Harsha L Rao MS DNB
Consultant
VST Glaucoma Center
Kallam Anji Reddy Campus
LV Prasad Eye Institute
Hyderabad, Andhra Pradesh, India

Jyotirmay Biswas MS FNAMS FIC (Path)
Director of Uveitis and Ocular Pathology
Medical and Vision Research Foundation
Sankara, Nethralaya
Chennai, Tamil Nadu, India

Kalpana Narendran MS CMO
Aravind Eye Hospital
Coimbatore, Tamil Nadu, India

Karobi Lahiri Coutinho MS
Consultant Vitreoretinal Surgeon
Bombay Hospital
Institute of Medical Sciences
Mumbai, Maharashtra, India

Lalitha Prajana MD DNB
Consultant Microbiologist
Aravind Eye Hospital and Postgraduate Institute
Madurai, Tamil Nadu, India

Meena Chakrabarty MS
Senior Consultant
Chakrabarti Eye Care Center
Thiruvananthapuram, Kerala, India

Murali Ariga MS
Director
Swamy Eye Clinic
Consultant
Glaucoma Services
MN Eye Hospitals
Senior Consultant
Sundaram Medical Foundation
Chennai, Tamil Nadu, India

Naresh Babu MS
Aravind Eye Hospital
Madurai, Tamil Nadu, India

Neha Sinha MBBS
Department of Ophthalmology
CSM Medical University
Lucknow, Uttar Pradesh, India

Nidhi Relhan MS
Srimati Kannuri Santhamma
Center for Vitreoretinal Diseases
Kallam Anji Reddy Campus
LV Prasad Eye Institute
Hyderabad, Andhra Pradesh, India

N Vankatesh Prajana FRCOphth
Professor
Aravind Eye Hospital and Postgraduate Institute
Madurai, Tamil Nadu, India

Paramdeep Singh MD
Assistant Professor
Department of Radiodiagnosis
Guru Gobind Singh Medical College and Hospital, Baba Farid University of Health Sciences
Faridkot, Punjab, India

Parthopratim Dutta Majumder MS
Junior Consultant
Uveitis and Ocular Pathology
Medical and Vision Research Foundation
Sankara Nethralaya
Chennai, Tamil Nadu, India

Pukhraj Rishi MS
Consultant
Shri Mahavir Vitreoretinal Service
Medical Research Foundation
Sankara Nethralaya
Chennai, Tamil Nadu, India

P Mahesh Shanmugam DO FRCSEd PhD
Head
Department of Vitreoretinal and Ocular Oncology Services
Sankara Eye Hospital
Bengaluru, Karnataka, India

R Ramakrishnan MS
Professor and CMO
Glaucoma Service
Aravind Eye Hospital
Tirunelveli, Tamil Nadu, India

Rajat N Agrawal
Adjunct Professor of Ophthalmology
USC School of Medicine
Los Angeles, California, USA
Founder and Managing Trustee
Retina India, Founder, Retina Global

Rashmin Gandhi
Senior Consultant
Cataract and Neurophthalmology
Sankara Nethralaya
Chennai, Tamil Nadu, India

Rupinderjeet Kaur MD
Senior Resident, Medicine
Guru Gobind Singh Medical College and Hospital, Baba Farid University of Health Sciences
Faridkot, Punjab, India

Sandeep Saxena MS
Professor
Retina Service
Department of Ophthalmology
CSM Medical University
Lucknow, Uttar Pradesh, India

Sandra C Ganesh MS
Aravind Eye Hospital
Coimbatore, Tamil Nadu, India

Shaloo Bageja DNB
Consultant
Department of Ophthalmology
Sir Ganga Ram Hospital
New Delhi, India

Shubhra Goel
Associate Consultant
Department of Orbit and Oculoplasty
Oculofacial Esthetics and Trauma
Sankara Nethralaya
Chennai, Tamil Nadu, India

Sonia S John DNB
Consultant
Chakrabarti Eye Care Center
Thiruvanthapuram, Kerala, India

Subhadra Jalali MS
Associate Director
Srimati Kannuri Santhamma Center for Vitreoretinal Diseases
Kallam Anji Reddy Campus
LV Prasad Eye Institute
Hyderabad, Andhra Pradesh, India

Supreet Singh Juneja MS
Aravind Eye Hospital
Madurai, Tamil Nadu, India

Suresh R Chandra MD
Professor
Department of Ophthalmology and Visual Sciences
University of Wisconsin School of Medicine and Public Health
University Avenue
Madison, Wisconsin, USA

Tarun Sharma MS
Director
Shri Mahavir Vitreoretinal Service
Medical Research Foundation
Sankara Nethralaya
Channai, Tamil Nadu, India

Yog Raj Sharma MS
Professor of Ophthalmology and Vitreoretinal Surgeon
RP Center for Ophthalmic Sciences
All India Institute of Medical Sciences
New Delhi, India

Preface

Advances in the field of ophthalmology are rapid and ever-increasing. It is impossible to cover all advances occurring every year in a small volume. Therefore, like previous series, *Recent Advances of Ophthalmology–11* contains some selected chapters on glaucoma, lens, retina, and systemic diseases. Approximately 50% of chapters deal with diseases of the retina, some are common and some rare. Two out of three editorials are on retina. Retinopathy of prematurity, macular hole, macular dystrophy, central serous chorioretinopathy, proliferative vitreoretinopathy, and retinal vascular occlusion are challenging problems. They may cause loss of vision if not managed properly.

Earlier macular hole was considered untreatable, but now with better surgical techniques, it can be managed with encouraging results. The subject is comprehensively reviewed by Meena and coworkers. Kulkarni and Chandra suggested certain tips to further improve the results of the macular hole surgery.

Readers may find the editorial on artificial retinal implants interesting. The ongoing pilot researches indicate that implantation of biomedical devices can restore some useful vision in patients with RP or AMO. Can the blind see again with the implant? Studies conducted on a large number of cases with long follow-up can provide a valid answer.

Every year, hundreds of research articles are published on the diagnosis and treatment of glaucoma. But how to assess and arrest the progress of glaucoma is not adequately explored, although it is an essential component of glaucoma management. Murali Ariga discussed the problem briefly in Chapter 3 on Progression of Optic Disk and Visual Field Changes in Glaucoma. Halting the progression of glaucomatous damage is likely to retain good visual acuity and visual fields in patients with glaucoma. The progression of glaucoma can be determined by periodic visual field recordings. Both event-based (glaucoma progress analysis) and trend-based analyses (rate of progression) should be determined with the help of Humphrey VF Analyzer. The progression analysis of the retinal nerve fiber layer parameters obtained from time domain OCT should also be taken into consideration. Harsha and Chandra Sekhar emphasized the importance of objective diagnosis of glaucoma with the help of modern technology not in isolation but in combination with complete clinical picture.

Two chapters on collagen disorders—Ocular Involvement in Systemic Rheumatic Diseases and Giant Cell Arteritis—and one on HIV and Opportunistic Infections of eye have been included in this volume. They provide enough insight about close interrelationship between the eye and systemic diseases.

Indeed recent developments in ophthalmology have revolutionized the treatment of eye diseases and considerably improved the quality of life of the patients. Hopefully, the postgraduate students in ophthalmology and general ophthalmic practitioners will find the present series helpful not only in the basic understanding of new developments in the subject but also in day-to-day clinical practice and care of the patients.

HV Nema
Nitin Nema

Acknowledgments

We are indebted to the contributors of *Recent Advances of Ophthalmology—11* for their timely and scholarly contributions.

We would like to record our sincere thanks to Dr Amol Kulkarni, Professor Suresh Chandra, Dr Harsha H Rao, Dr G Chandra Sekhar and Dr Rajat Agarwal for contributing enlightening editorials.

Shri Jitendar P Vij (Group Chairman), Mr Ankit Vij (Managing Director) of M/s Jaypee Brothers Medical Publishers (P) Ltd, New Delhi, India and especially Mr Tarun Duneja (Director- Publishing) deserve our sincere thanks for their continued interest in the publication of the Recent Advances in Ophthalmology series.

Contents

Editorial

Role of Technology in the Diagnosis of Glaucoma and Assessing its Progression

Harsha L Rao, Chandra Sekhar Garudadri

Glaucoma is the second leading cause of blindness worldwide.[1] As clinicians, we not only owe the best possible care to the patients who seek medical help but also a responsibility towards those undetected and improperly treated. The current status of glaucoma care in the world is aptly summarized as follows: more than 50% of glaucoma in the community is undiagnosed (in the developing countries, this would be higher than 90%),[2] more than 50% of those undiagnosed would have seen an eyecare provider in the recent past, more than 50% taking medications do not need them (over treated),[3] and finally 50% of those advised medication do not use them. Missed diagnoses in those previously examined by an eyecare professional, (in the "system") is attributable to lack of comprehensive evaluation and appropriate clinical skills.[4] The recent advances in the imaging of the optic nerve head seek to achieve an early and "objective" diagnosis of glaucoma. One of the reasons for overdiagnosis is using the results of these technologies exclusively and not in the context of complete clinical picture.[5]

DIAGNOSIS

Imaging of the optic nerve head and retinal nerve fiber layer are widely reported to be useful in glaucoma diagnosis. One could (naively) argue that the imaging tests are objective and can be performed easily in uncooperative patients (since they are quick and need little attention) as opposed to standard automated perimetry (SAP) that is the current standard but time consuming and difficult due to the subjective nature of the test. Further, as it is reported that 20–40% retinal ganglion cells could be lost before a visual field defect could be picked up by SAP, these new imaging technologies can theoretically aid in the early diagnosis of glaucoma. This rationale needs not necessarily convert to a clinical reality. The reported sensitivity and specificity of these technologies and their agreement with each other are far from ideal.[6] The sensitivity (ability to diagnose the disease correctly – PID: positive in disease) of the best parameter for each of the imaging technologies at a fixed specificity (NIH: negative in health or ability to declare a normal subject as not having the disease) of 95% (labeling only 5 as abnormal out of hundred normal subjects) varies from 36 to 72%. This means that the imaging technologies fail to diagnose glaucoma in as many as 28–64% of the eyes with established abnormality on SAP. While we perform these investigations with the idea of either establishing or ruling out a disease, we fail to realize that there is a cost-benefit ratio even in diagnostic testing. These tests are expensive, there are risks of overdiagnosis with the attendant effect of labeling, and there are problems with interpretation (the normative database of the machine used for diagnostic classification is often limited to small number of subjects and few ethnicities and hence may not be appropriate to apply for testing patients of all ethnicities). We have reported that the incorporation of the Indian normative database does not improve the diagnostic ability of HRT3.[7]

In addition to the above limitations, bias in the ability of imaging devices to diagnose glaucoma can arises from multiple other sources. Optic disk size has been shown to be a confounder in the diagnostic accuracy of HRT.[8,9] Delineation of the optic disk margin and measurement circle placement have been shown to be confounders in the diagnostic ability of these instruments.[10] Reporting the diagnostic ability in glaucoma patients while using a set of totally normal subjects as controls, also is shown to artifactually inflate the sensitivity of these instruments.[11] This is because a diagnostic test in clinical practice is used in situations, which arouse a suspicion of the disease and not in situations where the diagnosis of a disease is easy to either rule in or rule out by clinical examination.

Garway-Heath and Friedman appropriately stated, "Devices cannot diagnose our patients' conditions, but the findings they provide frequently alter the probability that a subject has a particular condition".[5] Thus devices cannot be a substitute for poor clinical skills but at best a complement to good clinical evaluation. If after a good and comprehensive clinical evaluation, the probability (pre-test probability) of the disease is around 20%, it is futile to perform any diagnostic test, as even a positive result cannot confirm the presence of the disease. On the other hand, if the probability of the disease is about 80% after a good clinical examination (the need for testing is not to diagnose but probably to establish a baseline for follow-up), even a negative test result cannot rule out the disease. It is in the intermediate range, when the probability of disease is around 50% that the diagnostic test result would strongly help in the diagnostic decision. Before ordering a diagnostic test, it is useful to ask ourselves as to how our course of action would change on the basis of the test result. The probability of the disease before and after the diagnostic test can be mathematically calculated using the likelihood ratio (LR) of the test result in consideration. If we want to use the results of the diagnostic tests appropriately, estimating the LR is the best way around. Thus, it is important for us to know the LRs associated with different test results before investing in a new diagnostic test.

The principle behind the use of the likelihood ratios is the calculation of the increase in the probability of a given diagnosis given the prior probability of the disease (based on complete clinical evaluation or the prevalence of the disease) and the result of the diagnostic test with its likelihood ratio. This principle is applicable not only for the diagnosis of a disease but also for any event. This principle in mathematical terms is called the Bayesian theorem. Keeping the mathematics aside, the concept is very intuitive and we keep using this in our daily lives extensively, albeit without the mathematical calculations or the complex terminologies.

For example, on a cloudy day during the rainy season, if it rains we say "it is bound to happen" and if it did not rain, one might say "that was very unlikely" or some such thing. If a 25-year-old healthy, prospective, army recruit ends up with an ST segment change on ECG, one would suspect the test or the machine, as the likelihood of this young, healthy man having ischemic heart disease (IHD) is very low. The same result in a 60-year-old gentleman with diabetes and hypertension with precordial discomfort on exertion would be diagnostic of IHD. The prior probability of IHD is very high in the latter and very low in the former. This explains why the same test result is interpreted differently in different situations.

PROGRESSION

Halting progression of glaucomatous damage during the lifetime of the patient, with minimum effect on the quality of life, is one of the main objectives of any glaucoma treatment. But judging glaucoma progression is a challenging task. Progression of glaucoma is known to occur at variable pace. The untreated arm of the Early Manifest Glaucoma Treatment (EMGT) trial is a great source information of the natural history of glaucoma. It was found in the EMGT trial that untreated normal tension glaucoma in the younger age group had the least rate of progression (never progressing to blindness from normal vision) and pseudoexfoliation glaucoma in the elderly group could progress to blindness from normal vision in a little less than 2 years.[12]

The standard method to detect glaucoma progression is to monitor the visual field (VF) defects periodically for change. Two commonly used approaches to detect change in VF defects over time are the event-based and the trend-based progression analyses. Event-based analysis determines VF progression to be either present or absent depending on a predefined change in the VF parameters. Trend-based analysis provides the actual rate of change of VF parameters. In clinical practice, information from both these analyses is important, because it is not only sufficient to identify VF progression in glaucoma but also to determine the rate of progression, so that the treatment can be more aggressive in patients that progress rapidly. The recently introduced Guided Progression Analysis by the Humphrey VF Analyzer (Carl Zeiss Meditec, Inc. Dublin, CA) provides both an event-based progression analysis and a trend-based analysis on the same printout. The event-based progression analysis, called the glaucoma progression analysis (GPA), is based on the criteria designed to identify VF progression in the EMGT.[13] Trend-based progression analysis is based on the rate of progression (ROP) of the visual function of the eye through a linear regression model using a new global index, visual field index (VFI).[14] The VFI is the aggregate percentage of visual function for a given field at each point where the visual thresholds are estimated. VFI is calculated from pattern deviations in eyes with a mean deviation (MD) of better than –20 dB and from total deviations in eyes with a MD worse than –20 dB. The central points in visual field have more weight than peripheral points. VFI is also shown to be less affected by media opacities like cataract.[15]

Though most of the imaging technologies have both event- and trend-based algorithms to judge structural progression in glaucoma, their usefulness needs to be validated, and there is no consensus on what constitutes a significant structural change clinically. HRT topographic change analysis (TCA) is the most well developed and tested progression detection analysis available for optical imaging techniques. Glaucoma progression algorithms on GDx are called GDx GPA. Time domain OCT also has progression analysis of the RNFL parameters. The agreement between the structural changes of these imaging technologies and the visual field parameters have been reported to be moderate to poor.[16-22] Longitudinal data of the anatomical changes on the imaging technologies subsequently converting to filed changes is available only for HRT from the OHTS.[23] We believe that the gold standard for assessing glaucoma progression continues to be the standard automated perimetry.

In conclusion, in establishing the diagnosis and progression of glaucoma, advances in the imaging technologies of the optic nerve are a complement to a good and comprehensive clinical evaluation and cannot be a substitute. The results of these tests need to be interpreted in the context of the remaining clinical picture and not in isolation.

REFERENCES

1. Quigley HA, Broman AT. The number of people with glaucoma worldwide in 2010 and 2020. *Br J Ophthalmol.* 2006;90:262-7.
2. Vijaya L, George R, Arvind H, et al. Prevalence of angle-closure disease in a rural southern Indian population. *Arch Ophthalmol.* 2006;124:403-9.
3. Vaahtoranta-Lehtonen H, Tuulonen A, Aronen P, et al. Cost effectiveness and cost utility of an organized screening programme for glaucoma. *Acta Ophthalmol Scand.* 2007;85:508-18.
4. Thomas R, Dogra M. An evaluation of medical college departments of ophthalmology in India and change following provision of modern instrumentation and training. *Indian J Ophthalmol.* 2008;56:9-16.
5. Garway-Heath DF, Friedman DS. How should results from clinical tests be integrated into the diagnostic process? *Ophthalmology.* 2006;113:1479-80.
6. Kanamori A, Nagai-Kusuhara A, Escano MF, Maeda H, Nakamura M, Negi A. Comparison of confocal scanning laser ophthalmoscopy, scanning laser polarimetry and optical coherence tomography to discriminate ocular hypertension and glaucoma at an early stage. *Graefes Arch Clin Exp Ophthalmol.* 2006;244:58-68.
7. Rao HL, Babu GJ, Sekhar GC. Comparison of the diagnostic capability of the Heidelberg Retina Tomographs 2 and 3 for glaucoma in the Indian population. *Ophthalmology.* 2010;117:275-81.
8. Medeiros FA, Zangwill LM, Bowd C, Sample PA, Weinreb RN. Influence of disease severity and optic disc size on the diagnostic performance of imaging instruments in glaucoma. *Invest Ophthalmol Vis Sci.* 2006;47:1008-15.
9. Garudadri CS, Rao HL, Parikh RS, et al. Effect of Optic Disc Size and Disease Severity on the Diagnostic Capability of Glaucoma Imaging Technologies in an Indian Population. *J Glaucoma.* 2011.
10. Gabriele ML, Ishikawa H, Wollstein G, et al. Optical coherence tomography scan circle location and mean retinal nerve fiber layer measurement variability. *Invest Ophthalmol Vis Sci.* 2008;49:2315-21.
11. Medeiros FA, Ng D, Zangwill LM, Sample PA, Bowd C, Weinreb RN. The effects of study design and spectrum bias on the evaluation of diagnostic accuracy of confocal scanning laser ophthalmoscopy in glaucoma. *Invest Ophthalmol Vis Sci.* 2007;48:214-22.
12. Heijl A, Bengtsson B, Hyman L, Leske MC. Natural history of open-angle glaucoma. *Ophthalmology.* 2009;116:2271-6.
13. Leske MC, Heijl A, Hyman L, Bengtsson B. Early Manifest Glaucoma Trial: design and baseline data. *Ophthalmology.* 1999;106:2144-53.
14. Bengtsson B, Heijl A. A visual field index for calculation of glaucoma rate of progression. *Am J Ophthalmol.* 2008;145:343-53.
15. Rao HL, Jonnadula GB, Addepalli UK, Senthil S, Garudadri CS. Effect of Cataract Extraction on Visual Field Index in Glaucoma. *J Glaucoma.* 2011.
16. Chauhan BC, Nicolela MT, Artes PH. Incidence and Rate of Glaucomatous Visual Field Progression After Optic Disc Change Measured With Scanning Laser Tomography [ARVO abstract]. *Invest Ophthalmol Vis Sci.* 2009;50:E-Abstract 2574.
17. Chauhan BC, McCormick TA, Nicolela MT, LeBlanc RP. Optic disc and visual field changes in a prospective longitudinal study of patients with

glaucoma: comparison of scanning laser tomography with conventional perimetry and optic disc photography. *Arch Ophthalmol.* 2001;119:1492-9.

18. Bowd C, Balasubramanian M, Weinreb RN, et al. Performance of confocal scanning laser tomograph Topographic Change Analysis (TCA) for assessing glaucomatous progression. *Invest Ophthalmol Vis Sci.* 2009;50:691-701.
19. O'Leary N, Crabb DP, Mansberger SL, et al. Glaucomatous progression in series of stereoscopic photographs and Heidelberg retina tomograph images. *Arch Ophthalmol.* 2010;128:560-8.
20. Alencar LM, Zangwill LM, Weinreb RN, et al. Agreement for detecting glaucoma progression with the GDx guided progression analysis, automated perimetry, and optic disc photography. *Ophthalmology.* 2010;117:462-70.
21. Grewal DS, Sehi M, Greenfield DS. Comparing rates of retinal nerve fibre layer loss with GDxECC using different methods of visual-field progression. *Br J Ophthalmol.* 2011;95:1122-7.
22. Leung CK, Cheung CY, Weinreb RN, et al. Evaluation of retinal nerve fiber layer progression in glaucoma: a study on optical coherence tomography guided progression analysis. *Invest Ophthalmol Vis Sci.* 2010;51:217-22.
23. Weinreb RN, Zangwill LM, Jain S, et al. Predicting the onset of glaucoma: the confocal scanning laser ophthalmoscopy ancillary study to the Ocular Hypertension Treatment Study. *Ophthalmology.* 2010;117:1674-83.

Editorial

Macular Hole

Amol D Kulkarni, Suresh R Chandra

Neil Kelly and Rob Wendell reported a relatively high success rate in the cure of macular holes previously considered beyond repair. Since that time, surgical techniques have improved and success rates have increased. The pathogenesis of macular holes is not well understood. Various theories exist regarding the etiology of macular holes including trauma, cystic degeneration and vitreous traction. It is likely that macular holes represent a heterogeneous group of conditions with a common final pathway and similar clinical manifestation. The vitreous exerts anteroposterior traction, tangential traction, or both which is thought to be critical in the pathogenesis of a macular hole. Gass classified macular hole into various stages precisely defined by OCT which is now the diagnostic modality of choice for this condition.[1] Furthermore, OCT is a useful aid in patient education to demonstrate the presence of the macular hole and the postoperative result. The current anatomic success rates range from 82 to 100%. There is relief of traction (tangential and A-P) and stimulation of fibroglial proliferation to plug the hole after vitrectomy and gas tamponade.

Dr Meena has written an excellent comprehensive review of pathophysiology, diagnosis, and management of macular holes. There is detailed description of OCT staging of macular hole. She specifically highlights the various controversies that exist regarding the surgical management of macular holes.

Our recommendations include:

1. *Timing of surgical intervention*: Surgical results are best for macular holes of less than 1 year duration. Given that chronic holes may do well, it is reasonable to offer surgery for macular holes of 1–5 years duration.
2. *Stage of the macular hole*: It is best to observe stage 1 and lamellar macular hole and monitor for progression. Surgical management is recommended with documentation of a stage 2 or higher, full-thickness macular hole.

3. *Internal limiting membrane peeling*: The removal of internal limiting membrane (ILM) is considered to be a contributing factor in the success of macular hole surgeries.[2] ILM peeling also removes any contractile epiretinal membrane (ERM), thereby, relieving tangential traction. In addition, membrane removal can enhance mobility of the hole edges, thereby, facilitating reapproximation. Several retrospective studies suggest that ILM peeling is beneficial in attaining improved visual acuity and anatomic closure in macular holes of less than six months duration. However, there has been some concern regarding damage to the retina secondary to membrane peeling. The absence of a large randomized clinical trial likely accounts for the lack of consensus regarding the efficacy of and indications for ILM peeling.[3]
4. *Use of vital dyes for internal limiting membrane peeling:* Indocyanine green (ICG) dye was the first vital dye used for macular surgery. There is considerable literature questioning the toxicity of ICG dye to the retina and retinal pigment epithelium (RPE). Despite the laboratory and literature cautioning the use of ICG dye, an equal amount of literature documented good surgical and visual results. ICG dye is still used by surgeons with care taken to limit the exposure of the retina and, potentially more importantly, the RPE to the dye. Trypan blue has been used to stain the ILM; however, it does not appear to stain as effectively as ICG dye. Triamcinolone acetonide has also been used to facilitate peeling of the ILM. Brilliant blue G is a newly introduced vital dye which is less toxic to the retinal pigment epithelium and stains both ERM and ILM as well.[4] It has been comparable to ICG in terms of ILM staining and ease of surgical removal.
5. *Adjuvants for macular hole surgery*: An assortment of adjuvant therapies has been used at the time of surgery in an effort to enhance glial proliferation. These include transforming growth factor beta (TGF-ß), autologous platelets, autologous plasmin, and plasmin. Prospective randomized studies of TGF-ß and autologous platelets have, however, shown little benefit in terms of anatomic closure or final visual acuity. Hence, their use has not gained much popularity.
6. *Intraocular tamponade*: The primary difference achieved using different gases is the duration of action of the gas bubble and, consequently, the amount of internal tamponade achieved within the first several days after surgery. Longer acting gas like C3F8 allows for 2–3 weeks of contact between hole and gas if supine position is avoided. Hence, there is more leeway in positioning. Shorter acting gas therefore requires more rigorous positioning to achieve hole/gas contact as bubble dissipates.

Positioning may actually be more critical as the bubble dissipates. Majority of surgeons uses C3F8 (64% C3F8 versus 33% SF6). Intraocular tamponade with C3F8 gas produces 6 weeks of visual debility, which is as cumbersome to the patient as the prone positioning.

7. *Duration for face-down prone positioning*: Historically, strict face-down positioning had been recommended for patients for up to 4 weeks, with consequent difficulties of compliance and patient's quality of life during that period. Majority of surgeons advocates at least 2 weeks of face-down positioning. The advent of ILM peeling has reduced the number of days for face-down positioning.[2] Extended periods of face down positioning often produce neck or back pain. There have been reports of complications, including ulnar nerve neuropathy and pressure sores. In addition to these medical complications, there are the financial costs of lost time from work, caregiver requirements, and expensive medical equipment. A shortened prone positioning period offers patients decreased risk of medical complication, increases patient convenience, and lowers the indirect costs of macular hole surgery.
8. *20-gauge versus small gauge vitrectomy systems*: While no one system poses a significant long-term advantage, smaller gauge vitrectomy systems, with frequently self-sealing wounds, avoid induced astigmatism from suturing sclerotomies, resulting in a more rapid recovery of vision.[5] An initial increase in endophthalmitis appears to have been addressed by changing the means of wound construction but may still be considered a disadvantage to small gauge vitrectomy systems.

In conclusion, the advent of vitreoretinal-microsurgical techniques has sparked a renewed interest in idiopathic macular hole and, particularly, its management. There is still a need to develop new techniques to improve visual outcomes, enhance patient convenience, and diminish complications. New diagnostic modalities, such as ultra-high resolution OCT and adaptive optics will improve our understanding of the cellular repair process following macular hole surgery. This may help us understand pathogenesis of macular hole at molecular level and consider the role of neuroprotection and photoceptor rescue to further improve the visual function.

REFERENCES

1. Wolf S, Wolf-Schnurrbusch U. Spectral-domain optical coherence tomography use in macular diseases: a review. *Ophthalmologica*. 2010;224(6):333-40.
2. Bainbridge J, Herbert E, Gregor Z. Macular holes: vitreoretinal relationships and surgical approaches. *Eye*. 2008;22(10):1301-9.
3. Lois N, Burr J, Norrie J, at al. Internal limiting membrane peeling versus no peeling for idiopathic full-thickness macular hole: a pragmatic randomized controlled trial. *Invest Ophthalmol Vis Sci.* 2011;52(3):1586-92.

4. Shukla D, Kalliath J, Neelakantan N, et al. A comparison of brilliant blue G, trypan blue, and indocyanine green dyes to assist internal limiting membrane peeling during macular hole surgery. *Retina.* 2011;31(10):2021-5.
5. Nam Y, Chung H, Lee JY, et al. Comparison of 25- and 23-gauge sutureless microincision vitrectomy surgery in the treatment of various vitreoretinal diseases. *Eye.* 2010;24(5):869-74.

Editorial

Artificial Retinal Implants: Can the Blind Really See Again?

Rajat N Agrawal

Improvement and restoration of a lost bodily function has always been a goal for physicians and researchers. From the philosophical works of Robert Hooke predicting use of mechanical devices, which would improve special senses to an English surgeon, CH Wilkinson, in 1799 advertising "medico-electric" rooms, where patients could be treated for a variety of ailments, including blindness, there have been various attempts at trying to offer some form of treatment and rehabilitation for people who become blind due to various etiologies.[1] These attempts, though conjectural, demonstrated the understanding from scientists' perspective that electricity may have therapeutic uses in a human body and have now resulted in using biomedical devices, such as cardiac pacemakers and cochlear implants routinely in medicine. Success of these implantable devices and improved technology provided the feasibility for the idea of the development of a visual prosthesis that could help blind people.

Löwenstein and Borchardt, in 1918, initially demonstrated that the position of electrically induced visual percepts within the visual field was systematically related to the area of the occipital lobe that received the electrical stimulation. This visual percept was described as a *phosphene*. This formed the basis of the field of cortical implants, leading to implantation of 80-electrode device by Giles Brindley and colleagues in London in 1968 in a 52-year-old woman blind from glaucoma. This was the first serious effort in the field of artificial vision.

Experiments in the early 1970s demonstrated that ocular stimulation, via a contact lens stimulating electrode, could allow blind humans to perceive electrically elicited phosphenes. These responses indicated the presence of at least some functioning inner retinal cells in the subjects. A number of retinal disorders that lead to blindness, such as retinitis pigmentosa (RP) and age-related macular degeneration (AMD) have been morphometrically studied and have been found to have significant numbers of inner retinal cells still present even in advanced stages of the disease.[2-5] On average, 78% of the inner nuclear layer cells and 30% of the ganglion cells were found to remain histologically intact in a patient with advanced RP, although this will obviously vary from subject to subject. Similar results were found in AMD patients. Thus, the remaining cells act as a "platform" for implantation of the artificial retinal prosthesis that is based on the premise that electrically stimulating the still functional inner retinal neurons in RP and AMD will help restore at least some level of vision.

There are currently many groups around the world involved in the development of retinal prostheses. The position of the electrode device and the stimulating array in relation to the retina defines the nomenclature of the groups. The two leading groups in *epiretinal prosthesis* (implant fixed in front of the retina) are the group from Doheny Eye Institute at the University of Southern California working with Second Sight Medical Products Inc. (USC-SSMP) in the United States and the other group is led by Intelligent Medical Implant GmbH (IMI) in Switzerland. Both are currently in clinical trials. The *subretinal prosthesis* (implant placed in the subretinal space between the neurosensory retina and the retinal pigment epithelium) work is led by the German Consortium coordinated by Zrenner in Tubingen, while Rizzo from Massachusetts Eye and Ear Infirmary along with Wyatt heads the other group. Another group in Japan has made significant progress on a *suprachoroidal transretinal* approach, which places the device in the suprachoroidal space for stimulation, while an Australian consortium is experimenting with the development of the device, and is likely to implant in their first patient in 2013.

Currently, the epiretinal work of USC-SSMP is at the most advanced stage, while most of the other groups are still in clinical trials. The device, ARGUS-II,™ has received CE mark in Europe, which signifies that it can be sold commercially in Europe. The device (and most other devices in development) is indicated only for very advanced stages of retinitis pigmentosa. Macular degeneration (AMD) is considered to be the other disease of interest, but due to the delayed or rare nature of complete loss of vision in those eyes, this device is not permitted for implantation in AMD patients.[6]

In general, the devices of most groups around the world work on the following principle: a video camera placed on a pair of glasses convert visual image into electrical impulses, which undergo processing before being sent to a surgically implanted device in the eye close to the retina. The electrodes release an electrical charge (which has been found to be safe to the retina)[7], which creates an electrical potential that gets carried through a functioning optic nerve to the occipital cortex, thus, allowing a blind patient to see phosphenes. The pattern of phosphenes allows a patient to make sense of what he/she is seeing in front of him, which needs a little amount of training, considering the fact that these patients have not had functional sight for more than 15–20 years at least.

The ARGUS-II™ technology consists of 60 electrodes, with the device being placed epiretinally via a surgical procedure that is akin to a vitrectomy-scleral buckle approach in retinal surgical. A conductive coil is placed on the sclera, that also contains telemetry equipment, which allows information to be sent and received, and power to be received from another coil placed on special glasses.

More than 30 patients with advanced RP have been implanted with this device with the surgical outcomes being achieved in majority of patients. Most of these patients are able to navigate independently, without assistance or with a cane, and are also able to perform activities of daily living, such as sorting washed laundry. The actual improvement in terms of vision and field of vision is difficult to grasp, since they are not quantifiable by the routine methods of investigation we use in the clinic.[8] In spite of that, we have noted a marked improvement in functionality of these implanted patients.

There has been an ongoing serious attempt to get the device to India soon, while also working on a proposal to develop an Indian bionic eye, built in India, specifically with the need and requirement of Indian patients in mind.

Dating from the time almost 50 years ago when it was first found that electrical stimulation of the retina would generate phosphenes in patients' eyes, the work has been able to demonstrate significant progress with the 60-electrode device. The USC-SSMP team is working on a 1000-electrode device that is likely to give significant visual information to a blind subject. In particular, it is hoped that face recognition and reading ability will be restored allowing for mainstreaming of many blind patients and vastly improvement in the quality of life.

REFERENCES

1. Weiland JD, Humayun MS. Past, present, and future of artificial vision. *Artif Organs.* 2003;27:961-2.
2. Stone JL, Barlow WE, Humayun MS, de Juan E, Jr., Milam AH. Morphometric analysis of macular photoreceptors and ganglion cells in retinas with retinitis pigmentosa. *Arch Ophthalmol.* 1992;110:1634-9.
3. Santos A, Humayun MS, de Juan E, Jr., Greenburg RJ, Marsh MJ, Klock IB, Milam AH. Preservation of the inner retina in retinitis pigmentosa. A morphometric analysis. *Arch Ophthalmol.* 1997;115:511-5.
4. Kim SY, Sadda S, Humayun MS, de Juan E, Jr., Melia BM, Green WR. Morphometric analysis of the macula in eyes with geographic atrophy due to age-related macular degeneration. *Retina.* 2002;22:464-70.

5. Kim SY, Sadda S, Pearlman J, Humayun MS, de Juan E, Jr., Melia BM, Green WR. Morphometric analysis of the macula in eyes with disciform age-related macular degeneration. *Retina.* 2002;22:471-7.
6. Weiland JD, Cho AK, Humayun MS. Retinal prostheses: current clinical results and future needs. *Ophthalmology.* 2011;118:2227-37.
7. Eng JG, Agrawal RN, Tozer KR, Ross-Cisneros FN, Dagnelie G, Greenberg RJ, et al. Morphometric analysis of optic nerves and retina from an end-stage retinitis pigmentosa patient with an implanted active epiretinal array. *Invest Ophthalmol Vis Sci.* 2011;52:4610-6.
8. Chader GJ, Weiland J, Humayun MS. Artificial vision: needs, functioning, and testing of a retinal electronic prosthesis. *Prog Brain Res.* 2009;175:317-32.

1

chapter

N Venkatesh Prajna
Lalitha Prajna
C Veerajayalakshmi

Fungal Keratitis

ABSTRACT

Fungal keratitis is an important cause of ocular morbidity in the developing world. It has replaced bacteria as the most common cause of suppurative keratitis. Characteristic clinical features include feathery edges, raised dry surface, satellite lesions, and a cheesy hypopyon. Microbiological investigations, such as KOH, Gram's stain and Sabouraud's dextrose agar culture confirm the diagnosis. Natamycin is the drug of choice for the treatment of fungal keratitis, while other drugs include voriconazole, econazole, itraconazole, and amphotericin B. Deeper lesions require a keratoplasty.

Introduction

The incidence of fungal keratitis has shown a dramatic increase in the recent years. In fact, in countries like India, fungi have nearly replaced bacteria as the most common cause of infectious suppurative keratitis. This increase is thought to be due to a combination of various factors, namely increased clinical suspicion, advances in diagnostic techniques, and paradoxically, the advancement in the field of antibacterial therapy, which has proportionately reduced the incidence of bacterial keratitis. Morbidity in fungal infections tends to be greater than that in bacterial keratitis, because the diagnosis is often delayed and the available drugs are not very effective.

Epidemiology

Fungal keratitis is most often encountered in rural populations, where agricultural workers are exposed to corneal injury contaminated with organic matter much more frequently than population at large.[1] It is relatively uncommon in the western world. Even, when it happens, it is usually caused by *Candida*. Filamentary fungi, especially *Aspergillus* and *Fusarium* are the common causes of mycotic keratitis in most of the developing world.

Classification of Fungi

Fungi are eukaryotic and heterotrophic organisms. Although numerous fungi have been implicated, the pathogenic fungi, which cause significant keratitis, can be divided into filamentous, yeast, and dimorphic forms.

FILAMENTOUS FUNGI

Filamentous fungi are also known as moulds. They occur as long filaments, called *hyphe*, which grow by apical extension and produce feathery aerial colonies above the culture media. They can be further divided into septate and nonseptate organisms. The septate filamentary fungi are the most common cause of keratomycosis. They are divided into nonpigmented monilial (which include *Fusarium* sp., *Aspergillus sp.,* and *Acremonium* sp.) and pigmented dematiaceous (*Curvularia sp., and Lasiodiplodia* sp.) varieties. The nonseptate filamentary fungi (*Mucor, Absidia* and *Rhizopus* sp.) are important causes of orbital disease and endogenous endophthalmitis but do not commonly produce corneal disease.

YEASTS

Yeasts are fungi with usual and dominant growth as unicellular organisms and form creamy, pasty colonies, which may be mistaken for staphylococcal colonies. They divide by asexual budding, forming pseudohyphae and do not form mycelium in culture. The most common fungi in this category are the *Candida* sp. and *Cryptococcus* sp., which are part of the normal flora of skin, respiratory tract, and conjunctiva and act as opportunistic pathogens.

DIMORPHIC FUNGI

Dimorphic fungi have two distinct morphologic forms: the yeast phase, which occurs in tissues and a mycelial phase, which occurs in media and natural surfaces. These fungi in this category are *Blastomyces, Coccidiodes, Histoplasma,* and *Sporothrix*, exhibit properties of molds, when cultivated at 25°C and of yeasts when grown at 37°C.

Risk Factors

Fungi are ubiquitous organisms present almost everywhere in the environment. Although the eye is continuously exposed to these pathogens, the normal defense mechanisms, such as the eyelids, tear components, and the corneal epithelium provide adequate protection. An epithelial defect is a prerequisite for these organisms to set up an infection.

The importance of trauma that is often trivial and frequently associated with plant material has been well documented in the initiation of fungal infection caused by filamentous fungi.

Contact lens wear is an uncommon risk factor in fungal keratitis. These organisms have been shown to grow within the matrix of soft contact lenses.[2] Filamentous fungi were more commonly associated with cosmetic lens wear and yeasts from therapeutic lens use.

Corticosteroids appear to activate and increase the virulence of fungi. The other factors uncommonly reported include vernal or allergic keratoconjunctivitis, neurotrophic ulcers, and penetrating keratoplasty. The predisposing factors for the development of fungal keratitis in patients after penetrating keratoplasty include suture problems, topical steroid therapy, chronic antibiotic use, contact lens wear, graft failure, and persistent epithelial defects. Fungal corneal ulcers have been reported following refractive surgical procedures like radial keratotomy, photorefractive keratotomy, and more recently following Laser *in situ* keratomileusis (LASIK) procedures, either in the immediate postoperative period (direct surgical contamination) or later (following trauma).

The principal risk factors for yeast or *Candida keratitis* are prolonged epithelial ulceration, penetrating keratoplasty, and therapeutic contact lens wear. In addition systemic diseases like Sjögrens syndrome, erythema multiforme, immunodeficiency, endocrinopathy, diabetes, and hypovitaminosis A have been shown to predispose to candidal infection.

Certain investigators have highlighted the association between the prevailing climatic conditions and the incidence of fungal keratitis. In India the incidence is highest in the harvesting seasons (September-October). There is less seasonal variation with regard to yeast infections.

Pathogenesis

The filamentous fungi affect normal eyes of immunocompetent hosts after corneal abrasion or trauma, from some kind of vegetable matter. The yeasts usually cause keratitis in immunocompromised individuals. Their pathogenicity is related to a decrease in the systemic or local defense mechanisms either by a direct effect on the immune system (topical steroids) or by an alteration in the normal epithelial barriers (i.e. persistent epithelial defects, bandage contact lenses, neurotrophic keratitis, topical anesthetics, etc.) with predisposing systemic and/or eye disease. The dimorphic fungi are a rare cause of keratitis.

The exact mechanisms underlying the pathogenesis of fungal infections are unclear. As compared to bacteria, the fungi are relatively nonimmunogenic, partly, because of their large size, which prevents them from being engulfed by the neutrophils, and partly because they do not secrete chemotactic factors, which attract inflammatory cells. After entering through a corneal epithelial defect, the fungi elaborate toxic substances and enzymes, such as proteases, hemolysins, and exotoxins. *Fusarium* sp, especially is known to possess specific cellular and molecular attributes, which aid to cause virulent reaction. They can adhere to biopolymers and have the ability to produce toxins and elaborate enzymes.[3]

A few strains of *Asperigillus* produce aflatoxins and ochratoxins.[4] The conidia of *Aspergillus fumigatus* have been shown to bind to and degrade basement membrane laminin, an extracellular matrix glycoprotein found in basement membranes. They have the capacity to penetrate an intact Descemet's membrane. The resultant host inflammatory response subsequently contributes to a part of the tissue damage. Activation of the complement system leads to concentration of polymorphonuclear inflammatory cells in the corneal cells that liberate proteolytic enzymes. Encapsulated *Cryptococcus neoformans, Candida albicans,* and the conidia of *A. fumigatus,* all activate the complement system by either classic or alternative pathways.

Fungi can penetrate deep into stroma and through an intact Descemet's membrane. It is thought that once fungus gains access into anterior chamber or to the iris and lens, eradication of the organism becomes extremely difficult. Likewise, organisms that extend from cornea into sclera become difficult to control.

Candida albicans strains have also been known to produce a variety of proteolytic enzymes. The most important of these is an aspartyl acid protease that can act on a wide variety of tissue proteins and is thought to contribute to the invasiveness of the organism. In addition, various virulence factors, such as a phospholipase A and lysophospholipase have been identified with *Candida* sp.

Clinical Features

FILAMENTARY FUNGI

Unlike bacterial infections, there is less pain, conjunctival congestion, discharge and chemosis early in the course of fungal infection and the symptoms are far less than what is expected of the size of the ulcer.

The earliest finding may be a small nonspecific stromal infiltrate with a surrounding unhealthy looking epithelium, in which case it is indistinguishable from a bacterial infection. Commonly the patient presents with a central or a paracentral ulcer with feathery stromal margins (Fig.1.1). The common misdiagnosis, which might be made at this stage, may be a dendritic keratitis caused by herpes simplex. These fungal pseudodendritic lesions are shorter, stockier and are associated with surrounding stromal infiltration. In addition, a mirror image of the pseudodendritic lesion in the deeper stromal layers can also be seen. The adjacent Descemet's membrane may be thrown into folds.

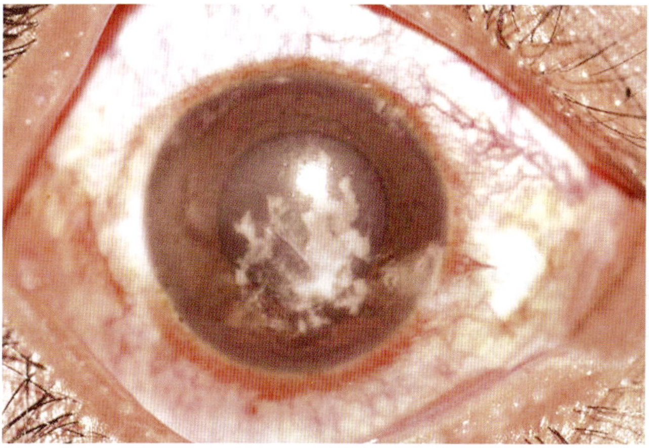

Fig. 1.1: Typical fungal ulcer with feathery margins

With time, the ulcer starts to become larger and elevated above the level of the corneal surface. The edges of the ulcer looks serrated, somewhat looking like a can opener capsulotomy. The surface looks dirty white and dry and has a rough texture. The serrated edges and the dry elevated rough surface can be considered pathognomonic of a fungal lesion (Fig.1.2). The stromal lesions are present beyond the size of the epithelial defect and have a feathery pattern. In rare instances, the lesion may be entirely in the posterior aspect of the corneal stroma without an accompanying epithelial defect. In these cases, the posterior stromal lesions also have a feathery edge like paint sprayed over a wall.

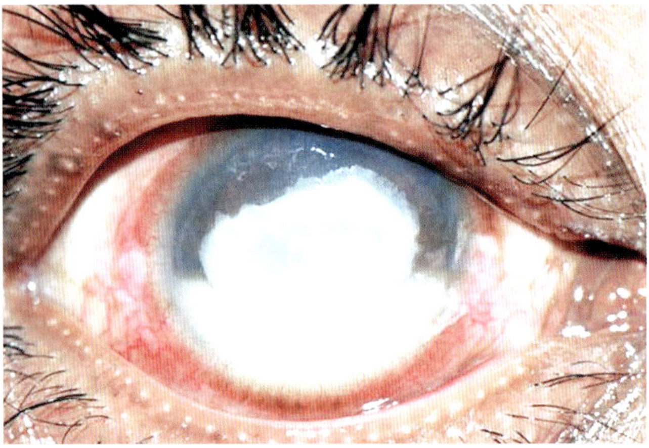

Fig. 1.2: Ulcer with raised surface

Foci of infiltration can be seen several millimeters away from the main area of involvement. These are called *satellite lesions,* and they may remain isolated from the main lesion or may be connected with the main ulcer by a thin line of stromal infiltration (Fig. 1.3). The epithelium can be intact over the infiltrate. An endothelial plaque may also be present. Like in many other keratitis, a ring infiltrate may surround the primary lesion, most likely representing an antibody response to fungal antigen (Fig. 1.4).

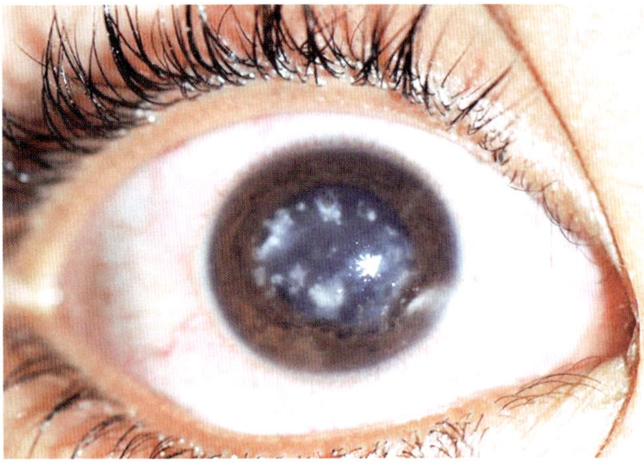

Fig. 1.3: Shows multiple satellite lesions

Hypopyon can be present in varying proportions and the amount is not directly proportional to the size of the ulcer.

As the lesions progress, the pain gets intense and the ulcer involves almost the whole of the cornea and starts to lose its characteristic pattern. The lesions look more suppurative and soupy. The edges of the ulcer may

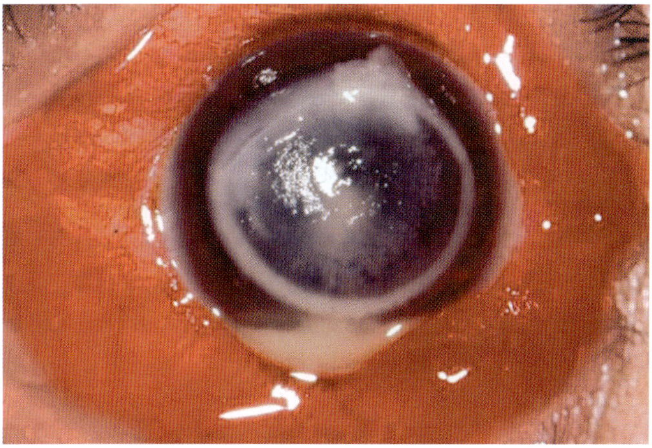

Fig. 1.4: Corneal ulcer with serrated margins and immune ring

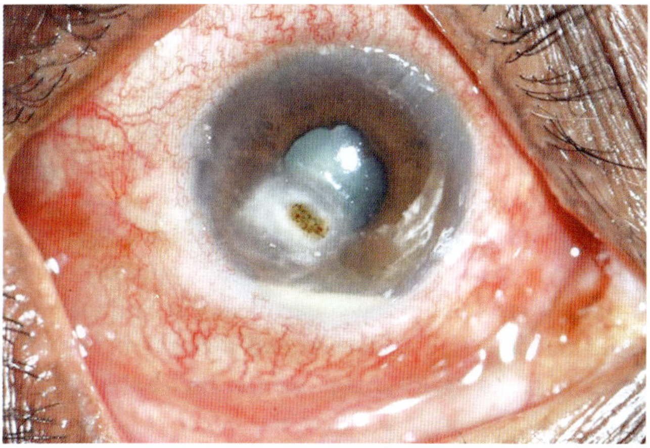

Fig. 1.5: Pigmented fungal ulcer with macroscopic pigments over the surface of the ulcer

start becoming rounded like a bacterial ulcer, but the edges of the deeper stromal lesions have the characteristic feathery pattern until the final course of the disease. As the size of the ulcer becomes larger, it becomes more flushed with the surface and assumes a smooth surface. A significant majority of the deeper stromal ulcers perforate over time.

In the ulcers caused by the dematiceous fungi, there may be macroscopic pigment deposition over the surface. The color may vary from a thick blackish-brown pigmentary lesion to a less mottled greenish-gray pigment dispersed over a whitish base (Fig. 1.5). The denser lesion can be mistaken for a uveal prolapse. The lesion caused by dematiceous fungi are more elevated than those caused by nonpigmentary filamentous fungi and has a characteristic mushroom head appearance. These lesions can be dissected from the surface using a Bard Parker knife and has a tough, leathery attachment to the ulcer surface.

In contrast to the filamentary fungal keratitis, the stromal keratitis caused by *Candida* may be more localized and have a collar-button configuration, often with a small ulcer and an expanding infiltrate. They are usually superimposed on a chronic debilitated ocular condition. The lesions tend to be oval, plaque like, and elevated. They are well outlined and surrounded by stromal edema and more closely resemble the bacterial keratitis. If untreated, the keratitis evolves to produce dense suppuration and necrosis of the deep stroma.

It should be emphasized that the differentiation between an advanced keratitis caused by bacteria and fungi is difficult to distinguish by clinical features alone. Future developments in the field of confocal microscopy may become a useful clinical tool for the diagnosis of fungal keratitis. The lack of experience and the cost of the instrument may be the limiting constraints for its widespread use.

Histopathology

Non-replicating fungi, and their mycotoxins, proteolytic enzymes and soluble fungal antigens are capable of inducing severe inflammatory reactions. These agents can result in necrosis of the corneal lamellae, and incite an antigenic response with immune ring formation and hypopyon. The inflammatory response tends to be less marked than seen in bacterial keratitis though the epithelium is often remain intact over the infective lesion. The classical histopathologic findings in fungal keratitis include fungal hyphal elements oriented perpendicular to the normal corneal lamellae and the tendency for the hyphal elements apparently to penetrate Descemet's membrane and spread into the anterior chamber (these two features are considered to be suggestive of progressive pathogenicity). When this occurs, it is seen as retrocorneal or anterior chamber inflammatory mass adjacent to an area of deep keratitis.

Laboratory Diagnosis

A standard microbiologic baseline work-up should be performed in every case of suspected infectious keratitis. This is even more crucial in the regions of the world, where fungi and bacteria cause keratitis, almost in equal proportions. In addition, combined infections with bacteria and fungi, or even with multiple fungi, can be detected through this routine examination.

Scrapings are made from the base and the edges of the ulcer under topical anesthesia using a Bard Parker knife or a Kimura spatula. The lesions caused by fungi often feel gritty and have a leathery attachment to the base of the ulcer. Calcium alginate swabs have been reported to increase the recovery rate of the organisms. In deeper lesions, a corneal biopsy may be required for obtaining adequate specimen.

Direct microscopic evaluation is the most valuable and rapid diagnostic tool for the detection of fungal elements in corneal scrapings. The initial smears can be examined using a potassium hydroxide mount (KOH) preparation and a Gram's stain. The KOH preparation is a simple, reliable and reproducible screening method for identifying filamentary fungi. KOH has been used as a 10–20% suspension, either plain or with ink or with lactophenol cotton blue. Proteinaceous components, such as host cells are partially digested by the alkali, leaving intact the polysaccharide containing fungal cell walls (Fig. 1.6). However, the sensitivity of this method is highly variable ranging between 33 and 94%. A recent study done by Sharma et al aimed to look at the sensitivity, specificity and predictive values of KOH preparation and to compare its efficacy with other methods of corneal scraping examinations used in the diagnosis of mycotic keratitis.[5] KOH is an excellent and simple tool and has a definite place in the armamentarium of diagnostic techniques.

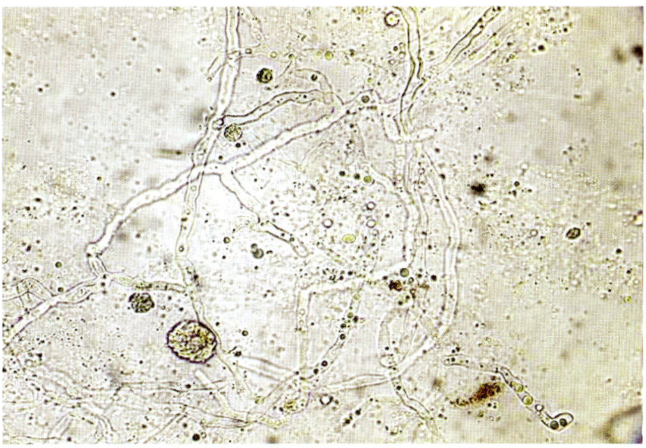

Fig. 1.6: Fungal filaments in KOH wet mount under 40x magnification

Giemsa and Gram's stain techniques are equally sensitive in detecting fungal elements. The Gram's stain does not stain the cell wall or septa of hyphal fragments but is absorbed by the protoplasm (Fig. 1.7). Yeasts typically stain dark blue and can be distinguished from bacteria, foreign

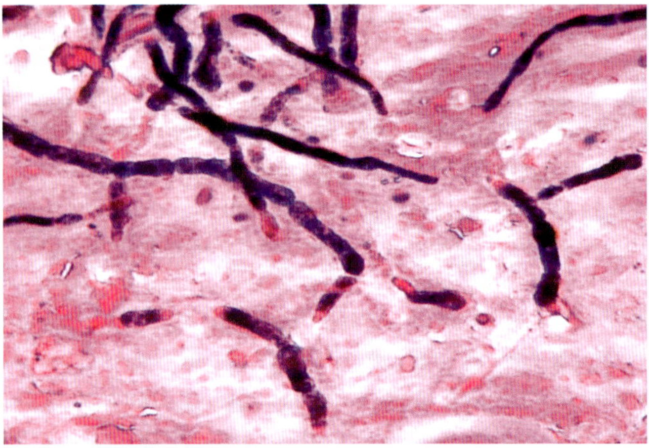

Fig. 1.7: Fungal filaments seen in Gram's staining under 100x magnification

material, precipitate and other artifacts. Hyphal fragments and yeasts appear dark blue or purple in Giemsa stain. Gomoris methenamine silver and periodic acid Schiff stains are other methods used when conventional staining techniques yield no results. However, these methods are time consuming, tedious and difficult to interpret.

Though the use of calcofluor white, acridine orange and fluorescein conjugated lectins yield rapid results, special infrastructural requirements make them inapplicable in most situations. However, these are the stains of choice for the detection of yeasts.

The findings of direct examination can be confirmed by culture. Sabourauds dextrose agar and brain-heart infusion broth are the most commonly used primary isolation media for fungi. Cycloheximide should never be incorporated in Sabourauds, because it inhibits the saprophytic fungi predominantly responsible for keratitis. The media are kept at room temperature (25°C) for the isolation of fungi. Since bacterial pathogens are always a consideration in the differential diagnosis of suppurative keratitis, additional material is inoculated in a row of C streaks on fresh sheep blood agar or chocolate agar media. Most fungi show mycelial growth on blood agar within 24-72 hours. Yeasts grow on these media at 30°C and are visible in 18-24 hours.

In our laboratory, we prefer to use potato dextrose agar as the principal culture media to isolate fungi, since this medium is thought to have a profound effect on the conidiogenesis and the surface character of *Fusarium* colonies. Colonies of *Fusarium* are usually white in the early stages of development, but often show reverse pigmentation. The classification is based on microscopic features of conidia that form on specialized hyphae called *conidiophores*.

Colonies of *Aspergillus fumigatus* are white at first, but as spores are produced, they become velvet green owing to the pigmentation of the conidia. *A. niger* colonies are also white during the initial growth phase but turn completely black on sporulation. The typical colony of *Candida* sp. on Sabourauds dextrose agar has a dirty white color. It is opaque with a smooth, flat, round contour and a pasty soft consistency. When grown on blood agar 35°C, they are slow-growing and nonhemolytic. *Candida* colonies have a distinctive fruity and yeasty odor.

Identification of *C. albicans* is usually based on the formation of germ tubes *in vitro* and further speciation is based on sugar fermentation. Classification of noncandidial yeasts is based on biochemical testing. Since most of the ocular fungal isolates grow quicker, it may not be absolutely necessary for the incubation period to be prolonged than a week.

Scraping also provides for debridement of organisms and the epithelium which may provide a barrier to antifungal drug penetration. When scrapings are negative, a diagnostic superficial keratectomy or corneal biopsy may be performed and sent for smear, culture and histopathological examination. In some cases of deep keratitis, a 27 G hypodermic needle or a 6-0 silk suture can be introduced into the infiltrate to obtain a specimen for culture.

A polymerase chain reaction (PCR) has been used in an animal model to develop a sensitive, specific and rapid test to diagnose *Fusarium keratitis*. Even as the availability of *in vitro* susceptibility testing for fungi have been reported, there is yet no agreement on the standardization and applicability of these tests and currently do not enjoy widespread usage.

Medical Treatment

All the available antifungal agents are fungistatic and not fungicidal. The penetration of the drugs is poor and has to be aided by repeated debridement, which acts by debulking of the pathogenic organism. The treatment schedules are usually prolonged and often leading to a poor compliance with medical therapy.

Most of the antifungal drugs exhibit their effect through their actions on the fungal cell membrane. In addition to its barrier function, the fungal cell membrane controls the movement of electrolytes and thereby controls the internal homeostasis of the cell. Ergosterol is the predominant sterol unique to the fungal cell membrane, while mammalian cell membranes are composed of cholesterol. Most antifungals capitalize on this important difference in plasma membrane constituents to damage the fungal cells, while minimizing damage to the host cells. There are three major classes of antifungal drugs available:

1. Polyenes.
2. Imidazoles, and
3. Fluorinated pyrimidines.

POLYENES

Polynes constitute the first line of the antifungal agents. They bind preferentially to ergosterol in the fungal plasma membrane, thereby, altering membrane permeability and disrupting the fungal cell. Larger polyenes (such as amphotericin B and nystatin) create channels that span the cell membranes and allow electrolyte movement. Small polyenes, such as natamycin are too small to bridge the width of the cell membrane and causes localized membrane disruptions thus altering permeability.[6]

Natamycin

Natamycin is a tetraene antibiotic. Discovered in 1958, it has proved itself to be the most valuable ocular antifungal agent available to date. The drug is available as a 5% suspension and must be shaken well before use. Natamycin has a broad spectrum of activity against filamentous fungi. When applied topically, it adheres to the ulcer site like a rope, which may act as a reservoir of drug. In general, topical natamycin is well tolerated and its corneal toxicity is rare. It may cause conjunctival necrosis when given subconjunctivally and, therefore, this route is not preferred.

Amphotericin B

Amphotericin B is a heptaene polyene. It is still considered the drug of choice for treatment of life threatening infections. It is also the drug of choice for candidal keratitis and *Cryptococcus*. The drug is variably active against filamentary fungi and is not recommended as the first line treatment for these organisms. Rifampin reportedly increases the effectiveness of amphotericin B against *Aspergillus* sp. but not against *Candida* sp. The drug is insoluble in water, unstable at 37°C and degrades rapidly if exposed to light. However, solubility can be improved by addition of deoxycholate. It is relatively toxic and cannot penetrate intact epithelium. The adverse effects of the topical application include a stinging sensation, chemosis and punctate epithelial keratitis. They are mostly though to be due to the presence of bile salt used to stabilize the drug in solution.

Amphotericin B is dispensed in 20 ml vials for intravenous use containing 50 mg powder. The powder is initially reconstituted to a concentration of 5 mg/ml in 10 ml of sterile water for injection. It should be prepared in distilled water because it precipitates in sodium chloride solution. An initial dose of 0.15% is applied for every five minutes for half an hour as a loading dose and then hourly. Subconjunctival injections can cause conjunctival necrosis and should be avoided. Systemic administration of amphotericin B is nephrotoxic and is ineffective in the treatment of keratitis.

Occasionally, intracameral injection of amphotericin B (5-10 μg in 0.1ml) can be a useful alternative treatment of severe fungal keratitis with intraocular extension that is resistant to conventional therapy.[7]

Nystatin

Nystatin is another polyene antifungal agent that is used as an ointment or formulated eyedrops (50,000 units /ml) and can be used for the treatment of superficial candidal keratitis. The ointment preparation causes severe stinging sensation and patient compliance is poor for prolonged usage. It is too toxic for parenteral administration.

IMIDAZOLES

This group constitutes the imidazoles and the structurally related N-substituted triazole. The imidazoles include clotrimazole, miconazole, econazole, and ketoconazole. The triazoles include fluconazole and itraconazole. These drugs exhibit their antifungal activity by having two mechanisms of action. In lower concentration, they are fungistatic by inhibiting sterol 14 alpha demythylase; a microsomal P-450 related enzyme, which is required in the demythylation of lanosterol in the synthesis of ergosterol.[8] At higher concentrations, they are fungicidal which is due to direct membrane damage to the phospholipids present in the fungal cell wall. However, they are never able to achieve fungicidal concentration in the human cornea

Clotrimazole

Clotrimazole is used extensively topically for the treatment of skin and genital candidal infection. A topical ophthalmic preparation of clotrimazole can be made with 1% clotrimazole in arachis oil. A dermatological cream containing clotrimazole 1% is well tolerated when applied to the eye. The drug is too toxic for systemic use. Though not preferred, it can be used in the treatment of *Aspergillus keratitis*.

Miconazole

Miconazole can be used through various routes— topically, subconjunctivally, or intracamerally. It can be prepared for topical application as a 1% drop in arachis oil or a 2% cream. The commercially available intravenous preparation can also be administered topically (10 mg/ml) or by sub-conjunctival injection (5–10 mg). The drug is relatively unstable in solution and has to be reformulated weekly. It is active against mainly yeasts and is variably active against filamentary fungi.

Econazole

Econazole is a dichlorimidazole and which exhibits a wide spectrum of activity against filamentous fungi. A topical preparation of econazole 1% can be prepared and is well tolerated.

Ketoconazole

Ketoconazole is more water-soluble and is better absorbed after systemic administration than other imidazoles. It is available as 200 mg tablets. The usual dose for adults is 200-400 mg/day, which can be increased to 800 mg or more. It can also be administered as a topical preparation in concentrations ranging from 1 to 5%. Clinically, the agent has been shown to be effective against *Candida, Aspergillus, Fusarium* and *Curvularia* sps in particular.[9]

The most common side effects are dose-dependent nausea, anorexia, and vomiting. Ketoconazole inhibits steroid biosynthesis in fungi. Several endocrinological abnormalities like decreased libido and testosterone levels, menstrual irregularities and suppression of the ACTH-stimulated plasma cortisol response have been reported. It blocks the hepatic microsomal system, interfering with the metabolism of several drugs, such as cyclosporine.

Fluconazole

Fluconazole, a water-soluble triazole is available in an oral dose of 100 mg capsules and intravenous solution (sterile solution in 0.9% sodium chloride, 2 mg/ml: 100 ml unit). Although the MICs of fluconazole are higher than other azoles in most susceptibility test systems, the *in vitro* activity of fluconazole does not parallel the efficacy in infections in animals and in clinical trials in humans.[10] The recommended dose of the drug is 200–400 mg/day and is the same for oral and intravenous route. It is useful in *Candida keratits.*

Itraconazole

The newer oral triazole antifungal agent itraconazole may also be a helpful adjunctive agent in the treatment of fungal keratitis, based on *in vitro* activity, pharmacokinetic properties and limited clinical trials in nonocular infections. However, its drawback is that it is quite hydrophobic, and being 90% protein bound in the serum, it does not permeate the tissues as well as fluconazole.

Voriconazole

Voriconaxole is one of the recent drugs useful in the management of fungal keratitis.[11,12] It is a synthetic derivative of fluconazole in which the triazole group is substituted with a fluoropyrimidine moiety and has an increased potency and *in vivo* efficacy. Addition of a methyl group to the propyl backbone increases the affinity of the drug for the target enzyme (14-α-sterol demethylase). It shows a broader spectrum of activity against *Fusarium, Aspergillus, Scedosporium, Paecilomyces,* and *Candida.* As with other triazole antifungal agents, voriconazole exerts its affect primarily through inhibition of cytochome P-450 dependent 14-sterol demethylase, an enzyme responsible for conversion of lanosterol to 14-demethyl lanosterol in ergosterol biosynthetic pathway.

Voriconazole is available in vials containing 30 mg lyophilized powder. It has excellent corneal penetration because of its low molecular weight (349 g/mol) and its lipophilic properties. It can be used topically in the form of 1% eyedrops and can be titrated based on epithelial healing. In deeper lesions, intrastromal voriconazole may be given in the dose of 50 μg/0.1 ml. Oral voriconazole may be supplemented in the dose of 5 mg/kg body weight. A baseline liver function test should always be performed before starting oral voriconazole therapy.

The adverse effects with systemic voriconazole therapy include transient visual disturbances (photopsias, photophobia, or color vision defects), formed visual hallucinations, and elevated liver enzymes.

FLUORINATED PYRIMIDINES

Flucytosine

Flucytosine is a fluorinated pyrimidine and is selectively taken by susceptible fungi and deaminated to fluorouracil which blocks thymidine synthesis. Since mammalian cells do not normally metabolize flucytosine, it does not inhibit metabolic processes in the mammalian cells. It is effective against *Candida* and *Cryptococcus,* and certain strains of *Aspergillus*, but is not effective against *Fusarium* and *Cephalosporium.* However, some fungal strains lack the specific permease to transport the drug into the cells and they are resistant to flucytosine. Topical flucytosine is used as drops in a 1% solution every hour and is well tolerated. Therapeutic levels can also be achieved in adults with the administration of a dose of 50–150 mg/kg /day in divided doses. Flucytosine should not be given alone in the treatment of keratomycosis for fear of inducing resistance. Its topical form is relatively nontoxic to the eye. When administered systemically, it may cause a transient depression of the bone marrow and diarrhea.

Principles of Therapy

As mentioned earlier, the treatment for fungal keratitis is usually prolonged. Improvement may not be visible for several days. Lack of progression of the stromal infiltrate is the first sign that the antifungal drug is effective. This is followed by a rounding of the feathery margins, blunting of the perimeters and reduction in cellular infiltrate and edema in surrounding stroma. Prolonged conjunctival injection, protracted epithelial ulceration, punctate corneal epithelial erosions and diffuse stromal haze imply drug toxicity. The appearance of a transient hypopyon in the face of an improving corneal picture has been attributed to hypersensitivity or a toxic reaction.

The initiation of treatment can be performed as soon as the results of the KOH mount and the Gram's stain are obtained. These tests can readily be performed at the office of the physician itself. Studies have questioned the reliability of the positivity of culture as the gold standard and have recommended that all smear positive cases of mycotic keratitis be treated accordingly despite negative culture reports.[13] If the smears and the culture results are negative, but the clinical features are strongly in favor of fungal keratitis, we recommend initiation of topical antifungal therapy, especially in countries where there is a high prevalence. Culture results are useful in certain situations and can play an effective role in identification of the species, which is useful for epidemiological purposes.

For suspected filamentous fungal keratitis, natamycin 5% drops should be administered hourly for the initial 24–48 hours and at 2-hour intervals. The dosage can then be gradually reduced depending upon the response. If natamycin is unavailable, then 1% econazole or 1% miconazole can be used.

For yeast keratitis, topical amphotercin B 0.1% to 0.25% drops are initally applied at 15 minute intervals for the first 24–48 hours and then frequency of application is gradually reduced for the next 4–6 days. If initial therapy was topical natamycin or amphotercin B drops alone and the stromal suppuration is progressing, oral ketoconazole or fluconazole should be added for either filamentous fungal or yeast keratitis. Subconjunctival miconazole (5 mg) or fluconazole (1 mg) can be given.

Prolonged treatments with systemic antifungals are reserved for deep keratitis associated with scleritis and endophthalmitis. The most frequently used oral antifungal has been ketoconazole. Recent evidence suggests that fluconazole may penetrate better into the cornea after systemic administration than some other azoles and associated with fewer side effects.[14] The other drugs, which have been tried for the treatment of fungal keratitis in past include silver sulfadiazine and sulfacetamide.

The issue of synergy or antagonism when the antifungal drugs are combined has given varying results. A combination of flucytosine and miconazole or natamycin was found to be synergistic *in vitro* against *Aspergillus keratitis*.[15] Certain investigators routinely use flucytosine topical (1% solution) and systemic (oral 150 mg/kg) in combination with amphotericin B in the management of *Candida keratitis*.[16] Antagonism has been reported when amphotericin B and the imidazoles have been used systemically.[17]

Supplementary therapy of keratomycosis includes a cycloplegic-mydriatic agent, such as atropine 1% twice a day, and topical beta blocker or oral carbonic anhydrase inhibitor to control secondary ocular hypertension. Corticosteroids do not have any role in the treatment regimen of fungal keratitis and is not recommended in any stage of the disease.

Surgical Treatment

Regular debridement of the ulcer using a scalpel or a Kimura spatula is an invaluable step to ensure adequate therapeutic levels of the antifungals into the deeper stromal layers. Some authors feel that surgery is seldom needed during the acute spread of the infection.[18] Studies conducted at the Bascolm Palmer Institute indicate that therapeutic keratoplasty was required seven times more frequently in fungal keratitis than in bacterial keratitis. We also feel that the surgical modality of excisional keratoplasty has an important role to play in the treatment of fungal keratitis and perhaps in some parts of the world, it may well be the primary choice of treatment.

Therapeutic keratoplasty has to be contemplated when the ulcer progresses despite specific antifungal therapy. The progression is characterized by increased area and depth of stromal suppuration, stromal ulceration to the point of extreme thinning of the cornea, dense fibrinos exudate in the anterior chamber and frank perforation. However, a small perforation developing during the course of the healing can be managed by the use of a tissue adhesive.

The goals of the therapeutic keratoplasty are to remove the infected part of the cornea, and restore the integrity of the globe. A recurrence of infection in a graft is more difficult to treat than a graft rejection. Even if one of these transplants is rejected, a second keratoplasty for optical rehabilitation can be performed at a later date. A large-sized graft should be used without any fear of rejection.

Local anesthesia may suffice in a majority of the cases. In these cases, O Brien's facial nerve block is given first prior to the ciliary block to prevent squeezing of the eyelid and resultant inadvertent perforation. The initial incision is performed using a hollow trephine needle. The anterior chamber is entered using a sharp razor blade. If the area of suppuration is large and asymmetric, decenteration of the trephination or a free hand dissection to encompass the infected areas should be done. The size of the trephination should preferably leave 1 to 1.5 mm clear zone of the uninvolved cornea to reduce the possibility of residual infective organisms peripheral to the trephination. Thicker fibrous membranes covering the surface of the iris or the lens can be peeled off using a forceps or in some cases excised using scissors. A peripheral iridectomy should be performed in all cases to prevent secondary glaucoma. If involvement of the posterior segment or endophthalmitis is suspected, an antifungal agent such as amphotericin B (5 microorganisms per 0.1 ml) is injected. The intact lens should not be removed as much as possible and localized cataracts should warrant an extraction at a later date in a separate sitting. The graft is then secured with 10 nylon interrupted sutures. The advantage of these interrupted sutures is that they can be removed selectively if future infiltrations develop. Results of therapeutic keratoplasty are often encouraging (Fig. 1.8). The recurrence of the infection in the graft starts from the periphery.

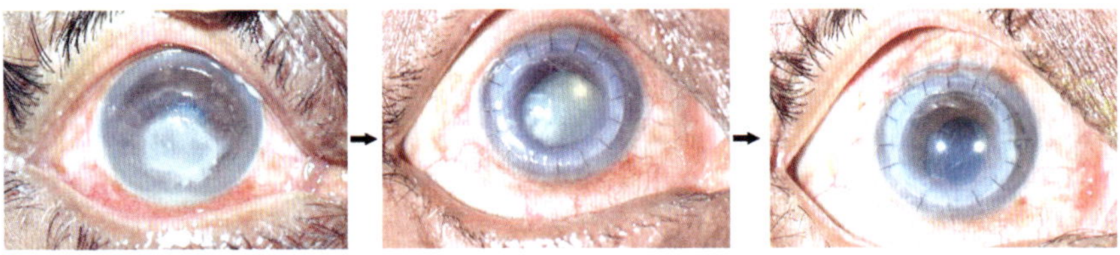

Fig. 1.8: A clear graft without any infiltrate after surgery

Postoperatively, topical natamycin 5% is continued for a period of 1-2 months. During this time, the usage of topical steroids is not recommended and supplementary topical nonsteroidal anti-inflammatory drugs may be used. Steroids can be used cautiously after the first postoperative month follow-up.

Conclusion

In conclusion, fungal keratitis is fast becoming a silent epidemic, especially in developing countries. A lot of research is clearly needed in the field of antifungal pharmacology to limit the morbidity caused by these infections. Until then, early surgical intervention may be the preferred mode to eliminate the infection.

References

1. Forster RK. Fungal keratitis and conjunctivitis. Clinical disease. In Smolin G, Thoft RA, (Eds): *The Cornea: Scientific foundation and clinical practice.* Bostom Little Brown; 1994:229-52.
2. Churner R, Cunningham RD. Fungal contaminated soft contact lenses. *Am J Ophthalmol* 1988;106:708-14.
3. Nelson PE, Dignani MD, Anaissie EJ. Taxonomy, biology and clinical aspects of *Fusarium* species. *Clin Microbiol Rev.* 1994;7:479-504.
4. Bennett JE. Mycoses: *Aspergillus*. In Mandell GL, Douglas RG Jr, Bennett JE (Eds): *Principles and practice of infectious disease.* New York: Churchill Livingstone; 1990. p. 1958-62.
5. Sharma S Silverberg M, Mehta P, et al. Early diagnosis of mycotic keratitis: predictive value of potassium hydroxide preparation. *Ind J Ophthalmol* 1998;46(1):31-5.
6. Medoff G, Kobayaski GS. Strategies in the treatment of systemic fungal infections. *NEJM.* 1980;302:145-55.
7. Saye Yilmaz, Ture M, Maden A. Efficacy of Intracameral Amphotericin B in the management of refractory keratomycosis and endophthalmitis. *Cornea* 2007;26:398-402.
8. Sud IJ, Feingold DS. Mechanisms of action of the antimycotic imidazoles. *J Invest Dermatol.* 1981;6:438-41.
9. Thienpont D, Van Cutsem J, Van Gerren F, et al. Ketoconazole, a new broad spectrum orally active antimycotic. *Experimentia.* 1979;35:606-9.
10. Saag MS, Dismukes WE. Azole antifungal agents: Emphasis on new triazoles. *Antimicrob Agents Chemothe.* 1988;32:1.
11. Hariprasad SM, Mieler WF, Lin TK, et al: Voriconazole in the treatment of fungal eye infections: a review of current literature. *Br J Ophthalmol.* 2008;92:871-8.
12. SponselW, ChenN, et al. Topical voriconazole as a novel treatment for fungal keratitis. *Antimicrob Agents Chemother.* 2006;50:262-8.
13. Jones DB. Initial therapy of suspected microbial corneal ulcers. II. Specific antibiotic therapy based on corneal smears. *Surv Ophthalmol.* 1979;24:97-116.
14. O'Day DM. Orally administered antifungal therapy for experimental keratomycoses. *Trans Am Ophthalmol Soc.* 1990;88:685-725.
15. Johns KJ, O'Day DM: Pharmacologic management of keratomycosis. *Surv Ophthalmol* 1998;33:178.
16. Abad JC, Foster SC. Fungal keratitis. *International Ophthalmol Clin.* 1998;36 3:1-15.
17. Brajtburg J, Kobayashi D, Medoff G, Kobayashi GS. Antifungal action of amphotericin B in combination with other polyenes or imidazole antibiotics. *J Infect Dis* 1982;146:138-46.
18. O'Day DM. Fungal keratitis. In Pepose JS, Holland GN, Wilhelmus KR (Eds): *Ocular infection and immunity.* St.Louis, Mosby. 1996;1048-1061.

2

chapter

Parthopratim Dutta Majumder
Jyotirmay Biswas

Episcleritis and Scleritis

ABSTRACT

Diagnosis of episcleritis and scleritis, one of the important causes of acute red eye, is important as these are the two separate clinical entities and often associated with systemic collagen vascular diseases. The management of necrotizing scleritis is very challenging and needs rapid and effective immunosuppression as this condition can lead to sight threatening complications.

Introduction

Episcleritis or scleritis is one of the important causes of acute red eye. Even though both are inflammation of the outer coat of the eyeball, they are clinically, etiologically, and morphologically distinct and different. Therefore, it is essential to differentiate between these two separate clinical entities, especially from treatment point of view.

Anatomic Considerations

The term sclera is derived from Greek word *scleros* meansing hard. Sclera is an opaque, elastic, and resilient tissue of the eye. It can be compared with an incomplete shell comprising approximately 90% (five-sixths) of the outer coat of the eye. Anteriorly, it begins at the limbus and terminates at the optic nerve canal posteriorly. It is predominantly composed of collagen and some elastin fibrils and is relatively avascular and acellular.

The episclera is the thin densely vascularized layer of connective tissue overlying the sclera and situated below the Tenon's capsule. Apart from the vessels and unmyelinated nerve fibers, it contains bundles of collagen. Anteriorly, episclera blends with subconjunctival tissues and Tenon's capsule 1 to 3 mm behind the limbus, and it becomes very thin and indistinct posterior to the equator. Scleritis is always accompanied by an overlying episcleritis. On the other hand, episcleritis *per se* is very rarely associated with scleritis. However, sclera is supplied with nerves particularly near the extraocular muscle insertions. Direct damage to or the stretch of these nerves is the cause for pain in scleritis. Scleritis occurs more commonly anterior to the equator because of the more abundant anterior vascular supply. The circulation overlying the sclera includes 3 vascular layers.[1,2] The location, configuration of vessels, and their clinical significance is tabulated in Table 2.1 and shown in the Figure 2.1.

TABLE 2.1: Layers of vessels of episclera and sclera

Conjunctival plexus	Most superficial in conjunctiva	Arteries are tortuous and veins straight	Can be easily moved on the underlying structure Blanch with 10% phenylephrine
Superficial episcleral plexus	Lies at the level of Tenon's capsule	Vessels are straight with a radial configuration	In episcleritis, maximal congestion occurs within this vascular plexus. Can be easily moved on the underlying structure Blanch with 10% phenylephrine
Deep vascular plexus	Lies deep to the Tenon's capsule and directly over sclera	Vessels are arranged in crisscross pattern	Maximal congestion in scleritis. Cannot be moved on the underlying structure. Does not blanch with 10% phenylephrine

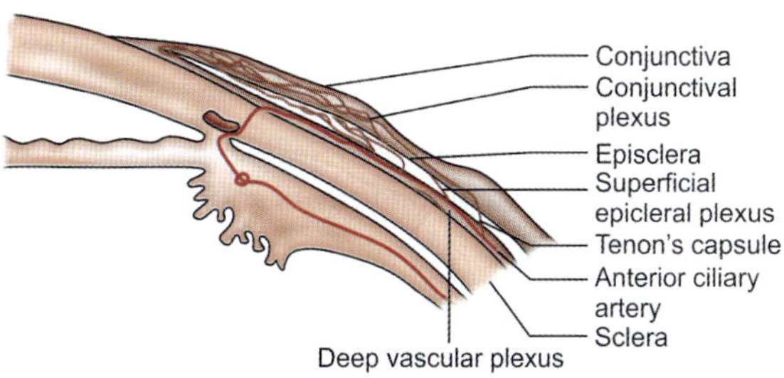

Fig. 2.1: Diagram showing vascular plexuses

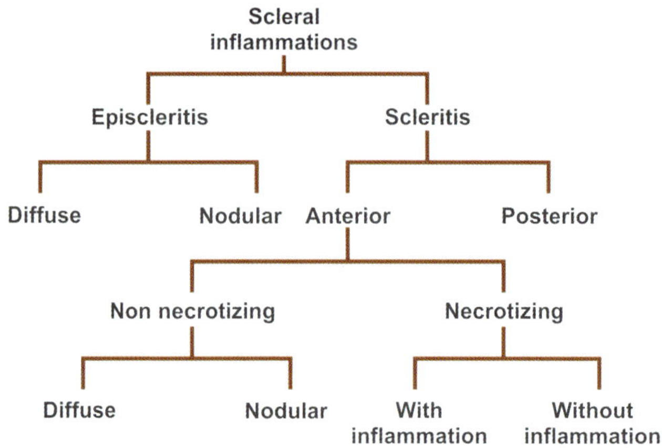

Flowchart 2.1: Classification of scleral inflammation

Nomenclature and Classification

The classification system proposed by Watson and Hayreh is widely accepted.[3] Scleritis can be divided into anterior and posterior scleritis. Anterior scleritis has been classified into four subgroups: diffuse, nodular, necrotizing with inflammation, and necrotizing without inflammation. (Flow chart 2.1) Necrotizing scleritis without inflammation is also called *scleromalacia perforans*.

Episcleritis

Episcleritis was first called "*subconjunctivitis*" by von Graefe, then subsequently "*Hot eyes*" by Hutchinson. The name "episcleritis" was first used by Fuchs, who described the condition as "*episcleritis periodica fugax*" in 1895.

Episcleritis is a transient, self-limited disease of adults. It is seen more frequently in young to middle-aged women. The chief complaint of patients with episcleritis is usually ocular redness with or without irritation. The redness typically persists for 24–72 hours and then resolves spontaneously. Rarely, patients may experience more severe redness and mild pain. Episcleritis occurs most commonly in the exposed zone of the eye and is generally recurrent in nature. More than one-third of patients have bilateral disease.

Half of the episcleritis cases are idiopathic in nature. Systemic diseases associated with episcleritis are rheumatoid arthritis, relapsing polychondritis, Cogan' syndrome, polyarteritis nodosa, etc.[4] The majority of patients with episcleritis recovers completely with treatment with NSAIDs[5] and has no residual changes. However, episcleritis can sometimes be associated with corneal involvement, uveitis, and glaucoma.

Episcleritis is diagnosed clinically by the presence of inflamed episcleral vessels, which typically radiate from the limbus, have a salmon pink color in natural sunlight, can be moved over the deeper sclera with a cotton tipped applicator and will blanch with topical phenylephrine 10%.[6,7] Episcleritis is classified as diffuse or nodular. A localized mobile nodule develops in nodular episcleritis.

Episcleritis can be differentiated from the scleritis on cetain clinical features. The distinguishing features between episcleritis and scleritis are tabulated in Table 2.2.

TABLE 2.2: Distinguishing features of episcleritis and scleritis

Episcleritis	Scleritis
Generally redness, irritation are the main presenting symptoms	Severe boring pain is the main presenting complaint of the patient.
No or minimal tenderness	Moderate to severe tenderness
Congested vessels are bright red in color and vessels can be moved easily with the help of a cotton bud.	Congested vessels are purple-red in color and vessels cannot be moved easily with the help of a cotton bud.
Blanching of the vessels occurs with 10% phenylephrine	Blanching of the vessels does not occur with 10% phenylephrine.

Scleritis

Scleritis is a relatively more severe ocular inflammation than episcleritis. It is a severe painful inflammatory process characterized by edema and cellular infiltration of the sclera and episclera. If not treated properly and well in time, it can be a significant threat to vision. Scleritis affects women more often than men, with a peak incidence in the fifth decade. It frequently starts in one eye and become bilateral in more than half of the cases.[3,7]

Half of patients with scleritis have evidence of an underlying systemic disease. Scleritis can be a presenting manifestation of a life-threatening systemic autoimmune disease. Rheumatoid arthritis is the most common systemic condition associated with scleritis. The incidence of rheumatoid arthritis in patients with scleritis ranges from 10 to 33%.[3,4,7]

Scleritis may be associated with the following systemic diseases:[3,4,7,8-13]

- Rheumatoid arthritis
- Relapsing polychondritis
- Systemic lupus erythematosus and antiphospholipid syndrome
- Wegener's granulomatosis

- Polyarteritis nodosa
- Cogan syndrome
- Juvenile rheumatoid arthritis
- Ankylosing spondylitis
- Ulcerative colitis
- Polymyositis
- Sarcoidosis
- Syphilis
- Tuberculosis
- Herpes zoster ophthalmicus
- Acanthamoeba keratitis.

Perhaps Galileo had sufferered with scleritis associated with rheumatoid arthritis. He became totally blind at the age of 74 years probably due to complcations of sclerits.[8]

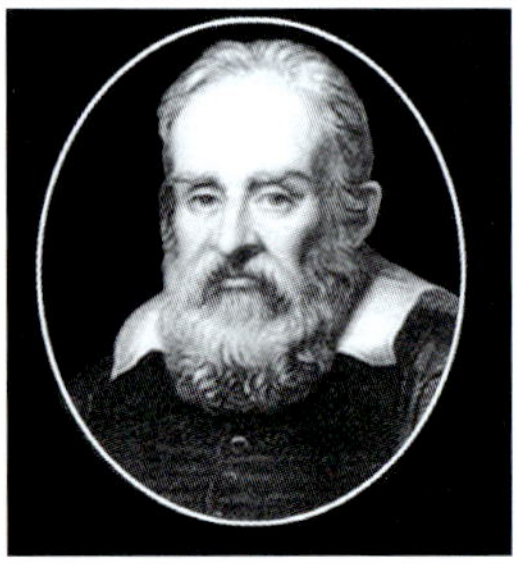

DIAGNOSIS

Diagnosis of scleritis is almost always clinical; however, when the posterior sclera is involved, clinical signs may be less obvious, and imaging studies are necessary to confirm the diagnosis. Patients with anterior scleritis presents with redness and pain. The onset is usually gradual, extending over several days. Ocular pain is severe and typically dull and boring (piercing) in nature, exacerbated by eye movement, and occasionally, may worsen at night and waken the patients from sleep. The pain often radiates to the ear, scalp, face, and jaw.

The *sine qua non of* scleritis is the presence of scleral edema and congestion of the deep episcleral plexus. Slit-lamp examination using red-free light is extremely helpful in determining the pattern and depth of episcleral vascular congestion and engorgement.

In diffuse scleritis (Fig. 2.2), the sclera assumes a violaceous hue in natural sunlight. It is very important to examine patients in daylight with the unaided eye to note the subtle color differences of the vessels. Also inflamed scleral vessels have a crisscross pattern. They are adherent to the sclera and cannot be moved with a cotton-tipped applicator. Engorged scleral vessels cannot by blanched with 10% phenylephrine, whereas phenylephrine easily blanches engorged vessels in the superficial episcleral and conjunctival plexuses.[6,7,9,10] There is tenderness of the globe.

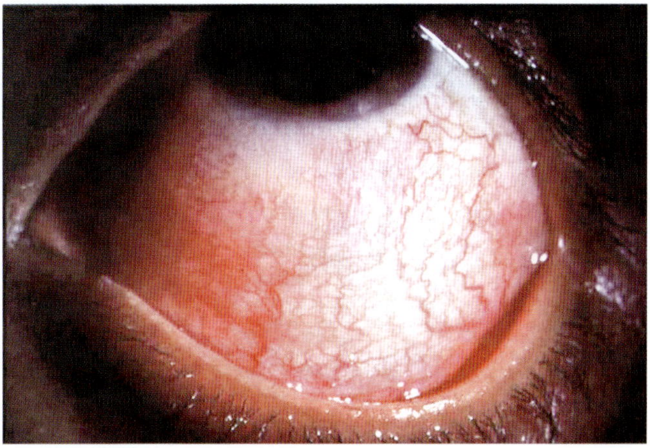

Fig. 2.2: Diffuse scleritis

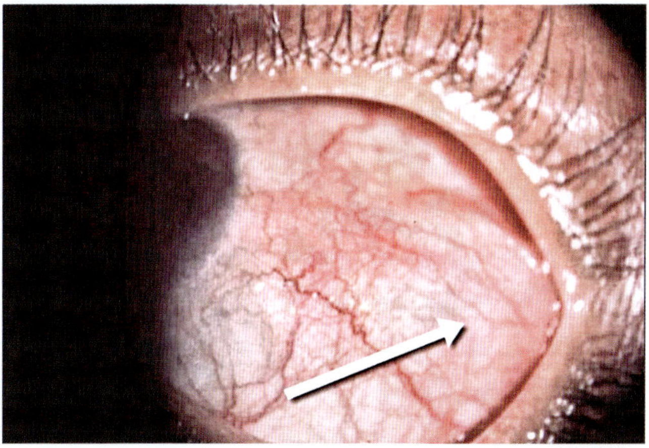

Fig. 2.3: Nodular scleritis

Nodular anterior scleritis (Fig. 2.3) is characterized by a localized area of scleral edema and congestion of the scleral vessels. The scleral nodule is deep red to purple in color, immobile, tender to palpation and separated from the overlying episcleral tissue, which is elevated by the nodule. These features distinguish the nodular scleritis from diffuse episcleritis. The lack of necrosis within the nodule and the localization of inflammation within the borders of the nodule differentiate this form from necrotizing anterior scleritis with inflammation. All of the vascular layers overlying the nodule are displaced forward. Sometimes, multiple nodules may be present and there may be an overlying episcleritis.[7-10]

Necrotizing anterior scleritis with inflammation (Fig. 2.4) is the most severe of all the type and is a potential threat to visual loss. It is seen in patients with rheumatoid arthritis (Fig. 2.5). It is bilateral in 60% cases.The

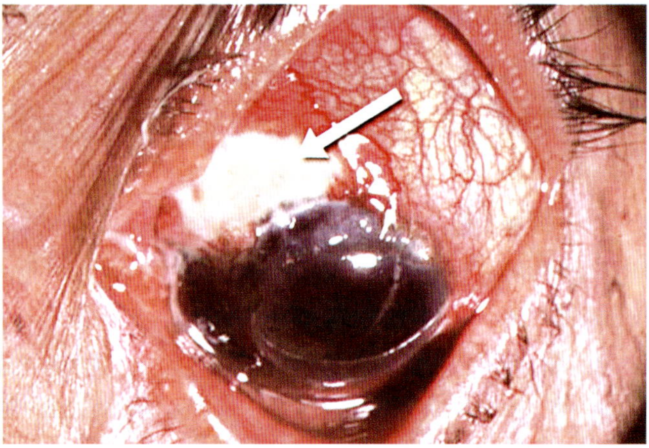

Fig. 2.4: Necrotizing anterior scleritis with inflammation (necrotizing scleritis). Note the avascular area (white arrow)

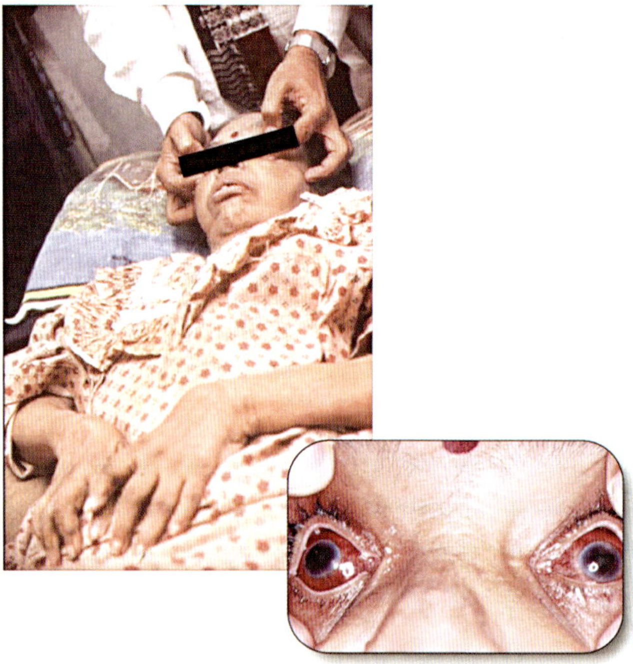

Fig. 2.5: Bilateral necrotizing scleritis in a patient of rheumatoid arthritis

patient presents with severe pain out of proportion to inflammatory signs. Examination reveals white, avascular areas of localized scleral edema and congestion, edges of these lesions are more inflamed than the center. Underlying uveal tissue becomes visible as the sclera becomes thin and translucent. If not treated, the necrotizing scleritis may spread to the equator and circumferentially and can involve the entire globe.[14,15]

NECROTIZING ANTERIOR SCLERITIS WITHOUT INFLAMMATION

Necrotizing anterior scleritis without signs of inflammation (scleromalcia perforans) occurs predominantly in patients with long-standing rheumatoid arthritis. There are minimal signs of inflammation and generally no pain accompanying with this type of scleritis. As the disease progresses, the sclera progressively thins and the underlying dark uveal tissue becomes visible (Fig. 2.6). Staphylomas can develop if the IOP is elevated. Though spontaneous perforation is rare, these eyes are prone to rupture with minimal trauma.[14,15] Occasionally, patients may present with blurred vision, because of astigmatism due to thinning and distortion of the globe.

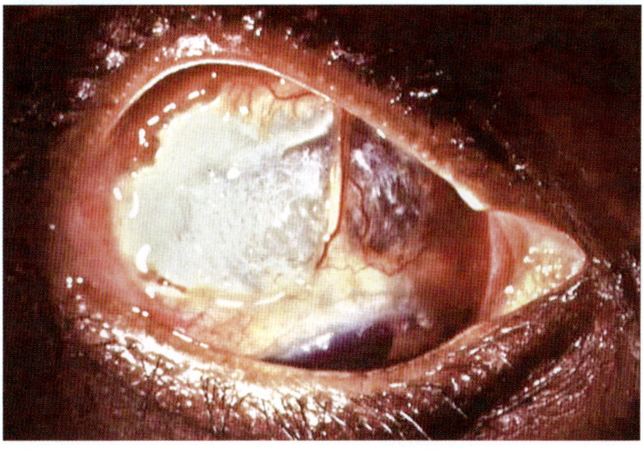

Fig. 2.6: Necrotizing anterior scleritis without signs of inflammation (scleromalcia perforans)

POSTERIOR SCLERITIS

Posterior scleritis is defined as an inflammation of the sclera, posterior to the ora serrata. Posterior scleritis may occur in association with anterior scleritis or may be isolated. Posterior scleritis without anterior scleritis is difficult to diagnose. Patients with posterior scleritis present with pain, tenderness, proptosis, visual loss, and occasionally, restricted motility, macular

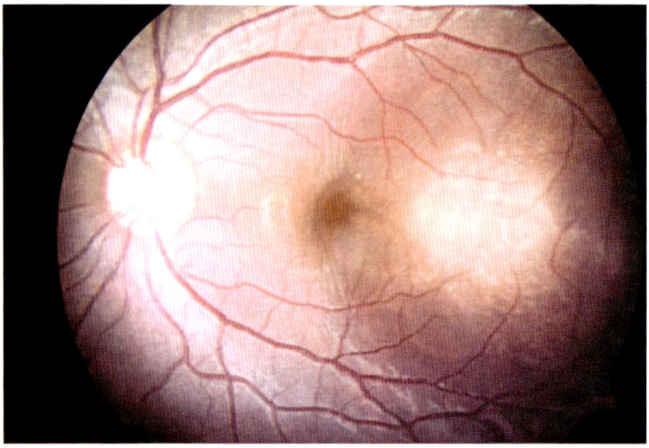

Fig. 2.7: A circular whitish-yellow patch of edema is seen temporal of the macula in posterior scleritis

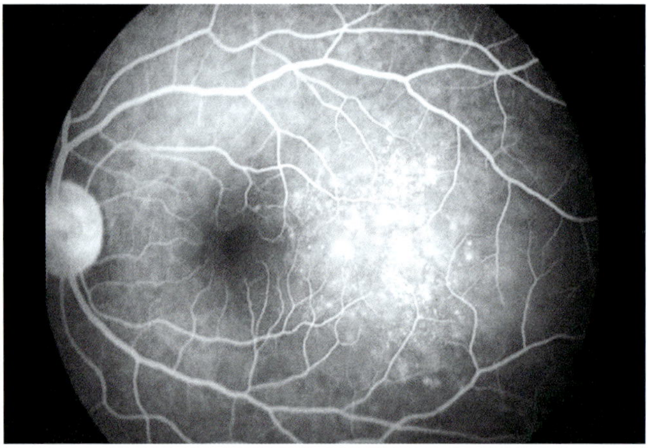

Fig. 2.8: Fundus fluorescein angiography (FFA): Angiography of the patient with posterior scleritis showing punctate leaks at the level of the retinal pigment epithelium and pooling into the subneurosensory retinal space

or paramacular edema (Figs 2.7 and 2.8) choroidal folds, exudative retinal detachment, papilledema, and angle-closure glaucoma secondary to choroidal thickening. Most cases of posterior scleritis need ancillary imaging modalities like ultrasonography (Fig.2.9) and a magnetic resonance imaging for confirmation of the diagnosis. An infiltration of extraocular muscles in the region of the posterior scleritis may lead to retraction of the lower lid in the upper gaze.[6,7,16,24]

Surgically induced necrotizing scleritis (SINS) can occur after any type of ocular surgery with excessive scleral manipulation, mostly after cataract

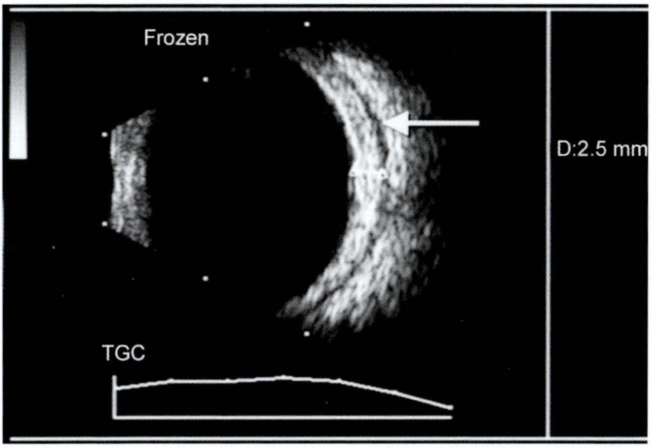

Fig. 2.9: USG scan of posterior scleritis. Note the characteristic T sign (white arrow) and thickened sclera

surgery [17,23] (Fig. 2.10), but may also be seen after glaucoma, RD, squint or pterygium surgery. SINS may occur from few days to few years after surgery. Inflammation is typically localized around the site of the surgical wound or adjacent to the site of surgery but may progress to involve the entire sclera. SINS is mostly necrotizing in nature and sometimes may even be the initial manifestation of serious systemic disease. So, all patients with SINS need to be investigated appropriately.

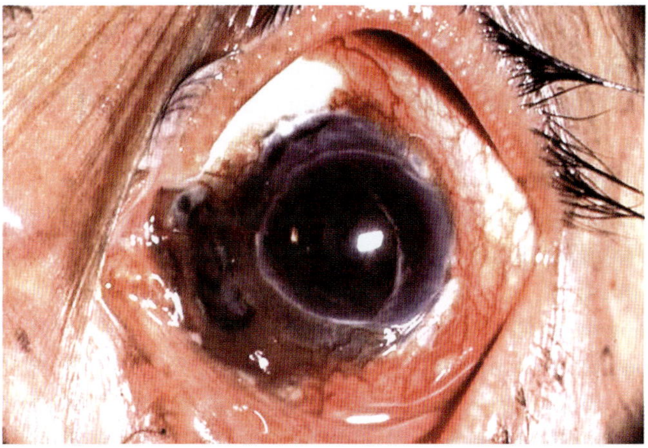

Fig. 2.10: Surgically induced necrotizing scleritis

INFECTIOUS SCLERAL INFLAMMATION

Scleritis with purulent exudates or infiltrates should raise the suspicion of an infectious etiology. Formations of granulomas or fistulas, painful nodules, conjunctival and scleral ulcers are often seen in infectious scleral inflammations. Endogenous spread of bacteria (*Staphylococci, H. influenzae, Treponema pallidum, M. tuberculosis*); fungi[23] (*Aspergillus*); viruses (*Herpes simplex* or *H. zoster*) or parasites (*Toxocara, Toxoplasma, Onchocerca*) are reported to cause infective scleritis.[6, 7] Also, in rare instances, infections of adjacent tissues like the conjunctiva, cornea may involve the sclera by contiguous spread. In chronic cases, possibility of a foreign body must be ruled out. Scleral infections can often follow buckling procedures for retinal detachment.

DIAGNOSTIC EVALUATION OF SCLERITIS

As we know that scleritis can occur in association with various systemic diseases. Sometimes, scleral inflammations can be the presenting signs of an underlying systemic disease. Thus work-up of scleritis should include a complete thorough physical examination, with attention to the joints, skin and cardiovascular and respiratory system. The following routine investigations should be performed:

1. Hemoglobin.
2. White blood cell count and differential count.
3. Erythrocyte sedimentation rate.
4. If connective tissue disease is suspected, full immunologic work-up should be undertaken, including levels of immunoglobulins and immunofluorescent studies for autoantibodies (including rheumatoid factor and antinuclear and anti-ds-DNA antibodies) and circulating immune complexes. If Wegener's granulomatosis and polyarteritis nodosa are suspected, the anti-nuclear cytoplasmic antibody (ANCA) tests should be performed. The C-reactive protein is a important laboratory parameter of an active generalized inflammatory response.[4,6]
5. Serum uric acid.
6. Full serologic tests for syphilis.
7. X-ray chest.
8. Ultasonography.
9. Ultrasound biomicroscopy.

B-scan Ultrasonography

B-scan ultrasonography should always be included in the examination of patients with scleritis. Many patients who were formerly thought to have only anterior segment disease have been found to have extensive and sight threatening posterior scleritis as well. It also has become known that many patients with posterior scleritis with minimum symptoms and signs may have much more extensive disease than had previously been considered possible. The hallmark features of posterior scleritis seen with B-scan ultrasonography are helpful in differentiating posterior scleritis from other conditions. B-scan ultrasonography may reveal the characteristic flattening of the posterior aspect of the globe due to retrobulbar edema. Abnormally increased thickening of the posterior ocular coats of the globe (>2 mm), optic disk swelling, distension of the optic nerve sheath, retinal detachments, and choroidal detachments can be detected. Fluid can accumulate in the posterior subtenon space and extend around the optic nerve, forming the characteristic "T-sign"on B-scan.[24]

Ultrasound biomicroscopy

This can bc valuable for better delineation of scleral thinning and evaluation of scleral edema (Fig. 2.11) and nodules. It is also an important boon for ruling out any malignancy. An underlying squamous cell carcinoma or a medulloepithelioma can extend to the sclera and can masquerade as scleral inflammation.

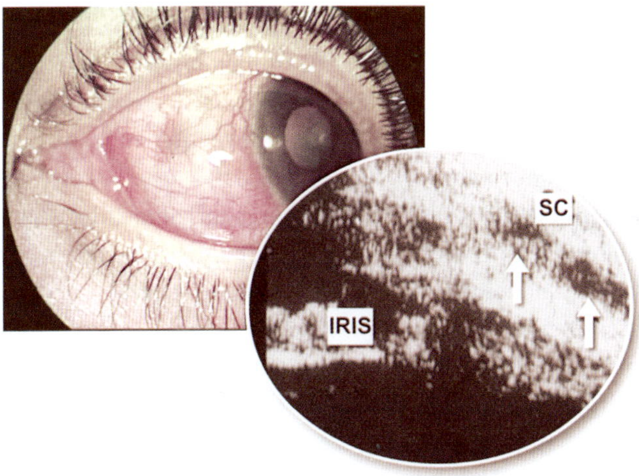

Fig. 2.11: UBM picture of a case of scleritis showing scleral edema (white arrows)

COMPLICATIONS OF SCLERITIS

Unlike episcleritis, scleritis is associated with potentially sight threatening ocular complications. Vision may be limited in scleritis due to keratitis, anterior uveitis, cataract, change of refractive status, macular edema, optic disk edema, or atrophy, and exudative retinal detachment. Decreased vision occurs most frequently with posterior scleritis followed by necrotizing scleritis, nodular scleritis and least often with diffuse anterior scleritis. During any stage of scleral inflammation, the intraocular pressure may be elevated due to several mechanisms, such as obstruction of the aqueous outflow channels, elevated episcleral pressure, angle-closure, or secondary to a steroid response. Signs of corneal infiltrate, thinning, or stromal keratitis may be present with corneal ulceration. Cataract formation may be accelerated by long-standing inflammation or secondary to steroid use.[6,7,15]

Necrotizing scleritis is a serious disease. Scleral thinning is most common, and it may progress to staphyloma in the presence of raised intraocular pressure. Though increased scleral transparency and thinning is a frequent complication of necrotizing scleritis but perforation is relatively uncommon Both ocular and systemic complications are reported in abot 60% of cases and approximately 40% of the patient suffer from serious visual impairment or visual loss. It can be fetal. About 29% die within 5 years of onset mainly due to complications of vasculitis.

TREATMENT

The primary aim of the treatment of scleral inflammation is to control the inflammatory process to relieve the symptoms and thereby reduce the damage to the eye. However, the effective management of a case of scleral inflammation involves timely diagnosis, prevention of complications and identification of underlying systemic or local cause, if any.

Generally, episcleritis is self-limiting benign inflammation, whether treated or not, it will resolve in 10 to 21 days. If the condition is recurrent, medications such as topical nonsteroidal anti-inflammatory drugs (NSAIDs) like flurbiprofen, bromofenac and nepafenac, or topical weaker corticosteroid (loteprednol, flurometholone) are often required to control the symptoms of irritation, foreign body sensation, etc. However, prolonged use of topical corticosteroid should be avoided, because of the side effects. It should be kept in mind that though simple episcleritis resolves spontaneously and rapidly, resolution of nodular episcleritis is much slower and may require oral medications. Systemic medications like oral NSAID and very rarely oral corticosteroids are required in the treatment of indolent episcleritis.[5,6]

Anterior non-necrotizing scleritis readily responds to topical steroid and systemic nonsteroidal anti-inflammatory drugs (NSAIDs). Both nonselective COX inhibitors (e.g., flurbiprofen, indomethacin, and to a lesser extent ibuprofen) and the more selective COX-2 inhibitors have been used successfully. Sustained-release indomethacin 75 mg twice a day has been found to be very effective in controlling the inflammation. However, prolonged use of NSAIDs should be avoided in view of their significant side effect on long-term use.

Corticosteroids are helpful in patients not responding to COX-inhibitors or those with posterior or necrotizing disease. A starting dose of 1 mg/kg/day is standard with weekly reduction by 10 mg/week until a dose of 40 mg/day is reached. After this dose is reached, the rate of reduction is individualized, according to the clinical findings and patients' response but is in the order of 5 mg /week until cessation or an acceptable maintenance dose is reached. Intravenous methylprednisolone is advocated in cases with threatened scleral or corneal perforation in necrotizing scleritis, which requires a rapid control of the inflammation.[3,5-7,9]

Necrotizing scleritis, particularly associated with autoimmune diseases is difficult to treat and almost always requires systemic immunosuppressive therapy, not only for ocular involvement, also for life threatening systemic complications. For example prompt and effective immunosuppression is required to control the necrotizing scleritis associated with systemic vasculitis like Wegener's granulomatosis because mortality is higher in this group of patients because of the systemic complications. This group of patients also requires a consultation with rheumatologist for their systemic ailments.[18]

Inications for immunosuppressive therapy in scleral inflammation:

- Anterior necrotizing scleritis
- Posterior scleritis
- Scleritis associated with a systemic disease.

Various immunosuppressants have been tried for treatment of scleritis and these include antimetabolites (methotrexate, azathioprine, and mycophenolate mofetil), alkylating agents (chlorambucil and cyclophosphamide), T-cell inhibitors (cyclosporine and tacrolimus). Newer biological agents like TNF-α inhibitors (infliximab or adalimumab), rituximab are reported to be used for the treatment of scleritis.

Methotrexate is commonly used to treat scleritis not responding to oral corticosteroid and less sever anterior necrotising scleritis with inflammation. Often the drug is used as a first-line treatment in patients in whom oral steroid cannot be started because of systemic ailments. Among steroid sparing immunosuppressives, methotrexate has gained the most widespread usage due to its relatively safe profile. Methotrexate, a folic acid analog, inhibits the enzyme dihydrofolate reductase and thus the production of thymidylate, which is essential for DNA replication. This results in the inhibition of rapidly dividing cells, including leukocytes. The drug is used with or without a short course of oral steroid in tapering dosage. Dosage of methotrexate is 0.1-0.5 mg/kg/week; low dose therapy is started at a dose of 7.5 mg/

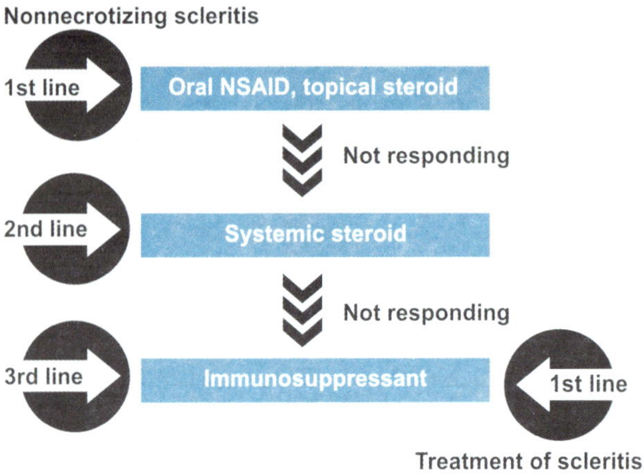

Flow chart 2.2: Treatment of scleritis

week and it can be increased up to 25 mg/week. Generally, it is given orally once a week. It has been observed that methotrexate immunosuppressive therapy is moderately effective. The drug takes months to achieve adequate tissue concentration for the therapeutic success. Severe side effects, such as hepatotoxicity, cytopenias, and interstitial pneumoni are not uncommon.[18,19]

Treatment of scleritis associated with necrotizing systemic vasculitis should be prompt and effective if immunosuppression is required. Treatment in such patients should be guided both by the ophthalmic response and control of the underlying disease. Cyclophosphamide is an effective immunosuppressive drug used in patients with necrotizing scleritis associated with systemic vasculitis like Wegener's granulomatosis (Fig. 2.12), relapsing polychondritis. Antineutrophil cytoplasmic antibody test is a useful laboratory parameter to monitor therapeutic response in patients with Wegener's granulomatosis. Concomitant administration of prednisone at a dose of 1 mg/kg/day may be needed. Oral corticosteroids can usually be tapered and often discontinued over the first 6–12 weeks of cyclophosphamide therapy. Cyclophosphamide in a dose of 100 mg per day (2 mg/kg/day)

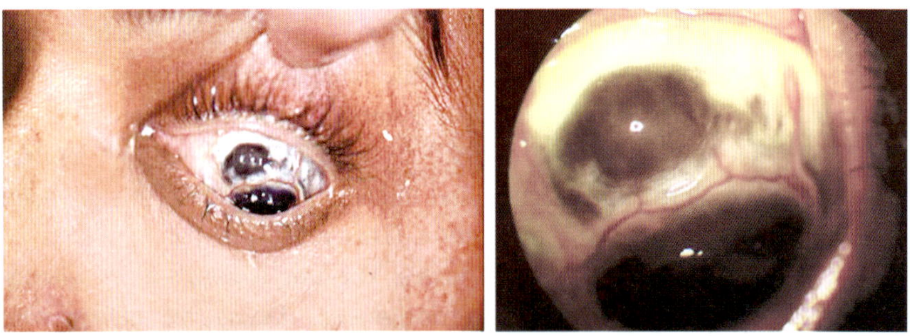

Fig. 2.12: Necrotizing scleritis associated with Wegener's granulomatosis

orally and tapered monthly, should be the first choice in treating patients with associated potentially lethal vasculitic diseases, such as Wegener's granulomatosis or polyarteritis nodosa. The patient should drink copious amounts of fluid to prevent hemorrhagic cystitis. In severe and nonresponsive cases, infusion of 500 mg of cyclophosphamide (given over 1 to 2 hours) is often required. Because of potential life threatening complications, it should be administered under the supervision of a rheumatologis. Other immunosuppressive agents, including methotrexate, azathioprine, cyclosporine, and newer biologicals agents have been successfully used for the treatment of necrotizing systemic vasculitis, but reports available are based on small case series.[6,18,20]

TREATMENT OF INFECTIOUS SCLERITIS

Systemic treatment with topical antimicrobial therapy is the mainstay of treatment of scleritis of infectious origin. Differentiating infectious scleritis from noninfectious scleritis is of paramount importance because corticosteroid therapy and immunosuppressive therapy (often used in noninfectious autoimmune scleritis) are contraindicated in active infections. Prior to microbiological determination of the causative organism and its antibiotic sensitivity spectrum, vancomycin or cephalosporins in combination with aminoglycosides usually are chosen. Any foreign body, if present, may need to be removed before the infection can be brought under control.[18,20]

SURGICAL TREATMENT

Tectonic surgical procedures rarely may be required to preserve the integrity of the globe. Scleral grafts from fresh sclera or glycerin-preserved sclera those are available through eye banks. Grafting (Fig. 2.13) may be performed

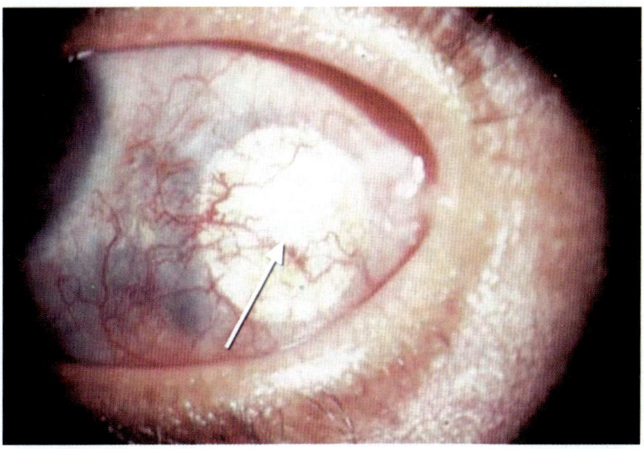

Fig. 2.13: Scleral patch graft

in cases of threatening perforation before the effects of systemic immunosuppressive agents manifest.[22]

Summary

Scleral inflammations are important causes of red eye and need to be differentiated from other causes. Though episcleritis is a benign self-limiting disease, scleritis is highly associated with potentially sight threatening ocular complications and serious systemic diseases. Early diagnosis and treatment of scleritis is important in preventing and diminishing ocular and systemic morbidity. Hence, attempts should be made to achieve good long-term prognosis with careful clinical history, detailed ocular examination, and use of immunosuppressant drugs whenever necessary without any delay.

References

1. Snell R, Lemp M. Clinical anatomy of the eye. Malden: Black-well Scientific Publications; 1989. p. 125-6.
2. Lee Ann Remington. Clinical anatomy and physiology of the visual system. Third Edition. Butterworth-Heinemann; 2011. pp 29-32.
3. Watson PG, Hayreh SS. Scleritis and episcleritis. *Br J Ophthalmol.* 1976; 60:163-8.
4. Carlos EP, Fabio MM. Systemic disorders associated with episcleritis and scleritis. *Curr Opin Ophthalmol.* 2001;12:471-8.
5. Lyons CJ, Hakin KN, Watson PG. Topical urbiprofen: an effective treatment for episcleritis? *Eye* 1990;4:521-5.
6. McCluskey P: Scleritis. BMJ Publishing Group;2001. pp 39-100.
7. Narciss O, Bola O, McCluskey P, Susan L. *Scleritis. Surv Ophthalmol* 2005;50:351-63.
8. Germani GM. Rheumatoid arthritis and the blindness of Galileo Galilei. *Ospedule Maggiore* 1964;59:193-6.
9. Watson PG. Treatment of scleritis and episcleritis. Trans Ophthalmol Soc U K. 1974;94:76-9.
10. Watson PG, Hazelman BL. The sclera and systemic disorders. Philadelphia, PA: WB Saunders;1976.
11. Sainz de la Maza M, Foster CS, Jabbur NS. Scleritis associated with rheumatoid arthritis and with other systemic immune-mediated diseases. *Ophthalmology.* 1994;101:1281-6.
12. McGavin DD, Williamson J, Forrester JV, et al. Episcleritis and scleritis. A study of their clinical manifestations and association with rheumatoid arthritis. *Br J Ophthalmol.* 1976;60:192-226.
13. Power WJ, Rodriguez A, Neves RA, et al. Disease relapse in patients with ocular manifestations of Wegener granulomatosis. *Ophthalmology.* 1995;102:154-60.
14. Sainz de la Maza M, Jabbur NS, Foster CS. Severity of scleritis and episcleritis. *Ophthalmology.* 1994;101:389-96.
15. Tuft SJ, Watson PG. Progression of scleral disease. *Ophthalmology.* 1991; 98:467-71.
16. McCluskey PJ, Watson PG, Lightman S, et al. Posterior scleritis: clinical features, systemic associations, and outcome in a large series of patients. *Ophthalmology.* 1999;106:2380-6.

17. Scott JA, Clearkin LG. Surgically induced diffuse scleritis following cataract surgery. *Eye.* 1994;8(Pt 3):292-7.
18. Thomas AA, Narsing AR, Ronald ES. The diagnosis and management of anterior scleritis. *Int Ophthalmol Clin.* 2005;45(2):191-204.
19. Kaplan M, Audrey, Barkana, Yaniv, Avni, Isaac, Neumann, Ron'Methotrexate as a first-line corticosteroid-sparing therapy in a cohort of uveitis and scleritis. *Ocular Immunol Inflamm.* 2003;11:2,131-9
20. Rachitskaya A, Mandelcorn ED, Albini TA. An update on the cause and treatment of scleritis. *Curr Opin Ophthalmol.* 2010;21(6):463-7.
21. Nguyen QD, Foster CS: Scleral patch graft in the management of necrotizing scleritis. *Int Ophthalmol Clin.* 1999;39:109-31.
22. O'Donoghue E, Lightman S, Tuft S, et al. Surgically induced necrotising sclerokeratitis (SINS)—precipitating factors and response to treatment. *Br J Ophthalmol.* 1992;76:17-21.
23. Sawant SD, Biswas J. Fungal scleritis with exudative retinal detachment. *Ocul Immunol Inflamm.* 2010;18(6):457-8.
24. Biswas J, Mittal S, Ganesh SK, Shetty NS, Gopal L. Posterior scleritis: clinical profile and imaging characteristics. *Indian J Ophthalmol.* 1998;46(4):195-202.

3
chapter

Murali Ariga

Progression of Optic Disk and Visual Field Changes in Glaucoma

ABSTRACT

Glaucoma progression can be assessed by clinical evaluation, visual fields, and imaging devices. This chapter reviews the clinical features that characterize progression besides the evolution of newer software in automated perimeters, such as the HFA and Octopus. The GPA and Eyesuite software are capable of detecting progression and also estimate the rate of progression.

Introduction

Glaucoma is defined as a progressive optic neuropathy, and therefore, optic disk examination and visual fields evaluation is of fundamental importance.

HOW TO EXAMINE AND DOCUMENT CHANGES IN THE OPTIC NERVE HEAD?

Clinical examination of the optic nerve head (ONH) can be done with direct and indirect ophthalmoscopes but is best performed in a dilated pupil on a slit-lamp biomicroscope using either 78 diopters or 90 diopters hand-held lenses. Advantages of this examination include the magnification provided by the slit-lamp and stereoscopic view provided by these lenses. Certain characteristic optic disk features are typical of glaucoma.

NEURAL RIM

Uniform pink color, contour and thickness of the neural rim are generally found in the normal eye (Fig. 3.1). The disk obeys 'ISNT' rule which

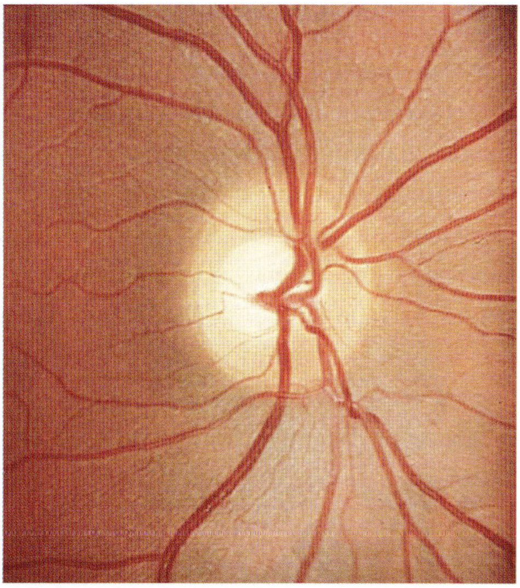

Fig. 3.1: Normal optic disk with healthy uniform neural rim

means that usually the inferior rim is the thickest followed by superior, nasal, and temporal rim. Glaucomatous changes noted are rim loss, notches in superior, inferior rim or both. Concentric enlargement of the cup with concentric rim thinning may also occur.

RETINAL NERVE FIBER LAYER

The retinal nerve fiber layer (RNFL) may show slit- or wedge-shaped defects. They are seen as dark areas in an arcuate pattern wider than the retinal vessels.

BLOOD VESSEL CHANGES

When neural rim loss occurs, the overlying circumlinear vessel may be 'bared'.

PERIPAPILLARY ATROPHY

Peripapillary atrophy (PPA) or a temporal crescent of chorioretinal and retinal pigment epithelial (RPE) layer atrophy is noted in two zones namely outer alpha and inner beta zones. The area of atrophy may correspond to the area of neural thinning. Beta zone atrophy occurs more often in glaucoma patients than in normal individuals and enlargement may indicate a progressive glaucoma.

CUP-DISK RATIO

An increase in cup-disk ratio (CDR) and asymmetry of CDR of 0.2 or greater between the two eyes have been considered as important signs of primary open-angle glaucoma. However, an assessment of optic disk size is important because smaller disks will have smaller cups. It has been noted that there is a tendency to over diagnose glaucoma in larger disks with larger cups and miss the diagnosis of glaucoma in smaller disks in which the rim changes may be subtle. A classical glaucomatous optic disk will usually present a rim loss, inferior notch, peripapillary atrophy and disk hemorrhage (Fig. 3.2).

The European Glaucoma Society[1] has suggested schematic guidelines for the glaucomatous changes in the optic nerve head (Fig. 3.3).

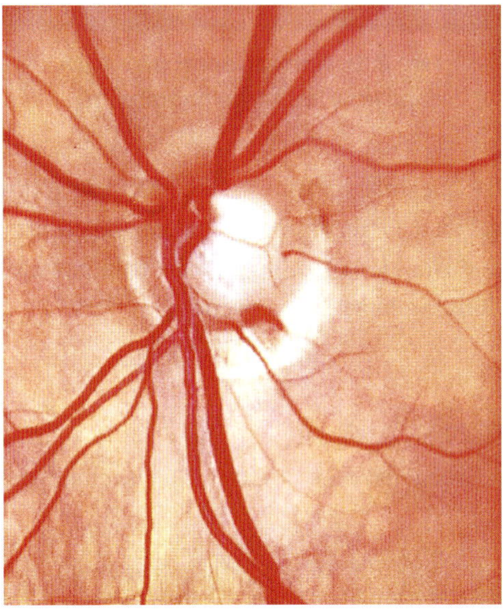

Fig. 3.2: Glaucomatous optic disk with rim loss, inferior notch, peripapillary atrophy and disk hemorrhage

DOCUMENTATION

Documentation of the ONH changes in glaucoma can be done by the following procedures:

1. Changes can be documented in the form of a diagram in the patient's chart.
2. Fundus photography/stereophotography/red free photography can provide details.
3. Imaging of the optic disc and RNFL using imaging devices like GDx, HRT or OCT.

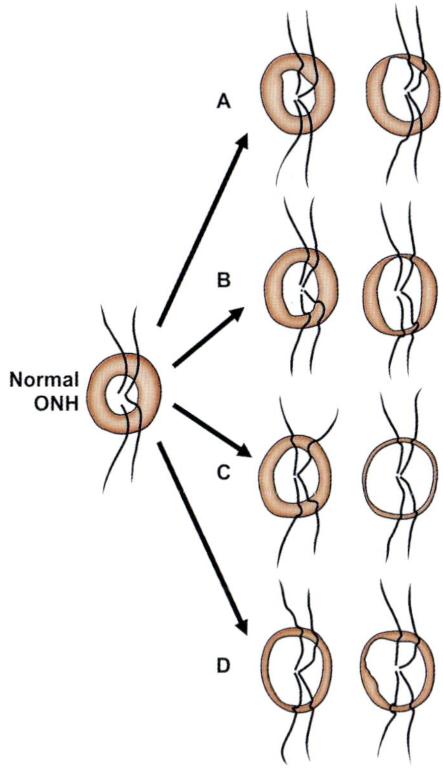

Fig. 3.3: Schematic changes in ONH (adapted from European Glaucoma Society guidelines)

DETECTING CHANGE OR PROGRESSION IN GLAUCOMA

- Objective (structural) changes seen in ONH/RNFL/Disk hemorrhages
- Subjective (functional) changes seen in visual fields
- Changes noted on serial testing with imaging devices (OCT, HRT and GDx VCC).

SIGNIFICANCE OF OPTIC DISK HEMORRHAGES (DRANCE HEMORRHAGES)

The prevalence of these hemorrhages is about 0.2 % in the normal population. However, a larger proportion of glaucoma patients have these hemorrhages, which are thought to be RNFL infarction. They are intermittent and tend to disappear over time. Very often they are missed on clinical examination and seen only in photographs. Recent publications have confirmed that the appearance of disk hemorrhages is associated with glaucoma progression.[6]

DETECTION PROGRESSION IN VISUAL FIELDS

Detecting progression in a chronic and slowly progressive disease like glaucoma is difficult. Monitoring visual fields is only one means of assessing progression. In following visual fields in glaucoma patients, it is often difficult to differentiate between normal short-term and long-term fluctuations and true disease progression. Due to variability, a new change on a visual field needs to be confirmed on repeat testing.

FLUCTUATION VERSUS PROGRESSION

The main problem in deciding whether or not a glaucoma patient's visual field loss is progressing is to separate true progression from changes due to variability or fluctuation between tests. Fluctuation[2] is defined as the variability in the response to the same stimulus that is not due to true disease progression. As visual fields testing is a subjective examination, variable responses may be obtained each time the test is performed (inter-test or long-term fluctuations) or during the same test (intra-test or short-term fluctuations). Fluctuation varies among patients and among sectors in the same visual field, and increases with severity of disease. To detect true progression, one has to evaluate whether the observed change exceeds the expected fluctuation in the tested area.

Visual field progression in glaucoma may be seen as:
1. Development of a new defect.
2. Deepening or enlargement of a preexisting defect.
3. Diffuse loss of sensitivity (less common).

Most often progression is identified as a deepening of a preexisting scotoma (as shown by various research studies), along with enlargement of the scotoma. In a study[3] evaluating visual field progression in glaucoma, most cases showed deepening (86%) or enlargement (23%) of a previous scotoma, while none of the eyes developed new visual field defects in previously normal areas. This highlights the importance of evaluating areas adjacent to existing scotomas when searching for visual field progression. However, these adjacent areas are also known to exhibit larger degrees of fluctuation, which makes identification of true progression more difficult. Diffuse sensitivity loss may also represent glaucoma progression, although it is usually accompanied by new defects or worsening of previous focal defects. Progressive diffuse loss should raise the suspicion of cataract progression and must be correlated with clinical examination.

The Humphrey field analyzer (HFA) has statistical software, STATPAC, which is capable of analyzing a single visual field for abnormalities or a series of fields for progression. The single field analysis provides a printout of a single visual field with most detailed information about that test. In the overview printout, several visual fields are arranged chronologically on the same page for the ease of comparison. The change analysis printout provides a chronologic box plot analysis, the time course of the four global indices (only MD and PSD in SITA), and the linear regression analysis of MD.

HOW FREQUENTLY SHOULD VISUAL FIELDS BE DONE TO ASSESS GLAUCOMA PROGRESSION

Most glaucoma patients under treatment will have slow rate of progression over the years, but there are those few who will have rapid progression rates. Published rates for mean deviation (MD) deterioration in glaucoma patients have varied and depend on individual susceptibility, severity of disease, and treatment strategies.[4] One should perform enough visual fields at the beginning of follow-up in order to detect cases that present with fast progression rates. It has been suggested that six visual field examinations be done in the first 2 years, in order to rule out aggressive disease and to establish a consistent baseline. Subsequently, the frequency of testing may be reduced to once or twice yearly as long as no change is detected. At any time during follow-up that a change is identified on the visual field, one should not wait another year to proceed with a confirmatory test, but instead the frequency of examinations should again be increased in order to confirm or exclude progression.

EVENT AND TREND-BASED ANALYSES

There are two main approaches to analyze progression—event-based and trend-based analyses. The first approach compares the current examination with a previous one (usually the baseline test). If the results are significantly worse on the follow-up examination, progression is indicated. This is called *event-based analysis*. In the second approach, instead of only comparing a few tests, one looks for progressive change by analyzing all the tests available in a specific period of time. This is called *trend-based analysis*, as a trend in the values is plotted over time, and significant deterioration can be assessed by observing the slope or decline of the regression line. Besides evaluating whether progression has occurred, trend-based analysis also allows an estimation of the rate of progression. It is well known that some patients deteriorate faster than others, and estimating each individual's rate of progression may help decide aggressiveness of treatment and the response to treatment.

The older software version is the glaucoma change probability (GCP) software. The GCP performs individual comparisons of each visual field point on follow-up examinations with a set of baseline fields. Progression is flagged if two or more adjacent points within adjacent to an existing scotoma show significant deterioration confirmed on two consecutive tests. The GCP performs individualized analysis of the sectors in the visual field; however, as it is based on the total deviation plot, it is affected by diffuse media opacities such as cataract.

The new guided progression analysis (GPA) software was developed to overcome the limitations mentioned above. Both the GCP and the GPA are event based analyses, but the GPA has following advantages when compared with the GCP:

- The GPA is based on the pattern deviation plot, as opposed to the total deviation plot used by the GCP. Therefore, the GPA evaluates progression adjusted for diffuse effects
- The GPA runs not only on SITA tests, but also accepts full-threshold tests for the baseline pair (the GCP did not), which is convenient as some patients with long-term follow-up have been tested with the full-threshold strategy during early follow-ups.

As detection of new or progressing visual field defects is performed by comparison to the baseline, it is imperative to have reliable baseline examinations. The software automatically selects the first two available examinations as the baseline tests. However, one can override this automatic selection to a more suitable time-point (e.g., change in therapy after progression), or to reject fields that are unreliable due to initial learning effects (which could reduce the sensitivity to detect progression). The GPA software then compares each follow-up test to the average of the baseline tests. It identifies points that show change greater that the expected variability (at the 95% significance level), as determined by previous studies with stable glaucoma patients (Fig. 3.4). If significant change is detected in at least three points, and is repeated in the same points over two consecutive follow-up tests, then the GPA software will flag the last examination as *possible progression*. If the same three or more points have significant change detected and repeated in three consecutive follow-up tests, the GPA software will flag the last examination as *likely progression*.

The latest version of the Humphrey field analyzer provides the visual field index (VFI) and VFI progression plot.[5] The VFI is a newly developed index that is proposed to evaluate the rate of progression. The aim of

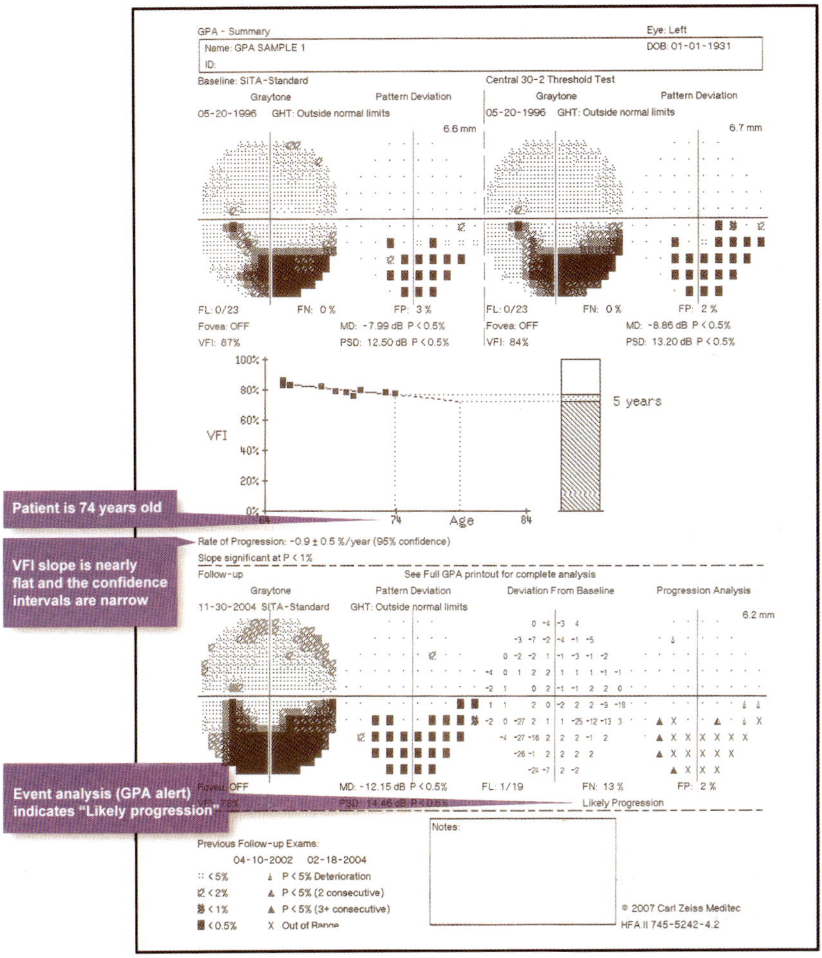

Fig. 3.4: Visual field loss progression using the GPA in sample analysis (*Courtesy*: Carl Zeiss Meditec brochure 2008)

this analysis is not to detect progression, which can be done with the GPA, but to provide valuable information on the rate of deterioration. The VFI is calculated as the percentage of normal visual field, after adjustment for age. Therefore, a VFI of 100% represents a completely normal visual field, while a VFI of 0% represents a perimetrically blind visual field. The VFI is shown on the GPA printout both as a percent value for each individual examination and as a trend analysis, plotted against age. While the MD is based only on the total deviation map, and thus is largely affected by cataract, the VFI is based both on the pattern deviation and the total deviation probability maps. The former (pattern deviation) helps in the identification of possibly progressing points, and the latter (total deviation) is used for the actual calculation of change of the total deviation value. In addition, the VFI algorithm gives weightage for different locations, giving more weight to the central points. The final VFI score is the mean of all weighted scores. For glaucoma patients with worsening cataract, however, the VFI showed a slower rate of progression than the MD, which would be a more accurate representation of the actual rate of glaucoma progression. Conversely, for glaucoma patients who had cataract surgery during follow-up, improvement in media clarity masked glaucoma progression when assessed by the MD. It did not happen when assessment was performed with the VFI. The VFI also provides an estimate of the visual field loss that will occur in the next 5 years, assuming that the same rate of progression is maintained. This is valuable for the treating ophthalmologist, as it estimates the number of years that a patient has before advancing to blindness. A summary of the progression of visual field loss analysis is presented in Table 3.1.

TABLE 3.1: Summary of progression analyses available in HFA

Tool used	Index used for analysis	Analysis	Progression
Mean deviation (MD) plotted against time	Mean deviation	Plots MD values over time	Decrease in MD over time
Glaucoma change probability	Total deviation	Compares individual field points at follow-up to baseline	Two or more adjacent points in or next to an existing scotoma show a significant deterioration on two consecutive tests
Guided progression analysis	Pattern deviation	Compares each follow-up tests to the average of the two baseline tests; identifies points that show change at the 95% significance level	Possible progression = significant change in at least three points that is repeated over two consecutive tests; likely progression = significant change in a least three points that is repeated over three consecutive tests
Visual field index	Mean deviation and pattern deviation	Provides information on the rate of progression; gives more weight to central visual field points	Provides an estimate of additional field loss that will occur over the next 5 years given a steady rate of deterioration

PROGRESSION ANALYSIS USING OCTOPUS EYESUITE PERIMETRY

The Octopus Eyesuite software provides a number of useful analyses, such as:

1. The overview analysis provides an overview of all previous examinations to show and look for changes (Fig. 3.5).
2. It can also provide bilateral viewing as a two on one report.
3. Trend analysis of the mean defect (MD) helps calculate the rate of progression per year including the probability level and fluctuations (Fig. 3.6).
4. The trend graph also shows areas for normal range (gray band), impaired (15 dB) and legal blindness (25 dB).
5. A red icon arrow will be displayed when significant worsening is noted (Fig. 3.7).
6. Trends can also be shown for sLV, DD, Cluster analysis and polar graphs.

MONITORING PROGRESSION WITH PHOTOGRAPHY AND IMAGING DEVICES

1. Optic disk and RNFL documentation using a fundus camera is an established method. This method has the advantage of being objective, simple and easy to interpret by a clinician. Changes in the rim, cup disk ratio,

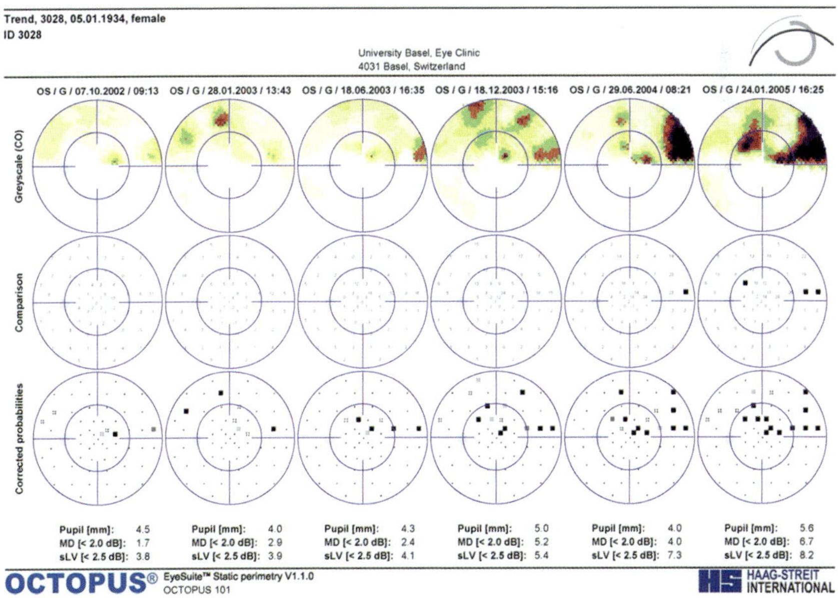

Fig. 3.5: Overview of visual fields using Octopus perimeter

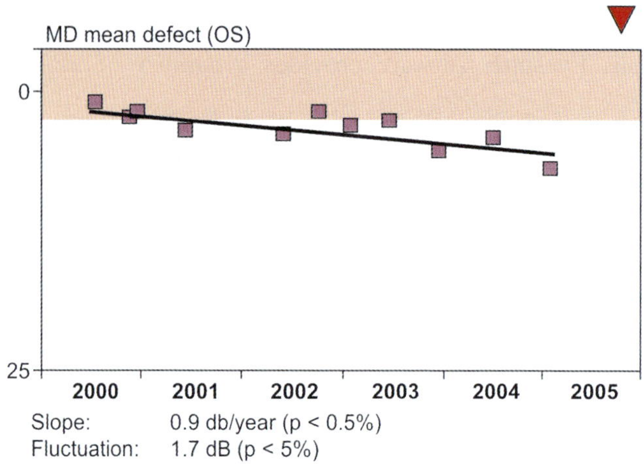

Fig. 3.6: Trend for MD indicates worsening of the field over time (red downward arrow)

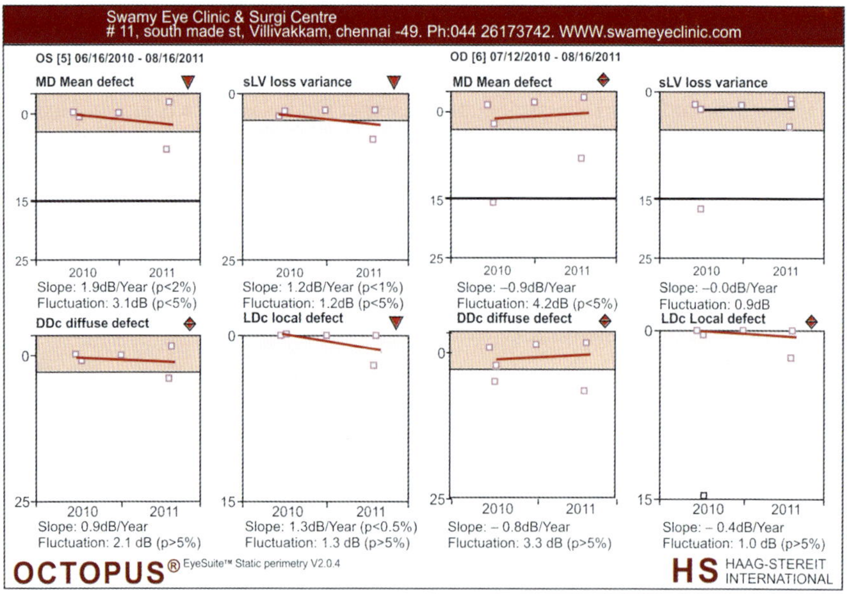

Fig 3.7: Global and local trends in a patient showing glaucoma progression

vessel changes, RNFL loss and progressive enlargement, development of new disc hemorrhages can be well documented. However, the disadvantages of photography include possible disagreement in diagnosis even between experts and also that change cannot be quantified. Data from the Ocular Hypertension Study (OHTS) show that in many cases glaucoma progression and optic disk hemorrhages were detected on photographs by trained observers and not on routine clinical examinations.[7]

2. Imaging devices: Imaging devices are in widespread use now and these include the GDx nerve fiber analyzer which is a scanning laser polarimeter that quantifies RNFL thickness by providing a map of the retardation of polarized light in the parapapillary retina. The recent GDx VCC has a variable corneal compensator to provide patient specific neutralization of corneal light retardation. The more recent GDx ECC provides accurate assessment in eyes with pale fundus and myopia. The Heidelberg retina tomograph is a confocal scanning laser ophthalmoscope and gives quantitative measurements of the optic disk, rim and cup size along with 3-dimensional height map. New software (glaucoma probability score) developed for HRT III gives ONH measurement without the need to draw a contour line. Optical coherence tomography (OCT) is available as spectral domain and time domain techniques. Although both give quantitative measurements of RNFL thickness (sector wise and overall average), the spectral domain is capable of 3D imaging and provides higher resolution.

These imaging based technologies for quantitative assessment are continuously evolving (software and hardware) and there are currently no clear cut guidelines (Which technology should be used and how often?) to monitor progression using these devices. HRT has been the instrument with the longest track record and published data are available on progression detection using HRT.

The Future

GDX Glaucoma Progression Analysis (GPA): It can help identify progressive RNFL loss, using terminology that is similar to what is used by GPA on the Humphrey field analyzer determine the rate of progression, in terms of microns per year and the confidence interval help assess treatment efficacy by comparing progression before and after treatment.

Progression monitoring using OCT: Currently, one can use the Stratus OCT's serial analysis function to follow patients. Basically, it is an overlay of the RNFL thickness at each of the 256 points along the scan. A different color represents each visit date. A new version of the software, GPA advanced serial analysis, will be available soon which takes into account measurement variability, scan quality and the patient's age. It displays an overlay of multiple thickness profiles and provides progression analysis of average RNFL thickness by quadrants and o'clock hours. It also provides trend (regression), event analysis and reports slope of change.

In studies evaluating the ability of imaging instruments to detect glaucoma progression, it is observed that a large proportion of patients show progression by imaging instruments only, but the clinical relevance of progression detected only by imaging instruments is still unclear. Several studies have evaluated the ability of optical imaging technologies to detect glaucomatous change over time. Although the clinical predictive value of longitudinal progression detected by imaging instruments has yet to be established, there is some evidence that abnormal results obtained on these tests are associated with future worse outcomes in glaucoma patients and that baseline measurements may be predictive of future development of visual field loss.

References

1. Terminology and Guidelines for glaucoma. 3rd Edition. European Glaucoma Society, 2008.
2. Kim J, Dally LG, Ederer F, Gaasterland DE, VanVeldhuisen PC, Blackwell B, Sullivan EK, Prum B, Shafranov G, Beck A, Spaeth GL; AGIS Investigators. The advanced Glaucoma Intervention Study (AGIS). Distinguishing progression of glaucoma from visual field fluctuations. *Ophthalmology.* 2004;111(11):2109-16.
3. Boden,C, Blumenthal EZ, Pascual J, McEwan G, Weinreb RN, Medeiros F, Sample PA. Patterns of glaucomatous visual field progression identified by three progression criteria. *Am J Ophthalmol.* 2004;138(6):1029-36.
4. Chauhan, B C, Garway-Heath DF, Goñi FJ, Rossetti L, Bengtsson B, Viswanathan AC, Heijl A. Practical recommendations for measuring rates of visual field change in glaucoma. *Br J Ophthalmol.* 2008;92(4):569-73.
5. Bengtsson B, Heijl A. A visual field index for calculation of glaucoma rate of progression. *Am J Ophthalmol.* 2008;145(2):343-53.
6. Prata TS, De Moraes CG, Teng CC, Tello C, Ritch R, Liebmann JM. Factors affecting rates of visual field progression in glaucoma patients with optic disc hemorrhage. *Ophthalmology*. 2010;117(1):24-9.
7. Keltner JL, Johnson CA, Quigg JM, Cello KE, Kass MA, Gordon MO, for the Ocular Hypertension Treatment Study Group: Confirmation of visual field abnormalities in the Ocular Hypertension Treatment Study. *Arch Ophthalmol.* 2000;118:1187-94.

4
chapter

R Ramakrishnan
Arjit Mithara

OCT in Glaucoma

ABSTRACT

OCT is an important tool for the diagnosis of glaucoma. The basic principles of OCT are described and the technique is compared with other Imaging modalities in glaucoma, namely the GDx, HRT, RTA, and UBM. The chapter mentions the importance of OCT in glaucoma. The different analysis protocols are described in detail and the interpretation of the scans discussed. The OCT images of ONH in normal and patients with unilateral and bilateral glaucoma are presented. Description of the Cirrus™ HD-OCT helps the reader gain an idea of the latest developments in the field. The advantages and disadvantages of OCT are discussed and the normative Indian data on OCT in the Indian population are presented.

Introduction

Optical coherence tomography (OCT) is a noncontact noninvasive technology providing high resolution, cross-sectional images of the eye. It is an optical imaging system providing *in vivo* imaging of the retina analogous to B scan. Its use in retina and glaucoma have been steadily growing. Many studies have been done showing its reproducibility and correlation with histological appearance. Its use for glaucoma diagnosis and *in vivo* capabilities of retinal nerve fiber layer (RNFL) and optic nerve head (ONH) analysis has revolutionized the previous uncertain diagnostic challenges into an accurate and precise diagnosis.

Although visual field assessment has been the gold standard for glaucoma diagnosis, it has been documented that up to 40% of the retinal nerve fiber layer may be lost before a defect is apparent on the visual field.

The Ocular Hypertension Study (OHTS) showed that 55% of eyes that converted to glaucoma did not have a field defect but only structural changes in the optic nerve head. Identification of structural optic nerve damage is thus very important in the early diagnosis of glaucoma and in monitoring its clinical course. Until recently, assessment of the optic nerve and retinal nerve fiber layer (RNFL) has been largely subjective. Variability in the size and appearance of the optic disk of normal eyes complicates the detection of early glaucomatous optic nerve damage. Standard techniques to diagnose and monitor structural changes in glaucoma, have included serial stereoscopic photographs of the optic disk and monochromatic photographs of the RNFL. While these methods provide objective information for comparisons, the interpretation of photographs remains subjective, and variation in photographic assessment among even experienced observers is well documented.[1] Furthermore, qualitative assessment of photographs may not be sensitive to small changes over time, and it is difficult to pick up diffuse damage on these photographs.

New technologies, such as confocal scanning laser ophthalmoscopy (HRT), scanning laser polarimetry (GDxVCC), and optical coherence tomography (OCT)[2] have become available that provide quantitative, reproducible, and objective measurements of optic nerve head and RNFL thickness.[3] The present chapter will focus on the principles of OCT and its role to diagnose and manage glaucoma patients.

Basic Principles of OCT

The OCT contains an interferometer that resolves retinal structures by measuring the echo delay time of light that is reflected and back scattered from different microstructural features in retina**.** Optical coherence tomography is based on the principle of Michelson interferometry. Low-coherence infrared (830 nm) light coupled to a fiberoptic travels to a 50/50 beam splitter and is directed through the ocular media to the retina and to a reference mirror, respectively. Light passing through the eye is reflected by structures in different retinal tissue layers. The distance between the beam splitter and reference mirror is continuously varied. When the distance between the light source and retinal tissue is equal to the distance between the light source and reference mirror, the reflected light from the retinal tissue and reference mirror interacts to produce an interference pattern. The interference pattern is detected and then processed into a signal (Fig. 4.1). The signal is analogous to that obtained by A-scan ultrasonography using light as a source rather than sound. A two-dimensional image is built as the light source is moved across the retina. One can think of the image as a series of stacked and

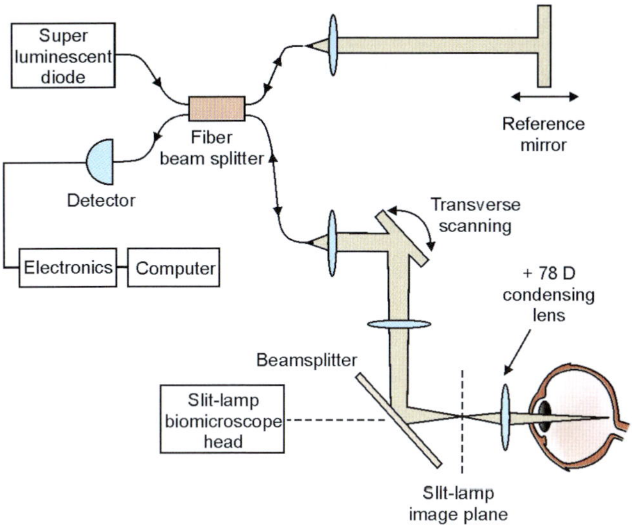

Fig. 4.1: Principle of OCT

aligned A-scans to produce a two-dimensional cross-sectional retinal image that resembles that of a histologic section. This imaging method thus can be considered a form of *in vivo* histology.

The newer Stratus OCT (OCT 3; Carl Zeiss Inc, Dublin, California, USA) can be used in the absence of dilation in many individuals, and usually requires a 3 mm pupil for adequate visualization. An infrared-sensitive charge-coupled device video camera documents the position of the scanning beam on the retina. The OCT image can be displayed on a gray scale where more highly reflected light is brighter than less highly reflected light. Alternatively, it can be displayed in color whereby different colors correspond to different degrees of reflectivity. On the OCT scanners, currently commercially available, highly reflective structures are shown with bright colors (red and yellow), while those with low reflectivity are represented by darker colors (black and blue). Those with intermediate reflectivity appear green.

Current commercial scanners employ a low coherence super luminescent diode source (820 nm). The presently available model Stratus OCT (OCT 3) has a theoretical axial resolution <10 mm. Ultra-high resolution research OCT scanners use a titanium sapphire laser that has an ultrabroad spectral bandwidth centered at approximately 800 nm. With these light sources, axial resolution can be increased to 2 mm to 3 mm, but these light sources are expensive and have a limited role in routine clinical applications.[4]

Comparison with HRT, GDx and RTA

Other technologies are available for optic nerve head in aging and nerve fiber layer analysis. The past decade has seen the emergence and refinement of confocal scanning laser ophthalmoscopy (HRT), scanning laser polarimetry (GDx) and the retinal thickness analyzer (RTA).

The major limitation of HRT is that the use of a reference plane is required. For this manual tracing of the optic nerve head margin has to be done by a trained technician or ophthalmologist. As compared to HRT II, OCT does not require a trained technician to mark the points for disk margin. The measurements may be affected by blood vessels. The HRT is useful for scanning the optic nerve head and its use for determining RNFL thickness is limited by axial resolution of the CSLO device.

The SLP device, GDx suffers from high variability in readings due to normal anatomical variations in different eyes as well as presence of pathological changes in different individuals. Some of these sources of error, which adversely affect reliability, include ethnicity and age variations, prior corneal surgeries like LASIK and corneal transplantation, vitreous opacities, motion artifacts and macular structural pathologies.

Comparison with Ultrasound

OCT is the optical equivalent of ultrasound using light reflection as opposed to sound detection of tissues. As compared to ultrasound it is a noncontact technology, providing for patient comfort and acceptability. As compared to UBM no special sterile materials are needed in OCT.

Importance of OCT in Glaucoma

The management of glaucoma has ideally been based on the combination of intraocular pressure, clinical examination of optic nerve head, and visual field testing. Advances in our understanding of glaucoma have contributed to the view that retinal ganglion cell layer death is an early process in glaucoma. This precedes the changes in the visual field by several years. IOP is the only variable currently amenable to treatment. However, owing to the variability, spikes and fluctuation of IOP throughout the day there is a doubt as to the reliability of the isolated IOP values measured days weeks or months apart. Also the correct value of IOP, as measured by the different types of tonometers, is subject to a lot of debate.

Stereophotographic evaluation as well as serial ophthalmoscopic examinations of the optic nerve head require a skilled observer. However, there is a significant amount of interobserver variation between different individuals, thus, grossly affecting the reliability. Coming to the visual field—the fields presently in vogue, use automated techniques and is a subjective test. The visual fields are prone to short and long-term fluctuations and thus require serial testing over a period of time to obtain reliable fields. Thus, the whole process is long drawn out and diagnosis is delayed resulting in loss of time in instituting management.

From the above, we can thus conclude that the diagnosis of glaucoma is delayed and the traditional tests do not provide a reliable diagnosis in time for providing appropriate care. Here comes the role of OCT in glaucoma. It can diagnose glaucoma early and with a certain degree of reliability whereby treatment can be instituted in time.

Optical coherence tomography provides high resolution measurements and cross-sectional imaging of the retina, optic disk, and the RNFL. For glaucoma applications, an operator-determined circular or linear path is scanned around the optic disk to generate a series of 100 axial reflectance profiles. From these, a real-time two-dimensional tomographic image is constructed. The first reflection measurement is the vitreous-internal limiting membrane interface. The highly reflective interface posterior to this is the retinal pigment epithelium-photoreceptor interface. A threshold of reflectivity between the two is set as the posterior boundary of the RNFL. Retinal nerve fiber layer and retinal thickness are calculated from these landmarks. Average measurements are given for 12, 30-degree sectors. The depth values of the scans are independent of the optical dimensions of the eye, and no reference plane is required. Useful measurements in glaucoma patients are normally made along a circle concentric with the optic disk.

Instrumentation

The OCT system hardware consists of the patient module, the computer unit, the flat screen video monitor, key board, mouse and color inkjet printer. The hardware mounts on a wheelchair accessible motorized power table.

Procedure

The patient is seated with the chin on the provided chin rest and the forehead against a curved strap. As it is a noninvasive procedure the patient enjoys a great degree of comfort throughout the duration of the test. A pupil diameter of 3.2 mm is recommended by the manufacturer. The room lights are dimmed and in most cases the scanning can be done without the need for dilatation. However, in Indian population sometimes the pupillary diameter is inadequate and thus pupillary dilatation is needed. In presence of media opacities pupillary dilatation is a must otherwise the signal strength will not be accurate to give a reliable reading. A pupillary size of 3 mm is however adequate for most purposes in presence of a clear optical media. An infra-red CCD camera monitors the position of laser beam on the retina. An internal fixation reference beam allows the patient to focus his vision, thereby, reducing unwanted movements. A circle of 3.4 mm is used for sampling the RNFL, as it has been shown to correlate best with changes in glaucoma (Schuman et al).[5] OCT 3 offers highest sampling density of 512 sampling points. The scans are made by linear scans in a spoke pattern configuration. The OCT generates a real-time tomographic section of the tissues from the collected reflectance interferometer data. The anterior reflectance is from the interface between the vitreous and the internal limiting membrane. The posterior limit of the RNFL is the boundary of retinal pigment epithelium (RPE).The ending of RPE at the edges of the optic disk automatically determines the disk margins eliminating observer variations inherent in HRT due to requirement for manually marking disk edges. The cup diameter is measured on a line parallel to the disk line and offset anteriorly by 150 microns and various optic nerve head parameters are automatically calculated. Mean RNFL thickness is calculated using the inbuilt RNFL thickness average analysis protocol.

Clinical Uses

- To evaluate the RNFL for early (preperimetric) glaucoma detection[6]
- To detect, study and follow the macular changes in hypotony induced maculopathy after glaucoma surgery
- To evaluate cystoid macular edema after combined cataract and glaucoma surgery and use of anti-glaucoma medications[7]
- To evaluate optic nerve head tomography in glaucoma patients.

Scans

There are two basic scan patterns—lines and circles. The OCT 3 constructs all 18 scan protocols from line or circle scans. The 3 most commonly used scans are:

1. *Fast optical disk:* This protocol acquires six 4 mm radial line scans which are designed for the optic nerve head analysis.
2. *Fast RNFL thickness:* This protocol acquires three 3.4 mm diameter circle scans, which are designed for use with the RNFL thickness analyses.
3. *Fast macular thickness map*: It consists of six 6 mm radial lines scans through common central axis. This protocol is designed for examination of macular thickness as an indicator of glaucoma. It

is designed for use with the analyses that measures retinal thickness and to obtain maps of retinal thickness in a circular area centered on the macula.

The analysis protocols assist us with diagnostic analysis of scan images of the posterior segment of the eye. There are 11 quantitative analysis protocols for glaucoma and retina and 7 image processing protocols.

Different Analysis Protocols in Glaucoma

Basically three different analysis protocols are used in glaucoma evaluation.These are the retinal nerve fiber layer analysis, the optic nerve head analysis and the macular thickness analysis. The sums of these three analysis protocols provide a comprehensive glaucoma evaluation and help the observer arrive at a diagnosis with a high degree of reliability.

1. **Retinal Nerve Fiber Layer (RNFL) Analysis**

   The analysis of RNFL aids in the identification of early glaucomatous damage.

   Circular scans of 3.4 mm in diameter around the optic nerve head provide measurement of the RNFL in the peripapillary region. This has been shown to correlate best with changes in glaucoma.[5] The RNFL measurement is graphed in a TSNIT orientation and compared to the age matched normative data.

2. **Optic Nerve Head Analysis**

   Radial line scans through the optic disk provide cross-sectional information on the degree of cupping and the neuroretinal rim area. The disk margins are objectively identified using signal from end of RPE. The key parameters include cup-to-disk ratio and horizontal integrated rim volume.

3. **Macular Thickness Analysis**

   This analysis is based on the fact that a thinning of the macula may reflect glaucomatous loss. The structural analysis of the retinal sublayers reveals macular complications. Cross-sectional view provides visualization and measurement of retinal layers.

RETINAL NERVE FIBER LAYER THICKNESS ANALYSIS

Interpretation of RNFL Thickness Average Analysis

OCT offers a variety of RNFL thickness measurement and analysis protocols for use in glaucoma. A fast protocol is used for a rapid analysis but the drawback of a fast protocol is that it may miss out on the finer critical points. The other protocol is a detailed one and is useful for diagnosis and follow-up of ongoing RNFL damage.

- **RNFL thickness protocol** (3.4 mm): It acquires a scan with radius 1.73 mm, centered on the optic disk
- **Fast RNFL thickness protocol** (3.4 mm): It acquires three fast circular scans. This is a time efficient scan alignment and placement is required only once
- **Proportional circle protocol**: This protocol allows measurement of RNFL thickness (RNFLT) around the optic disk along a circular scan, the size of which can be tailored as per individual's need taking into account the size of optic nerve head
- **Concentric 3 rings protocol**: This protocol enables us to measure RNFLT along three equally placed default circular scans of 0.9 mm, 1.81 mm, and 2.71 mm radii. However, the scan radius can be altered according to the need
- **RNFL thickness protocol** (2.27 × disk): This circular RNFLT scan size is 2.27 times the size of the optic nerve head as determined by OCT (ending of RPE is automatically defined as ONH margin by the program). This may be useful as a standardization in research studies for comparison in disparate population, providing normative data and comparing RNFL thickness in various ONH sizes. This may help us measure RNFLT with accuracy is various disk sizes[6]
- **RNFL** map protocol: This protocol comprises six circular scans of 1.44 mm, 1.69 mm, 1.90 mm, 2.25 mm, 2.73 mm, and 3.40 mm radii. This gives an overlay view of the RNFLT, around the peripapillary area. Retinal nerve fiber layer measurement with a circular scan of 1.34 mm radius, centered on the optic nerve head has been shown to have a maximum reproducibility in glaucomatous patients.[8] Mean RNFL thickness is calculated using the inbuilt RNFL thickness average analysis protocol.

Clinical Interpretation of RNFL Thickness Average Analysis

For understanding purpose the RNFL thickness average analysis printout can be divided into various zones (Fig. 4.2) that include:

1. Zone 1: Patient ID data.
2. Zone 2: Individual TSNIT curves for each eye presented in comparison with the age matched normative database.
3. Zone 3: Overlap of TSNIT curve showing a comparison of two eyes.
4. Zone 4: Circular diagram showing quadrant wise and clock hour wise distribution of average RNFL thickness in both eyes.
5. Zone 5: Data table: It shows various ratios, quadrant averages, and difference among the quadrants and between the two eyes. Each value is marked in color to show its level of deviation from the normal values.

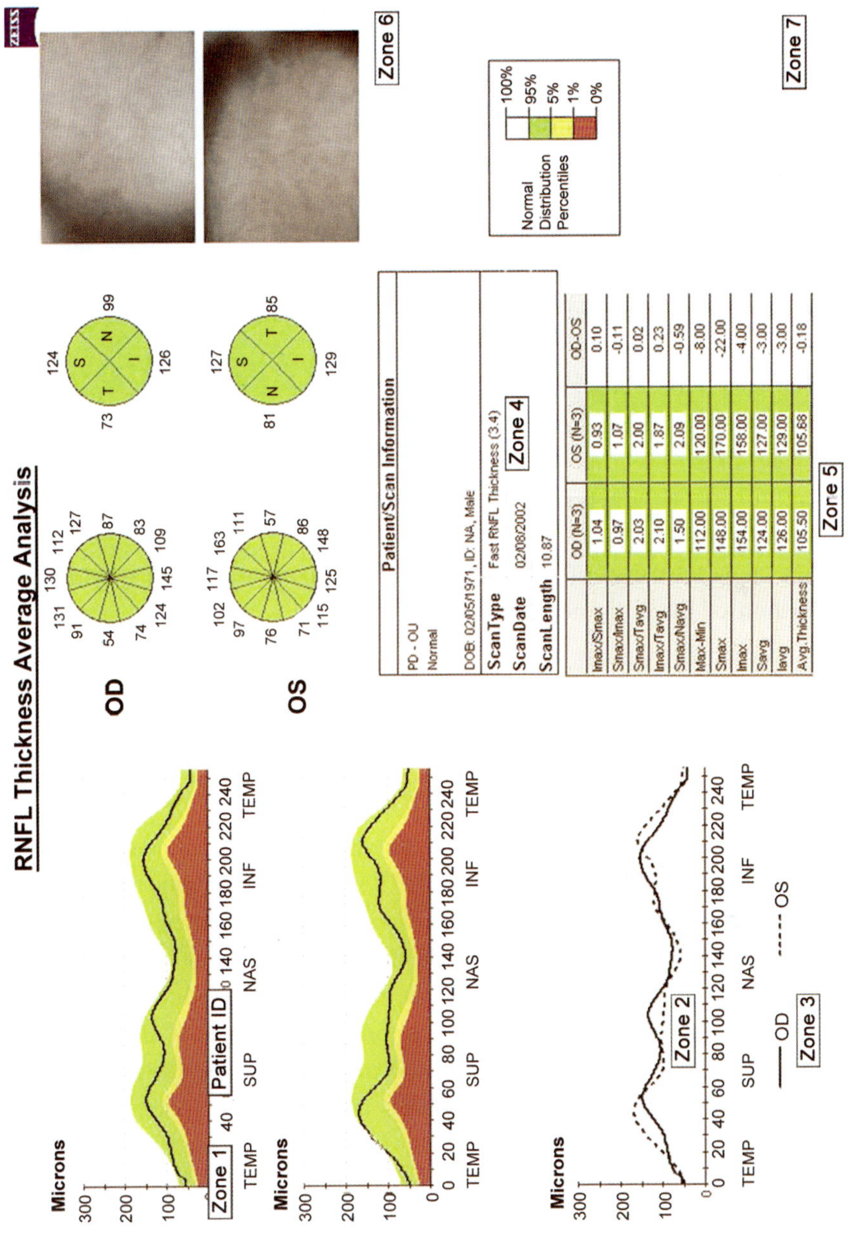

Fig. 4.2: RNFL thickness average analysis scan

Average thickness: The average RNFL thickness along the entire circular scan: Savg and Iavg (Superior average and inferior average): The average RNFL thickness in the respective 900 of the circular sSmax and Imax (Superior maximum and inferior maximum): Maximum RNFL thickness recorded in the respective 90° quadrant of the scan

Max-min: Difference between the maximum and minimum RNFL value along the circular scan.

6. Zone 6: Red free photograph: B&W photographs of two eyes taken with the infrared camera are available on the printout. These denote the position of scan circle on the fundus.
7. Zone 7: Percentile distribution color coding: A small box denoting the color coding of percentile distribution of normative database is provided. White and green color represent the distribution within 95%, yellow color representing the areas of RNFL thickness below 5th percentile, and red color representing the areas of RFNFL thickness below 1 percentile. Similar color coding is applicable for the individual quadrant (ISNT) of nerve fibers in the ONH.

The four ratios provided in the data table are self explanatory. OCT3 also enables us to perform a RNFL thickness serial analysis can serially compare up to 4 scan groups and provide an overview of RNFL thickness change overtime. Interpretation of optic disk scan provides optic nerve head analysis.

The newer version of the OCT, OCT 3 allows a detailed quantitative evaluation of the optic nerve head. It is provided with two scan protocols.

OPTIC NERVE HEAD ANALYSIS

Optical disk scan consists of equally placed line scans 4 mm in length, at 30° intervals, centered on the optic disk. The number of lines can be adjusted between 6–24 lines.

Fast optical disk scan compresses six optical disk scan into one scan and acquires scan in short time of 1.92 seconds. The optic nerve head (ONH) analysis and various ONH parameters are calculated using the inbuilt ONH analysis protocol. This analysis detects the anterior surface of the retinal nerve fiber layer (RNFL) and the retinal pigment epithelium (RPE). The cup perimeter is determined by automatic detection of the reference points. The inbuilt algorithm detects and measures all the features of disk anatomy based on anatomical landmarks, (disk reference points), on each side of the disk where the RPE ends. It locates and measures the disk diameter by tracing a straight line between the disk reference points. The cup diameter is measured on a line parallel to the disk line and offset anteriorly by 150 microns and various optic nerve head parameters are automatically calculated. These parameters include optic disk tomography included average disk area, cup area, rim area (disk area minus the cup area), vertical integrated rim area (VIRA), horizontal integrated rim width (HIRD), cup volume, average cup/disk ratio and horizontal and vertical cup-disk ratios.

Vertical integrated rim area (Volume): This estimates the total volume of RFNL tissue in the rim.

Horizontal integrated rim width (Area): It estimates the total rim area and other measurements.

The ONH analysis print-out can be divided into four zones (Fig.4.3).

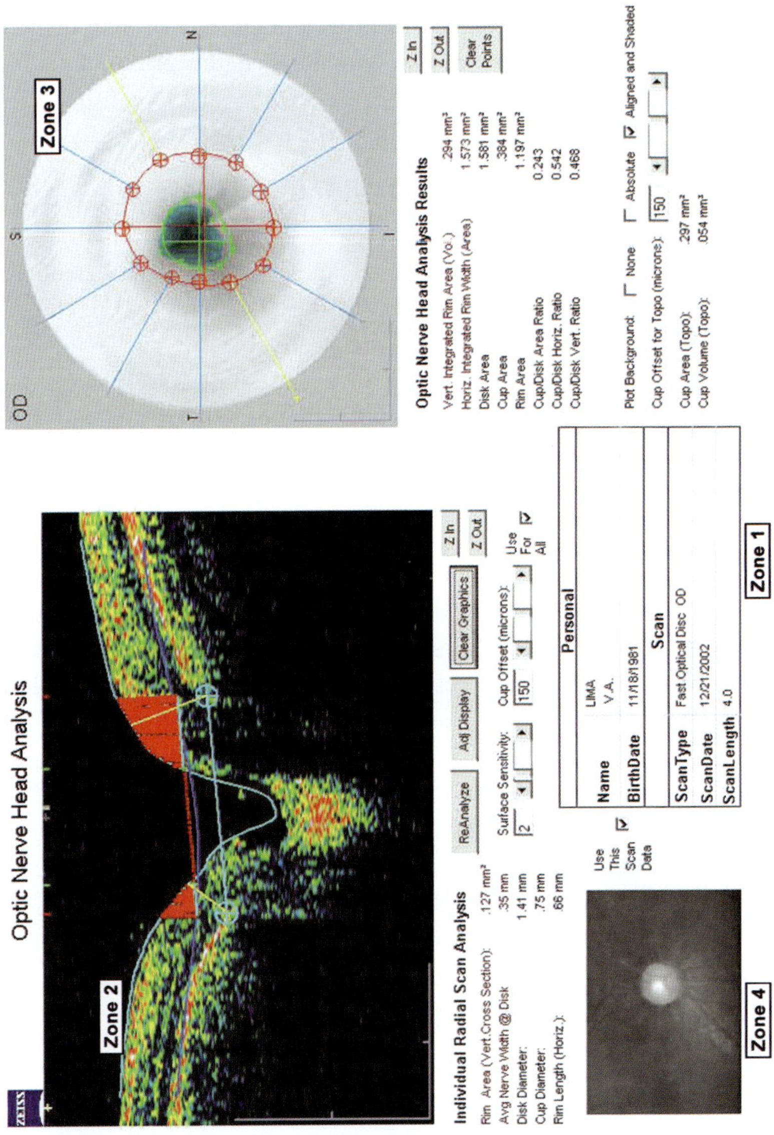

Fig. 4.3: Optic nerve head analysis scan

- Zone 1: Patient ID data
- Zone 2: It gives the overview of ONH head analysis along with the composite image figure constructed from all scans and all the important ONH parameters
- Zone 3: Individual radial scan analysis, along with scan image it gives the disk diameter, cup diameter, rim area, and rim length in that particular meridian. Overlap of TSNIT curve showing a comparison of two eyes
- Zone 4: Red free photograph; B&W photograph of the optic disk taken with the infrared camera is also available on the print-out.

MACULAR THICKNESS ANALYSIS

Macular Thickness and Macular RNFL Thickness in Glaucoma Eyes

Macula NFL thickness and macular thickness is significantly reduced in glaucoma. Mean macular volume is 7.01 ± 0.42 mm^3 vs 6.57 ± 0.85 mm^3 for normal vs glaucoma eyes, respectively.

The OCT scans are highly informative and show a very high degree of correlation with the slit-lamp –90D fundus evaluation and fundus photographs and the Humphrey automated perimetry single field analysis printouts as evident from the following examples (Figs 4.4 to 4.7).

SD OCT

The first generation OCTs enabled us to get the measurement of the thickness of the retinal nerve fiber layers (RNFL). Numerous studies have since then shown a correspondence between OCT measurements and histological measurements.[11-13] This is the reason why clinicians are studying the RNFL thickness more frequently to aid in early diagnosis of glaucoma and to obtain an accurate assessment of disease progression. The Cirrus™ HD-OCT spectral domain technology is further advancing the study of glaucoma. It employs a simple, easy to use system that allows us to precisely capture and clearly display information about the peripapillary area and the RNFL. The Cirrus™ HD-OCT provides the print-out of the two different maps on the same page—The neuroretinal rim thickness map and the RNFL thickness map (Figs 4.8 to 4.10).

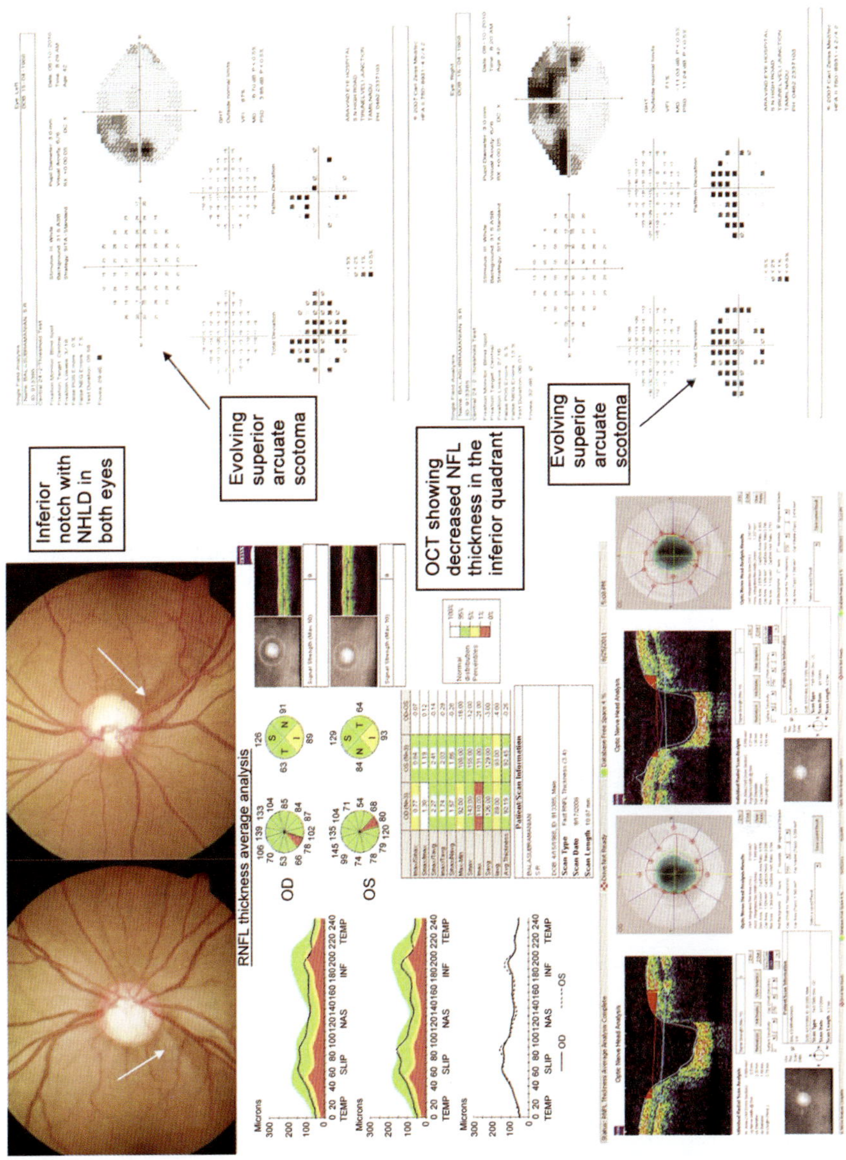

Fig. 4.4: Correlation of fundus photographs, OCT, and HFA in a glaucoma patient

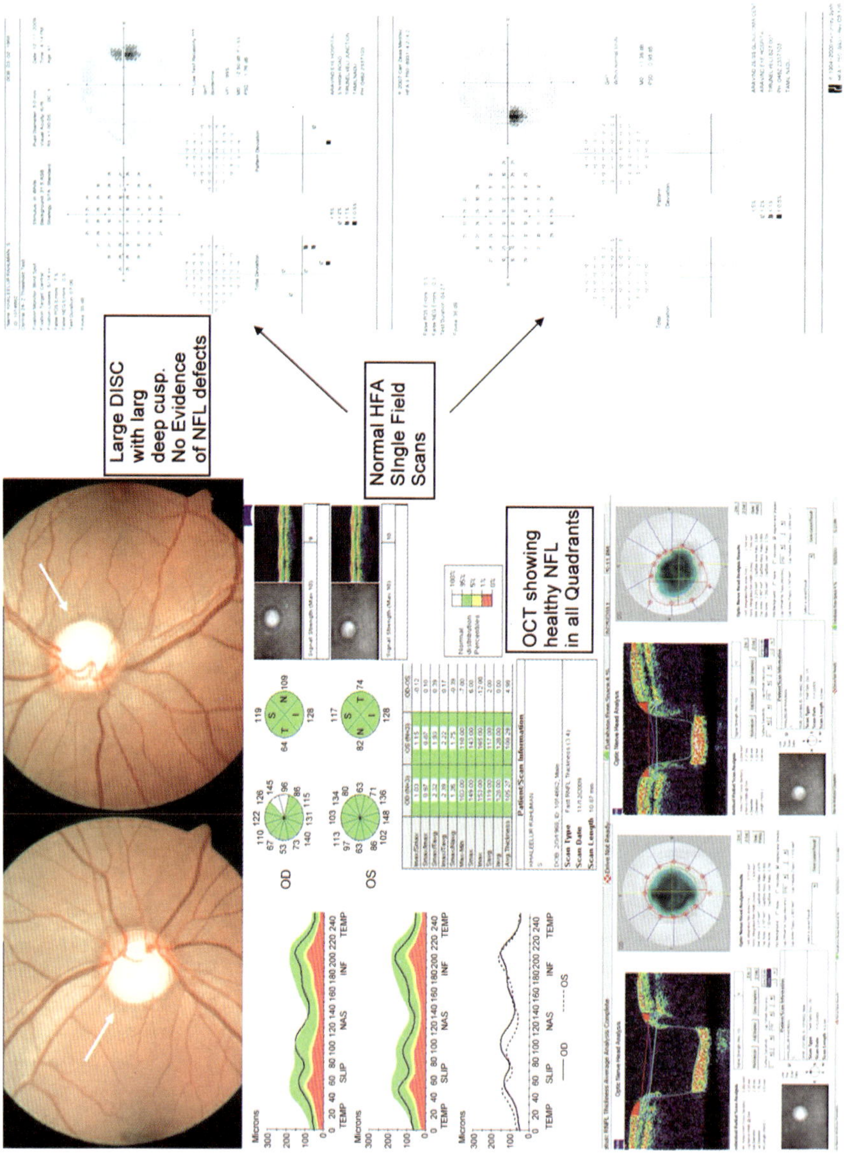

Fig. 4.5: Correlation of fundus photographs, OCT, and HFA in a normal patient

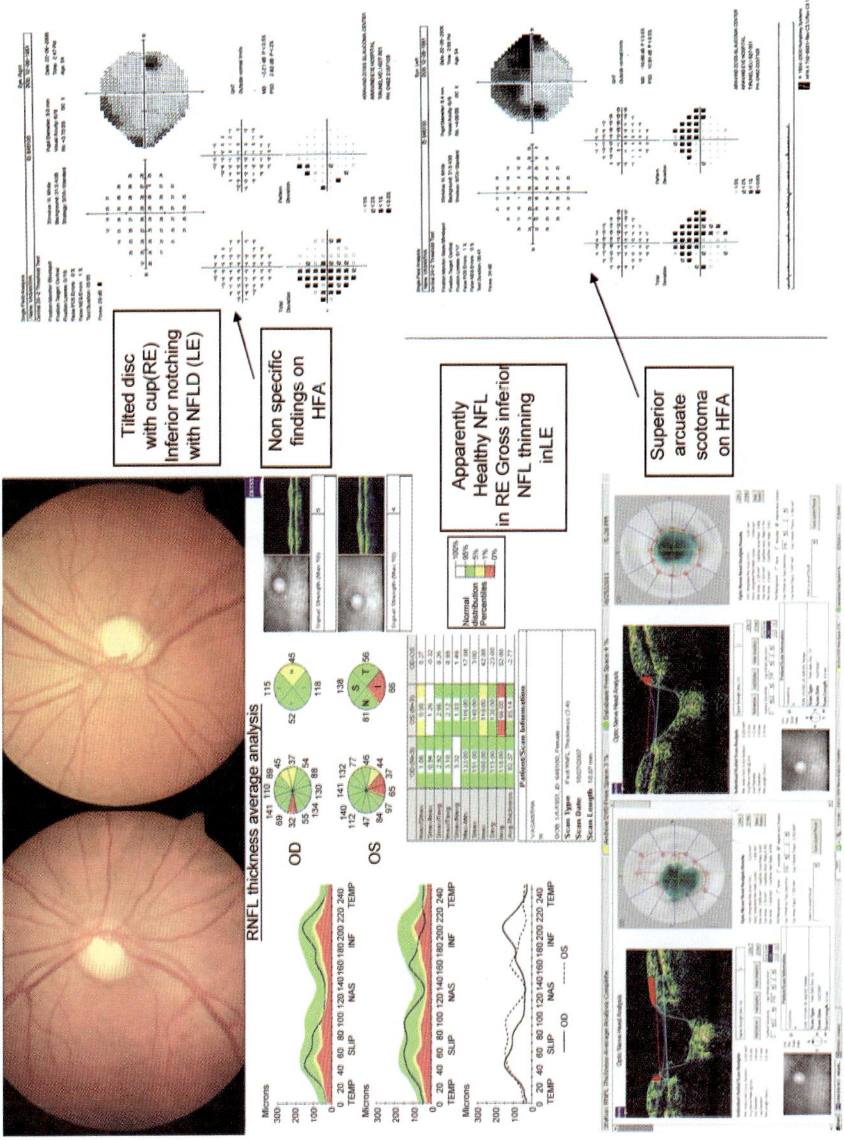

Fig. 4.6: Correlation of fundus photo, OCT, and HFA in a patient with inferior rim loss

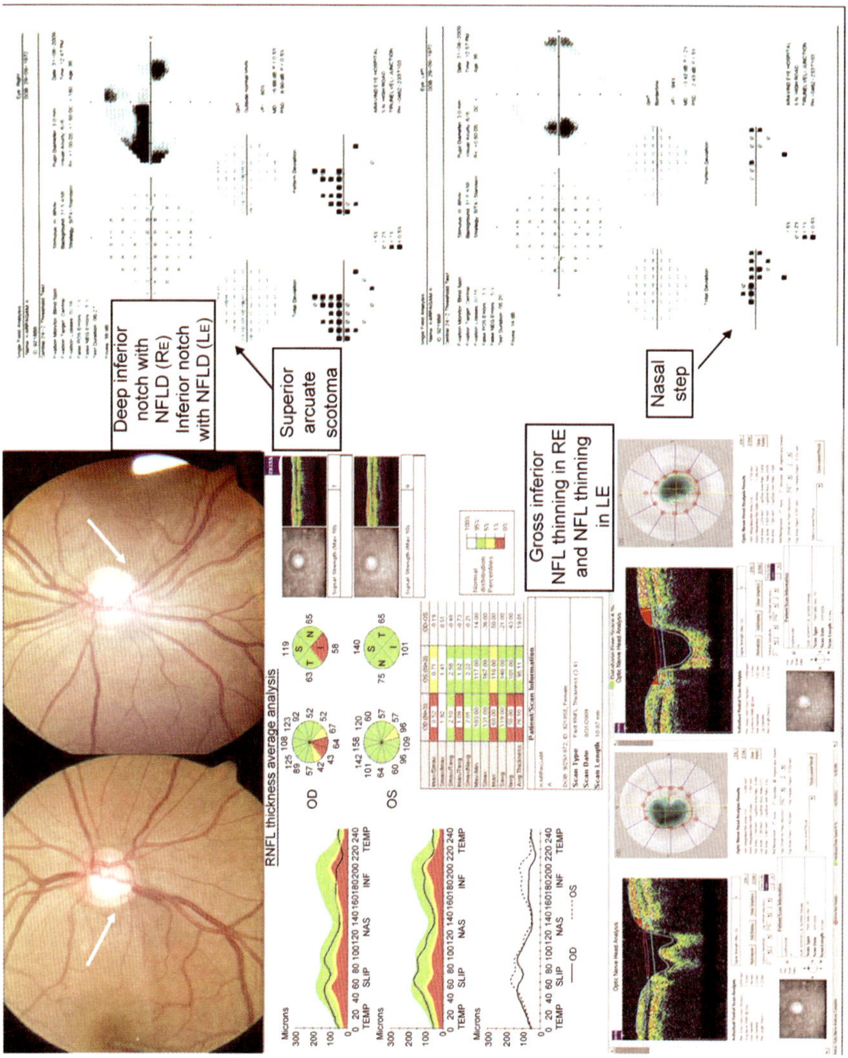

Fig. 4.7: Correlation of fundus photo, OCT, and HFA in a patient with bilateral inferior notching

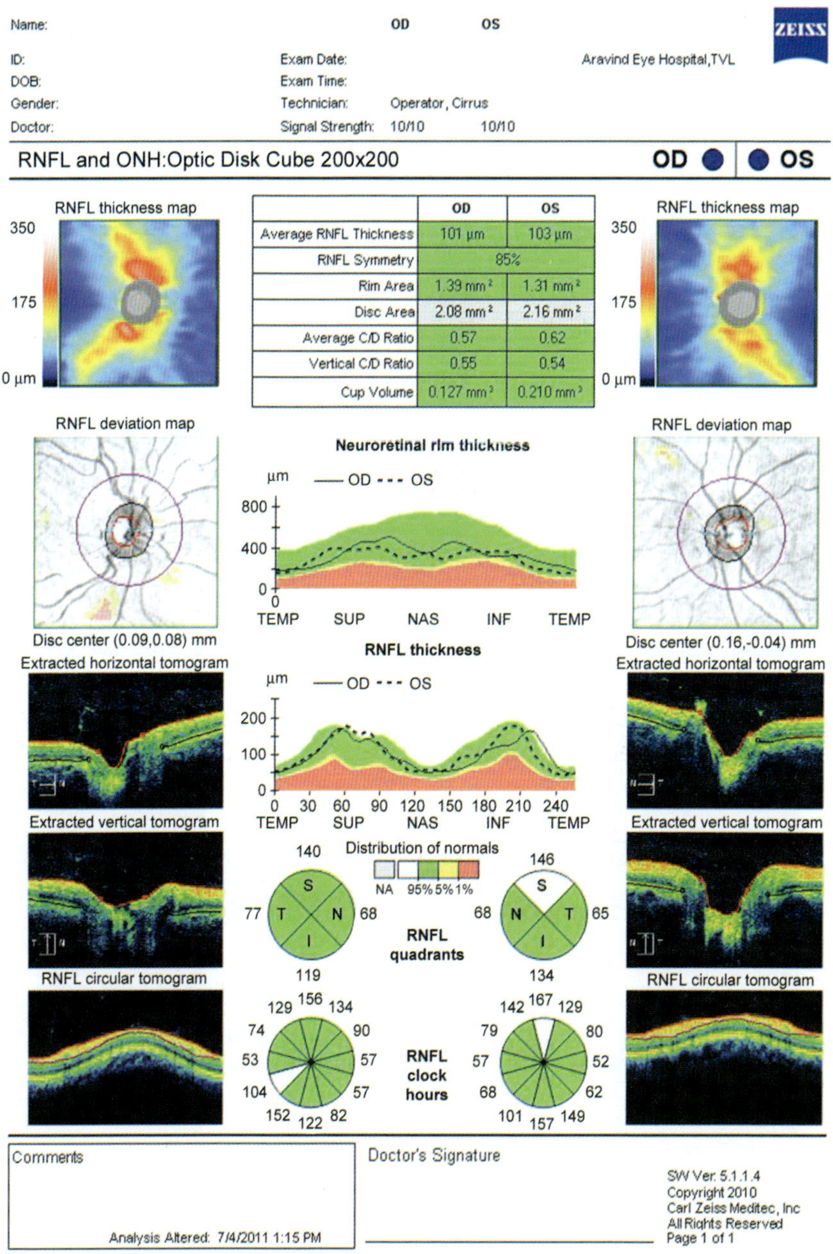

Fig. 4.8: SD OCT scan of a normal patient

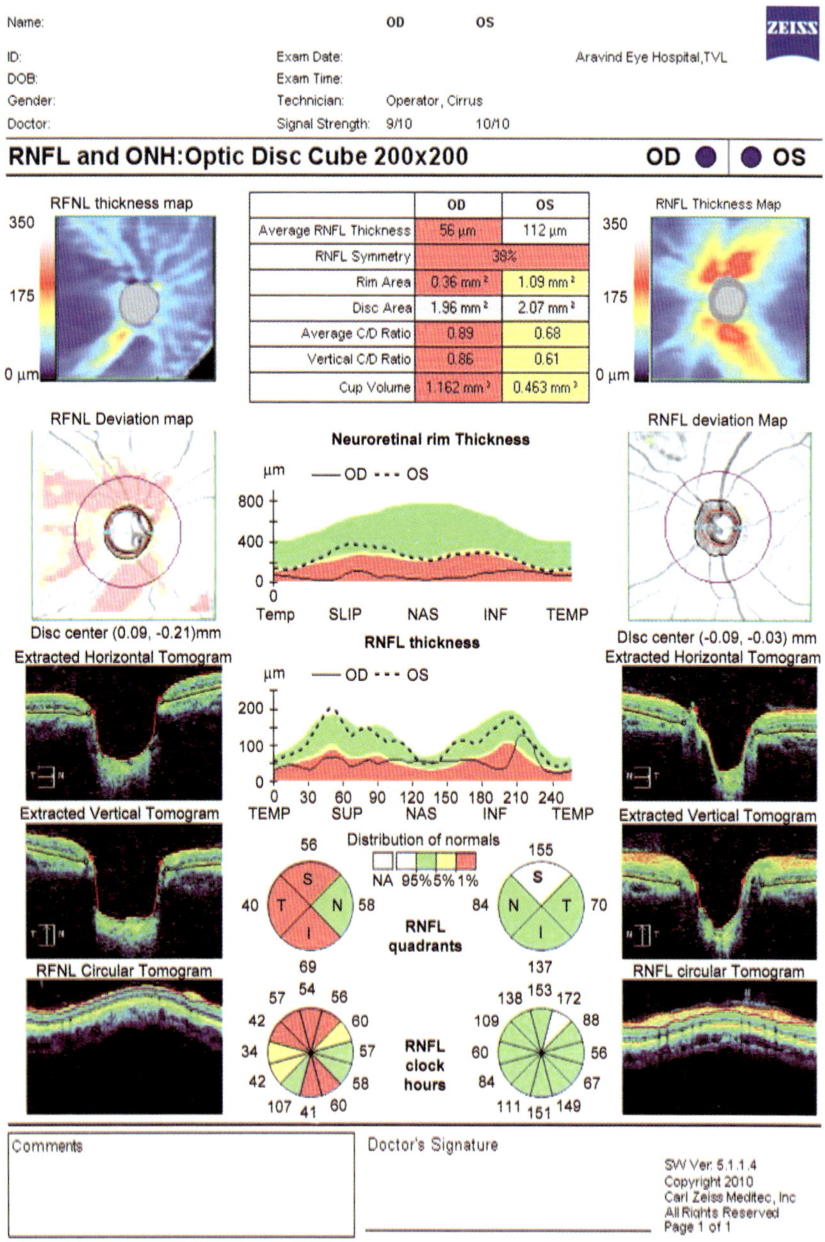

Fig. 4.9: SD OCT scan of a patient showing advanced glaucomatous damage in the right eye

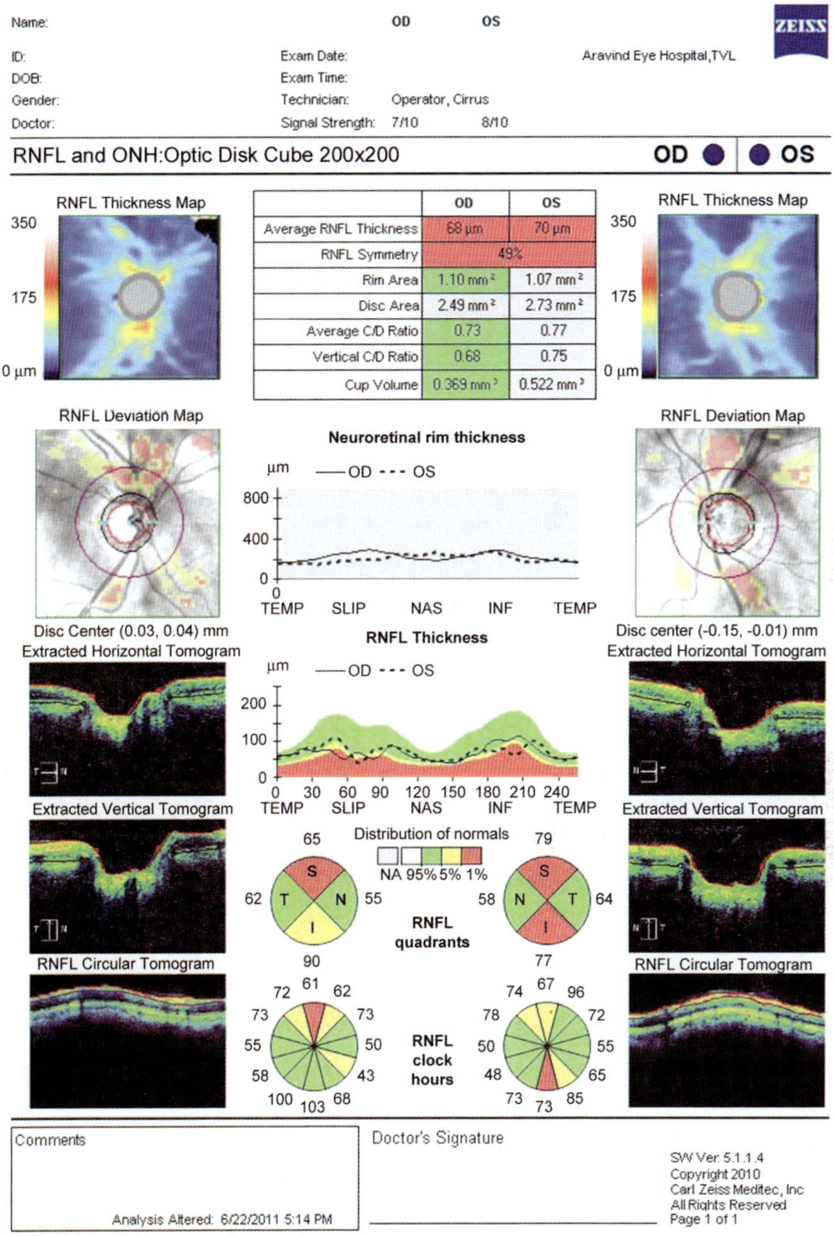

Fig. 4.10: SD OCT scan showing glaucomatous damage in both eyes

OPTIC DISK SCAN

The Cirrus HD-OCT scan of the optic disk captures a 6 × 6 mm cube which is formed from 200 A-scans for each of 200 B-scans. The area within the 6 × 6 mm area is segmented for analysis. From this cube of data the machine automatically identifies the center of the disk and creates a 3.46 mm calculation circle around the disk. The RNFL thickness along the peripapillary circle is analyzed and compared to normative data. Even if the scan was not centered on the optic disk, the RNFL circle analysis will be centered automatically assuring precise registration and excellent repeatability.

FUNDUS IMAGE

The laser scanning ophthalmoscope (LSO) fundus image with OCT fundus image overay is displayed at the top of the RNFL analysis screen or printout. The location of the calculation circle for the temporal superior or nasal, inferior temporal analysis is shown in red. The operator can reposition the circle for analysis after scan acquisition, but this is usually not necessary because the automatic centering is adequate.

RNFL THICKNESS MAP

The RNFL thickness map is based on data calculated over the entire cube. Using a color scale similar to that of a topographical map, cool colors represent thinner areas and warm colors represent thicker areas. It shows RNFL thickness at each point within the 6 × 6 mm area. The maps exclude the optic disk, which is displayed in dark blue. The color code expresses the thickness from zero (blue) to 350 microns (white).

Deviation Map

The deviation map compared the patients RNFL thickness versus normative data. Data points that are outside normal limits are shown in red and yellow.

Average Thickness Values

The RNFL thickness along the TSNIT calculation circle is also illustrated numerically in chart format. The average thickness for all points along the calculation circle is shown for both eyes. Average thickness is also shown for each quadrant and for the clock hours. In each of these charts the patient's values are compared to normative data. The data table calls out symmetry, which is also compared to normative data.

ISNT THICKNESS PROFILES

The ISNT profiles show RNFL thickness at each position along the peripapillary analysis circle and compare these measurements with a normative database. They are color coded (white, green, yellow, red) for comparison with the normative RNFL data for subjects of the same age.

NORMATIVE DATABASE

The normative database uses color to indicate the normal distribution percentiles among individuals of the same age as follows:

Red: The lowest 1% of normal measurements fall within the red zone. These readings are considered outside normal limits.

Yellow: The lowest 5% of normal measurements fall within or under the yellow zone.

Green: 90% of all normal measurements fall within the white area.

While interpreting the normative data, we must remember that for each measurement, 1 in 20 normal eyes (5%) will fall below the green zone.

The RNFL normative database helps us identify areas of clinical interest by comparing patient's RNFL thickness measurements with age matched normal subjects. The normative data comparison is available for patients over 18 years of age.

Advantages of OCT

- Optical coherence tomography provides objective, quantitative, reproducible measurements of the retina and RNFL thickness
- In contrast with other imaging techniques, direct measurements of the RNFL are calculated from cross-sectional retinal images
- Measurements are not affected by refractive status, axial length of the eye, or the presence of early-to-moderate nuclear sclerotic cataracts
- Structural information is independent of any arbitrarily defined reference plane
- A single device gives information about the macula, optic disk and retinal nerve fiber layer. While OCT provides an objective measurement of nerve fiber layer structure, its clinical use in the early detection and follow-up of glaucoma patients is still under evaluation.

Disadvantages

- As with other ocular imaging technology, high cost currently precludes generalized use of the OCT

- The presence, of posterior subcapsular and cortical cataracts impairs performance, and pupillary dilation is required to obtain acceptable peripapillary measurements
- Optical coherence tomography images contain significantly fewer pixels than both SLP and CSLO. Recent evidence suggests that increasing sampling density of OCT scans from 25 points/quadrant to 100 points or more/quadrant provides a less variable representation of RNFL thickness
- The follow-up for glaucoma requires change analysis techniques that require further development and testing.

NORMATIVE INDIAN DATA

Tewari et al[7]determined the normative values for macular thickness and volume by optical coherence tomography (OCT3) in healthy Indian subjects. They evaluated the macula of 170 consecutive, randomly selected normal subjects who were imaged on OCT 3 in this cross-sectional study. OCT parameters of macular thickness were analyzed with baseline variables including age, gender, axial length and refractive error. The average foveal thickness in the population under study was 149.16 ± 21.15 microns. Macular thickness and volume parameters of OCT correlated significantly (Pearson's correlation coefficient) with age ($r = 0.23$, $P < 0.01$), but not with gender, axial length and refraction.

Sony et al[9] studied 146 Indian eyes showing that the average RNFL thickness in the sample population under study was 104.27 ± 8.51 (95% CI 87.25–121). They also reported that the RNFL was thickest in the inferior quadrant followed by the superior quadrant and progressively less in the nasal and temporal quadrant.

Budenz et al[10] have recently reported that the retinal nerve fiber layer thickness as measured by stratus OCT varies significantly with age, ethnicity, axial length and optic disk area. In summary they reported that the mean RNFL thickness for the entire population was 100.1 μ (SD 11.6).Thinner RNFL measurements were associated with older age ($P < 0.001$): being Caucasian versus either Hispanic or Asian ($P = 0.006$); greater axial length ($P < 0.001$); or smaller optic disc area ($P = 0.010$). For every decade of increased age, mean RNFL thickness measured thinner by approximately 2.0 μ (95% confidence interval (CI),1.2–2.8). For every 1 mm greater axial length the mean RNFL thickness measured thinner by approximately 2.2 μ (95% CI,1.1–3.4). For every increase in square mm of optic disk area, mean RNFL thickness increased by approximately 3.3 μ (95% CI,0.6–

5.6). Comparison between ethnic groups revealed that Caucasians had mean RNFL values (98.1 ± 10.09 μ) slightly thinner than those of Hispanics (103.7 ± 11.6 μ) or Asians (105.8 ± 9.2 μ). There was no relationship between RNFL thickness and gender. Close relationship between OCT images of retina and retinal histology has been reported.[11-13]

In the study done by Ramakrishnan et al[14] 118 Indian patients were evaluated with the help of the Stratus OCT 3000 V 4.0.1. The results revealed that the Mean ± Standard deviation retinal nerve fiber layer thickness for the various quadrants: superior, inferior, nasal, temporal and along the entire circumference along the optic nerve head were 138.2 ± 21.74, 129.1 ± 25.67, 85.71 ± 21, 66.38 ± 17.37, and 104.8 ± 38.81μm, respectively. There was no significant difference in the measurements between males and females and no significant correlation with respect to age.

The Future

The preperimetric diagnosis of glaucoma is going to be the real challenge for the future. The ultrahigh resolution (UHR) OCT is the thing to look forward to for the diagnosis of glaucoma at the earliest. It utilizes $Ti:Al_2O_3$ laser and achieves a much lower resolution of around 2 μ, which is not possible with the currently available OCTs. The studies with UHR OCT have been encuraging.

References

1. Varma R, Steinmann WC, Scott IU. Expert agreement in evaluating the optic disc for glaucoma. *Ophthalmology.* 1992;99:215-21.
2. Daniel M Stein. Imaging in Glaucoma. Ophthalmology Clinics of North America Imaging. Joel S. Schuman, Vol 17, March 2004, Elsevier Saunders, 41-6.
3. Bowd C, Zangwill LM, Berry CC, et al. Detecting early glaucoma by assessment of retinal nerve fiber layer thickness and visual function. *Invest Ophthalmol Vis Sci.* 2001;42:1993-2003.
4. Irene Voo , Clinical applications of OCT. Ophthalmology Clinics of North America Imaging Joel S. Schuman, Vol 17, March 2004, Elsevier Saunders; 21-31.
5. Schuman et al. *Arch Ophthalmol.* 1995;113:586.
6. Jones AL, Sheen NJ, North RV, Morgan JE. The Humphrey optical coherence tomography scanner: quantitative analysis and reproducibility study of the normal human retinal nerve fiber layer. *Br J Ophthalmol.* 2001;85(6):673-7.
7. Tewari HK, Wagh VB, Sony P, Venkatesh P, Singh R. Macular thickness evaluation using the optical coherence tomography in normal Indian eyes. *Indian J Ophthalmol.* 2004;52(3):199-204.
8. Quigley HA, Addicks EM, Green WR. Optic nerve damage in human glaucoma: III Quantitative correlation of nerve fiber loss and visual field defects in glaucoma, ischemic optic neuropathy, papilledema, and toxic optic neuropathy. *Arch Ophthalmol.* 1982;100:135-46.

9. Sony P, Sihota R et al. Quantification of the retinal nerve fiber layer thickness in normal Indian eyes with optical coherence Tomography. *Indian Journal of Ophthalmology.* 2004;52(4):303-9
10. Budenz DL, Anderson DR, Varma R et al. Determinants of normal retinal nerve fiber layer thickness measured by stratus OCT. *Ophthalmology.* 2007;114:1046-52.
11. Abbott CJ, Mc Brien NA, Grunert U, Pianta MJ. Relationship of the optical coherence tomography signal to underlying retinal histology in the tree shrew (Tupaia belangeri). *Invest Ophthalmol Vis Sci.* 2009;50:414-23.
12. Chen TC, Cense B, Miller JW, et al. Histologic correlation of in vivo optical coherence tomography images of the human retina. *Am J Ophthalmol.* 2006;141: 1165-8.
13. Gloesmann M, Hermann B, Schubert C, Sattmann H, Ahnelt PK, Drexler W. Histological correlation of the pig retina radial statification with ultra high resolution optical coherence tomography. *Invest Ophthalmol Vis Sci.* 2003;44:1696-703.
14. R Ramakrishnan, Saurabh Mittal, Sonal Ambatkar, Mohideen A Kader. Retinal nerve fibre layer thickness measurements in normal Indian population by optical coherence tomography. *Indian J Ophthalmol.* 2006;54:11-5.

5

chapter

Frank Joseph Goes

Multifocal IOLs

ABSTRACT

Recent advances in materials and designs of IOL have converted cataract surgery to a more or less refractive surgery. Implantation of multifocals can result in achieving emmetropic status improving good visual acuity for distance, near and intermediate distances. The use of Tecnis ZM900 and ReZoom lenses provided good functional vision without spectacles in young patients. Mixing and Matching Tecnis and ReZoom IOLs are unique concept though requires further studies.

Introduction

The second generation of multifocal intraocular lenses (IOLs) has led to renewed interest in their use to correct refractive errors, particularly those who require higher levels of refractive correction and are not good candidates for corneal refractive surgery.[1-7]

The need for optimal refractive results in younger presbyopic patients has also opened the door to a new concept with multifocal IOLs-that of mixing and matching different designs—refractive and diffractive based on the needs of the individual patient, in order to provide a full range of vision: near, distant and intermediate. In particular, the use of the Tecnis ZM900 and the ReZoom lens often provides the younger patients with reasonable functional vision without the need for spectacles.

Our interest in multifocal IOL's is not new, we have gathered experience with several types of multifocal lenses over many years. It was started in 1985 with the use of the 3-piece, 6-mm, polymethylmethacrylate (PMMA)

3M multifocal intraocular lens. This technology was bought by Alcon later years and we were involved in the one-piece refractive PMMA Storz True Vista study from 1992. Later we began to implant the Alcon ReStor lens, and the Crystalens. Interestingly, we have in 2004 switched to the Tecnis ZM900 multifocal IOL and in 2006 and started combining Tecnis with the ReZoom IOL (Figs 5.1 and 5.2).

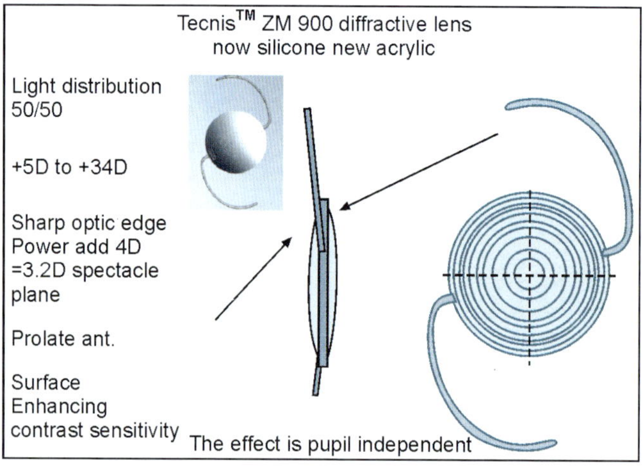

Fig. 5.1: Characteristics of the diffractive Tecnis multifocal IOL

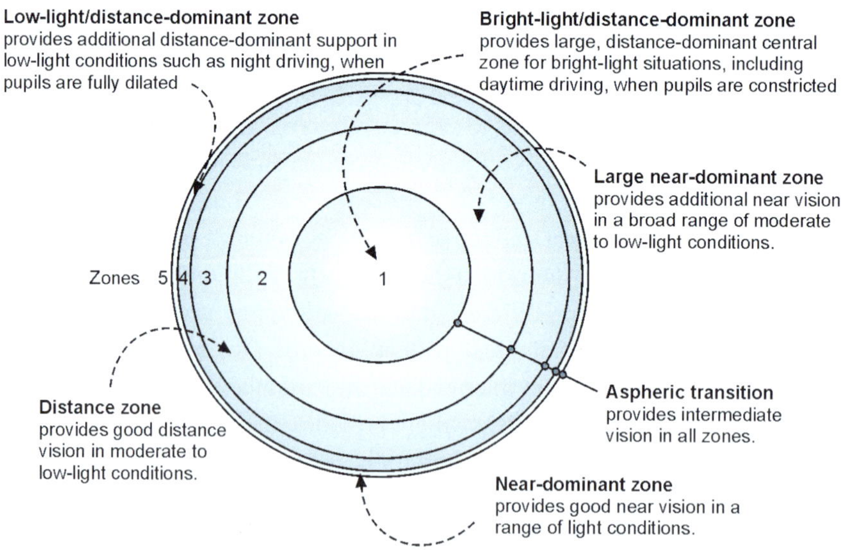

Fig. 5.2: Characteristics of the refractive ReZoom multifocal IOL

This chapter is based on our experience in implanting 400 Tecnis lenses bilaterally and additionally, 90 Tecnis combined with the ReZoom. All these eyes have a follow-up of at least 6 months.

TECNIS ZM 900

The Tecnis ZM 900 IOL is a 3-piece foldable diffractive IOL of high quality silicone with a near/far light distribution of 50/50. The diffractive component consists of 32 concentric rings on the back surface of the lens and provides an optical power add of 4 D corresponding with 3.2 D at the corneal plane. The lens comes in a power range of +5 to + 34 D in 0.5-D steps. The -0.27-prolate anterior surface compensates for the positive spherical aberrations of the typical cornea hence resulting in improved functional vision as reported for the monofocal model (8-9-10-11-12-13-). This technical feature is particularly relevant under low luminance condition because the amount of spherical aberration increases as the pupil size becomes larger. The light coming into the eye is distributed between the near and far focus, allowing a full range of vision independent of pupil size. The lens has the Z-SHARP optic edge technology, delaying early posterior capsular opacification (PCO) while minimizing edge glare. The overall diameter of the lens is 13 mm, with a 6.0-mm optic. The lens is available in hydrophobic acrylic material in Europe from 2008.

REZOOM MULTIFOCAL IOL

The ReZoom is a 3-piece acrylic multifocal IOL with UV blocking and an OptiEdge design that is said to minimize edge glare while reducing the potential for posterior capsular opacification. The IOL is designed to provide for 100% light transmission in order to provide the full range of vision.

The ReZoom multifocal, with its refractive design, has five focusing zones. From the outer edge of the lens towards the centre, these are: a low light/distance dominant zone, a near dominant zone, a distance zone, an additional near dominant zone and a bright light/distance dominant zone. Transitions between these zones are designed to provide intermediate vision with a design the company calls "Balance View Optics". Patients implanted with a ReZoom multifocal are intended to have 100% light transmission over all five optical zones.[1]

Selection of Patients

There are two groups of candidates or interested patients who seek implantation of multifocal IOLs:

The first group consists of cataract patients. Some have heard about the possibility of multifocal lenses that correct both far and near vision; some have friends or relatives who had the procedure done with successful outcomes. These people, specifically if they are in the 60-75 years old group, are very interested in discussing this option. Some cataract patients have never heard about this refractive lens concept. If we do not mention the option of a multifocal concept, some of our patients will be upset later on when they find out that they have missed the opportunity to have one.

The second group consists of refractive patients who specifically come in for refractive surgery: high hyperopes (greater than +4 D), moderate to low hyperopes with incipient reading problems at the age of 45 years or above, and presbyopic patients who have good distance vision but want to eliminate their reading glasses.

We would not advise refractive surgery in presbyopic myopes with a clear lens since sooner or later a YAG laser capsulotomy will have to be done, and we feel that the risk of complications (e.g., retinal detachment) is higher in myopes. It can be advised for myopes when there is some cataract. We have experience in performing at least 700 YAG laser capsulotomies in moderate to high hyperopes and have never seen a retinal detachment following a YAG capsulotomy. Rarely, RD occurs following laser capsulotomy in hyperopic patients.

Generally speaking, the cataract patient group is less demanding than the refractive group. The ideal candidate to start with is a moderate hyperope (2 to 5 D) between 50 and 60 years old. One should be cautious about presbyopic individuals with good distance vision because they are usually very demanding.

Patient Expectations

General advice such as "underpromise and overdeliver" and "more chair time before surgery means less chair time after surgery" are well known, but what do these statements actually mean? It is a fact that our patients will always remember the very first things we say during our discussion. They should feel that we are confident but that we do not want to "oversell" the product; otherwise it will backfire and discredit the technology. It is better to present your result on the basis of surgeries conducted in past one or two years and discuss the percentage of the spectacle free patients after the procedure for all distances—far, intermediate, and near.

It is always better to tell them that some will need time (1 to 3 months) to adjust to seeing at all distances. Some will have to get used to working closer to their desktop and/or laptop computer and only a minority will

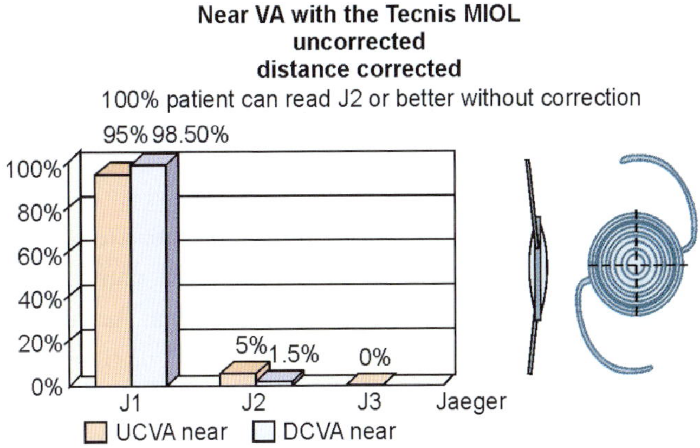

Fig. 5.3: Results of near vision with Tecnis MF

need to wear glasses for intermediate distances, such as specific hobby tasks (Fig. 5.3). Of course, patients should be motivated and interested in becoming spectacle free or less spectacle dependent. Motivation is the key point; they should be willing to be patient with the process, recognize that it may take time to adapt to the new visual system, and have the means to pay for the added cost of MIOL surgery.

We are working together with AMO and my International Colleagues on a project to filter out those patients who will be unhappy at the end of the journey? This may have more to do with the patient's personality than with the type of accommodative or multifocal lens implanted or the specific anatomical conditions of the eye.

Much has been said regarding neuroadaptation of the brain but at this point we do not have a total understanding or a way to measure this function before implanting a lens. Some patients may experience problems like halos and glare, one cannot predict who will experience them, and that most patients often get used to them and may not be bothered after 1 to 3 months. We also tell our patients that the lens can later be exchanged if necessary. Of course one should also discuss the patient's hobbies and activities such as driving and computer work. Patients should enter the process with a firm understanding of possible side effects, and the final decision must come from the patient himself. Two bus drivers were recently operated with custom mixing of ReZoom-Tecnis multifocal and they experienced no problem with night driving because they were advised to be seated high and look down at the upcoming car headlights and not right into it.

Also, the disturbing subjective complaints may decrease in many patients after a touch-up for residual refractive errors, after implantation of an IOL in the second eye, or with time due to neuroadaptation. Halos and unwanted images will remain significant in approximately 5% of patients and this is the same for all types of multifocal IOLs. This group of patients can still drive at night although they may not like to do so.

PREOPERATIVE TESTING

It is logical that prospective candidates for a multifocal lens should have normal and healthy eyes. Diabetes (under medical control) and other systematic general conditions are not exclusion criteria. Accurate biometry (preferentially with the IOL Master) and IOL power calculation is a "*conditio sine qua non*" especially for long myopic eyes where there is a staphyloma, and in short eyes where differences of 0.1 mm have an enormous impact on the IOL power calculation.

At least 2, and preferentially 3, formulae should be used for multifocal IOL calculation. Haigis formula, combined with Holladay II formula is excellent for all axial length calculation. The SRK T is excellent for long myopic eyes and the Hoffer Q formula is outstanding for short hyperopic eyes.

The constants are constantly updated on his website by Haigis and are 119.8 for the Tecnis ZM900 and 118.8 for the ReZoom lens (Fig. 5.4). With the Tecnis IOL, the target should be +0.25 D to plano since a myopic outcome will bring the reading distance too close. The refractive target should be plano with the ReZoom IOL. Preoperative astigmatism of more than 1.5 D should be a relative exclusion criterion for novices since the immediate effect of the multifocal lens would be diminished. Laser in situ keratomileusis (LASIK) enhancement or limbal relaxing incisions (LRIs) can solve this problem, but the patient should be informed about it beforehand.

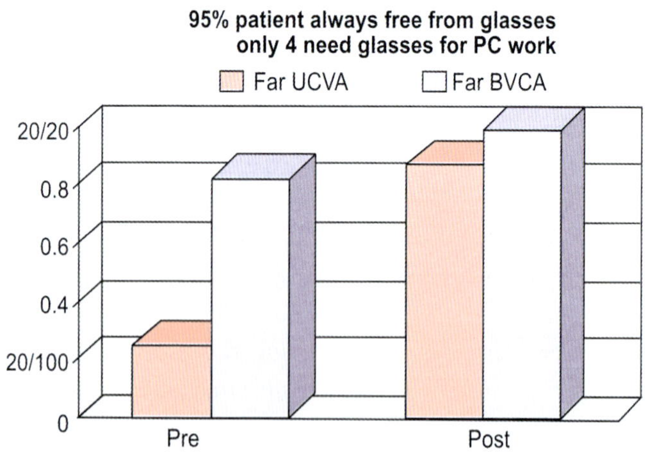

Fig. 5.4: Distance VA with the Tecnis MIOL uncorrected best corrected

SURGICAL TECHNIQUE

The surgery is performed under topical anesthesia. The patient is examined the day 1, day 14, and day 30 postoperatively. The site of incision is given according to the pre-existing astigmatism; superiorly when the astigmatism is 0.75 D or more with-the-rule, and temporally for all other cases. The corneal incision is more anteriorly when astigmatism is 2D. Since limbal relaxation incisions (LRIs) are not predictable enough, we perform them only when the pre-existing astigmatism is significant (more than 4 D). Generally, a 3.0-mm clear corneal incision is made with a diamond knife. The anterior chamber is filled with Healon GV or Healon 5 (AMO).

The capsulorhexis should be 5.5 to 6.0 mm in diameter and preferably central and circular. Routine phacoemulsification was sometimes limited to aspiration only because of the soft structure of the patient's natural lens.

IMPLANTATION TECHNIQUE OF TECNIS OR REZOOM

IOL loading of these multifocal IOL's, should be done by the surgeon under the microscope using the Silver Series unfolder. The different steps are nicely highlighted in the company brochure that comes with the lens. Always have a back-up lens available; a novice surgeon will have to discard, because of damage during the loading procedure some lenses (around 5 to 10%Tecnis MF in the first 20, this will drop to 1% with experience). Carefully ensure that the lens presents itself nicely with the leading haptic protruding toward the tip when you advance the knob.

Use sufficient viscoelastic material such as Healon GV or Healon 5 to fill the capsular bag. Slowly release the IOL as you would turn a pancake around. Once the optic becomes visible, proceed very slowly and the lens will unfold itself. Once the optic is in the capsular bag, retract the plunger of the unfolder and use a Sinskey hook to deliver the trailing haptic into the capsular bag. Since viscoelastic is used in a large amount, take care to thoroughly aspirate it out and go beneath the IOL with the irrigation-aspiration tip as well.

The corneal wound is hydrated at the end of surgery and one drop of Prednisolone acetate 5mg/ml and polymyxin B sulphate /3500 IE-Predmycine P is administered. Afterwards these drops are continued for three times a day for 4 weeks day.

The Tecnis ZM centers remarkably well by itself due to the broad C-haptics, even with an oval or asymmetric capsulorhexis. We never suture the wound unless we have had to enlarge it.

ENHANCEMENT AND LENS EXCHANGE

When a touch-up for residual refractive error (spherical or astigmatic) may be advisable, we prefer to use LASIK or EpiLasik (in case of a thin or irregular cornea) and wait until at least 3 months after surgery. Our present enhancement rate is 10%, going down from 20% for the initial cases.

INTRAOCULAR LENS EXCHANGE

We have never been forced to explant either the Tecnis or ReZoom. When faced with an extremely unhappy patient, one should exclude all other possibilities before considering an IOL exchange.A subjectively unsatisfactory outcome for the patient may be the result of residual refractive error, posterior capsule opacification that can be cured with YAG laser capsulotomy, or a retinal abnormality that can be demonstrated with optical coherence tomography. Even when you are convinced that the multifocal optic is the cause of persistent complaints, try to postpone doing an IOL exchange for as long as possible, at least 6 months.

STAGED IMPLANTATION AND CUSTOM MIXING OF IOLS

Diffractive lens Tecnis ZM900 provides good distance vision and excellent near vision and a refractive lens ReZoom provides an excellent distance and intermediate vision but performs weaker for near vision. We should select the multifocal lens by considering hobbies and professions of patients. Therefore, we prefer a staged implantation of the 2 eyes (Fig. 5.5). Considering the profession of the patients, it is found that:

1. A frequent computer user may be better off with bilateral ReZoom to provide good intermediate range.
2. A professional car or truck driver who must also drive at night will be best off with a Tecnis aspheric monofocal IOL in both eyes.
3. An avid reader, such as a librarian, will be better off with a Tecnis multifocal in each eye.

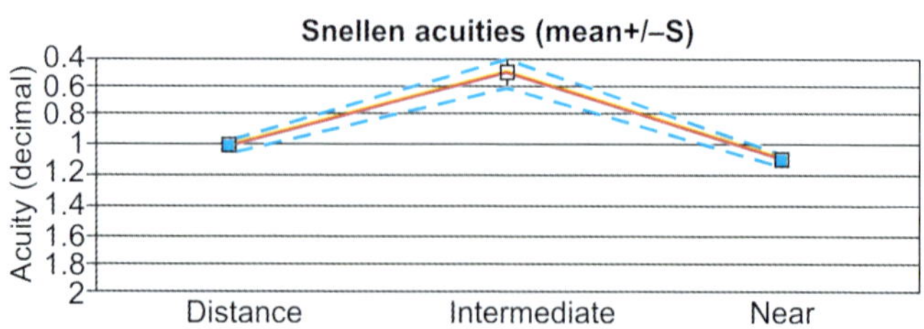

Fig. 5.5: Mean near, intermediate and distance binocular visual results

4. An outdoor enthusiast or golfer might feel better with a ReZoom in each eye.
5. A person with strong motivation for complete spectacle dependence will be a candidate for a mix and match.

Surgery is done first in the dominant eye, with the plan of operating on the second eye within 1 to 2 weeks.

WHICH LENS IN WHICH EYE?

1. If the major activities are distance dominant, ReZoom is implanted in the dominant eye.
2. If the major activities are near dominant, Tecnis multifocal is implanted in the dominant eye.
3. We evaluate the first eye outcome after 7 to 10 days and query the patient about his or her satisfaction. If he or she is completely happy, we chose the same lens for the other eye.
4. If a ReZoom patient complains of inadequate near vision, we implant a Tecnis multifocal in his or her second eye.
5. Finally, if a Tecnis multifocal patient complains of inadequate intermediate vision, we may implant a ReZoom in his or her second eye.

Refractive Lens Exchange Customizing-Mixing and Matching Tecnis-Rezoom

The concept behind "Mix and Match" is to provide patients with the best possible range of vision without significant visual trade off. The most appropriate patients for the "Mix and Match" approach are those who are motivated to become spectacle free. The best candidates will also be able to understand the concept of the "Mix and Match" approach and that it may take a number of months to adapt to this new visual system.

We report on the initial visual outcomes in 140 eyes of 70 patients implanted with a ReZoom multifocal in their dominant eye and a Tecnis ZM900 in their non-dominant eye 1-2 week later. One hundred twenty eyes were hyperopic (Range: +0.50 to 6.75 D, Mean SE = 2.62 D, SD ± 1.085 D), 12 eyes had a myopic spherical equivalent (-0.25 to -2.50 D) and 8 eyes were 0.00 D. For all eyes, the preoperative SE was 2.17 D (SD ± 1.417 D). The mean pre-op BCVA was 0.84, while the mean pre-op binocular BCVA was 0.94. All patients except 10 underwent refractive lens exchange (RLE) with the remaining patients undergoing cataract surgery with lens replacement. Exclusion criteria included corneal or retinal pathology and history of glaucoma or retinal detachment.

IOL POWER CALCULATION AND SURGERY

All IOL power calculations and surgeries were carried out by the same surgeon (FG). Biometry was done with the IOL Master (Carl Zeiss, Carl Zeiss-Meditec, Jena, Germany). The targeted refraction was emmetropia to 0.25 D in the Tecnis eye and emmetropia in the ReZoom eye.

Patients underwent either RLE or cataract surgery on an outpatient basis using a standardized procedure under topical anesthesia. Both eyes were operated within 2 weeks.

After surgery, patients were sent a subjective lifestyle questionnaire. Binocular acuities were recorded at distance, intermediate and near using appropriate test cards. Six months after surgery results were analyzed using the LogMAR acuities.

MEASUREMENTS AND ANALYSIS

Clinical data was collected preoperatively, at 1 week and 1 to 2 months and, again, at 6 months following surgery. The testing carried out included refraction, binocular uncorrected near, intermediate (60 cm = 24 inch) and distance vision, as well, preferential reading distance. Patients were asked to report any visual complaints or difficulties they experienced, as well as their level of spectacle independence.

Results

In terms of visual symptoms reported by patients, 40 out of 70 patients reported no subjective disturbance by glare or halos in both eyes, 28 reported some glare and halos in both eyes. The halos and glare were severe in 8 patients. They were present but easily accepted in the other 20 patients. Three patients required slightly tinted sunglasses in order to reduce glare.

The second most frequently reported visual symptom was day glare. Three patients reported with day glare in both eyes. The majority of patients reporting visual side effects indicated that visual disturbances were more apparent at night but, in general, were not a significant problem and improved over time.

The mean binocular distance vision was 1.06 (±0.6 SD), the mean intermediate was 0.5 (±0.9 SD) and the mean binocular near vision was 1.1 (±0.4 SD) (Table 5.1 and Fig. 5.6).

Only one patient required spectacle correction for reading. One patient did undergo a Lasik enhancement procedure in both eyes to correct a residual cylinder of -1.5 D and one needed YAG in two eyes.

TABLE 5.1: The mean binocular UCVA results for near, intermediate and distance shows that the best visual outcomes for near and distance was 1.2, with no patient worse than 0.8 at the 2-month follow-up

Decimal	Mean	SD	Best	Worst	Median
Distance	1	0.6 Lines	1.2	0.8	0.8
Intermediate	0.5	0.9 Lines	0.8	0.4	0.5
Near	1.1	0.4 Lines	1.2	0.9	1.1

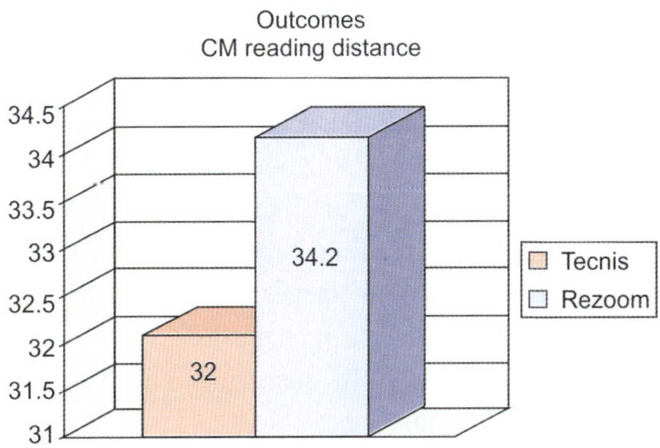

Fig. 5.6: Preferred reading distance with Tecnis eye (RED) and ReZoom eye (GREEN)

A follow-up questionnaire was sent to all patients following surgery to gather subjective information regarding lifestyle after "Mix and Match" multifocal implantation. Of the 70 patients enrolled in the study, 46 completed and returned the questionnaire. Topics on the questionnaire included reading, television viewing, computer and driving habits, as well as questions about the amount of time needed for adapting to multifocal vision, preferred eye (if any) and overall degree of satisfaction.

Analysis showed that the majority of patients with some complaints of glare and halo are adapted very fast (1-3 months). They did see the rings but it did not disturb them as such. Only 6 patients could comment on a difference of subjective complaints between both eyes; 4 out of 6 more disturbed by ReZoom 2 out of 6 more by the Tecnis eye.

Interim analysis showed that the average amount of time needed to adapt to their new vision was 33 ± 7 days). Twenty six patients reported that they had no preference of one eye over the other, while 6 based their preference on the UCVA results. Ten patients preferred the vision in their ReZoom eye, while the remaining 4 preferred the vision in their Tecnis ZM900 eye. There did not appear to be a correlation between patient preference and any residual refractive error.

In terms of degree of satisfaction, 38 of the 46 respondents rated their satisfaction very good, while 6 rated it good and 2 rated it fair. When asked if they would recommend a "Mix and Match" approach to friends or relatives, 40 said yes, while 5 said yes, with some restrictions regarding expectations, and one no. In the meantime this patient is improving since he needed reading glasses. One patient had still problems with intermediate vision.

The differences between ReZoom eye and Tecnis eye were analysed. The preferred reading distance in the ReZoom eye was 34, 2 cm (13.7 inches) while it was 32 cm (12.8 inches) for the Tecnis eye. This is understandable since the effective reading add for ReZoom is lower (2.8 D) compared to Tecnis (3.2 D). Figure 5.7 considering the reading at intermediate distances, 83% of ReZoom eyes could read Jaeger 5 at 60 cm (24 inches) but only 41% of Tecnis eyes could do the same at that this distance. The mean reading capability at 60 cm was different between both eyes; the mean was Jaeger 4.5 for Tecnis and Jaeger 6.7 for ReZoom. It is because of the design, the ReZoom which allows better reading at intermediate distances. To date, only one patient in this series required Nd: YAG capsulotomy.

Improvement in the material and modifications in the design of optics have improved the retinal image contrast and functional visual performance.[8,9] It has been reported that functional visual showed improvement with an anterior surface modified prolate intraocular lens implantation.[10,11]

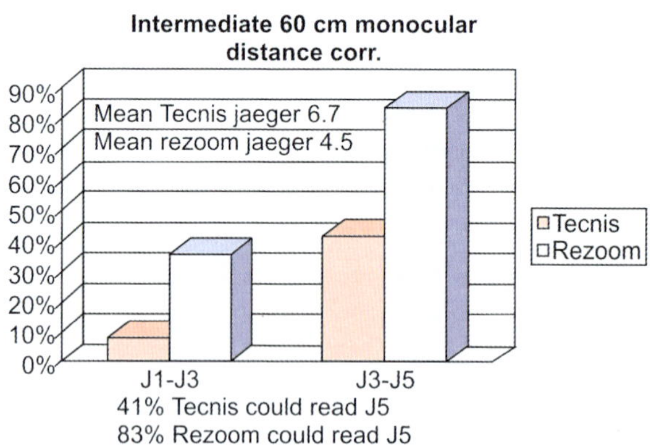

Fig. 5.7: Results intermediate distance monocular 60 cm= 42 inch: Tecnis (RED)

References

1. Lane SS, Morris M, Nordan L, Packer M, Tarantino N, Wallace RB 3rd. Multifocal intraocular lenses. *Ophthalmol Clin North Am.* 2006;19:89-105.
2. Hütz WW, Eckhardt HB, Rohrig B, Grolmus R. Reading ability with 3 multifocal intraocular lens models. *J Cataract Refract Surg.* 2006 ;32:2015-2021.
3. Kohnen T, Allen D, Boureau C, Dublineau P, Hartmann C, Mehdorn E, Rozot P, Tassinari G. European multicenter study of the AcrySof ReSTOR apodized diffractive intraocular lens. *Ophthalmology* 2006;113:584.
4. Blaylock JF, Si Z, Vickers C. Visual and refractive status at different focal distances after implantation of the ReStor multifocal intraocular lens. *J Cataract Refract Surg.* 2006;32:1464-1473.
5. Chiam PJ, Chan JH, Aggarwal RK, Kasaby S. ReSTOR intraocular lens implantation in cataract surgery: quality of vision. *J Cataract Refract Surg.* 2006 ;32:1459-1463. Erratum in: *J Cataract Refract Surg.* 2006 Dec;32:1987.
6. Sallet G. Refractive outcome after bilateral implantation of an apodized diffractive intraocular lens. *Bull Soc Belge Ophtalmol.* 2006;299:67-73.
7. Souza CE, Muccioli C, Soriano ES, Chalita MR, Oliveira F, Freitas LL, Meire LP, Tamaki C, Belfort R Jr. Visual performance of Acrysof ReStor apodized diffractive IOL: a prospective comparative trial. *Am J Ophthalmol.* 2006 ;141:827-832.
8. Kershner RM. Retinal image contrast and functional visual performance with spheric, silicone, and acrylic intraocular lenses. Prospective evaluation. *J Cataract Refract Surg* 2003; 29:1684-1694.
9. Mester U, Dillinger P, Anterist N. Impact of a modified optic design on visual function: clinical comparative study. *J Cataract Refract Surg* 2003; 29:652-660.
10. Packer M, Fine IH, Hoffman RS, et al. Improved functional vision with a modified prolate intraocular lens. *J Cataract Refract Surg* 2004; 30:986-992.
11. Ricci F, Scuderi G, Missiroli F, et al. Low contrast visual acuity in pseudophakic patients implanted with an anterior surface modified prolate intraocular lens. *Acta Ophthalmol Scand* 2004; 82:718-722.

6 chapter

Naresh Babu, Supreet Singh Juneja

Scleral Fixated Intraocular Lenses

ABSTRACT

Though placement of IOL in the capsular bag is the standard of care, situations arise where there is inadequate support for the IOL in the bag or in the sulcus; and scleral fixated IOLs are a viable option to this predicament, sans the complications associated with ACIOLs. The techniques and materials used for SFIOLs are diverse. Sutured SFIOLs though having anatomic and functional advantages are surgically challenging and associated with complications, especially suture related. Sutureless SFIOLs on the other hand provide good IOL stability and freedom from suture related complications. We herein describe our preferred "no glue no sutures technique", which once mastered is an excellent method of scleral fixating IOLs with good short- and long term stability and visual outcomes.

Introduction

Implantation of an intraocular lens (IOL) in the capsular bag during routine cataract surgery is the standard of care; however, surgeons must be comfortable with alternative techniques in the event of complications that preclude this placement. Loss of posterior capsule integrity is a well-documented complication of cataract surgery with an incidence of 0.69 to 6.7% in recent studies.[1,2] If this occurs, surgeons must assess intraoperatively whether sufficient support for IOL placement in the capsular bag or ciliary sulcus exists. If capsule support is inadequate, neither option is viable.

Several IOL types can be used in the absence of capsule support, including angle-supported and iris-fixated anterior chamber (AC) IOLs and iris-fixated and sclera-fixated posterior chamber IOLs. Due to the ease of insertion, angle-supported AC IOLs have been the predominant IOL choice in patients with compromised capsule support. Unfortunately, early closed-loop IOLs had a high complication rate, including fibrosis of the angle with subsequent glaucoma, corneal endothelial cell loss with resultant bullous keratopathy, pupil block, and cystoid macular edema.[3] Nowadays the flexible open-loop AC IOL has proved to be well tolerated and has fewer complications than its predecessor. Because of the AC IOLs' earlier problems, the scleral-fixated IOL is thought to be tolerated better long-term given its more anatomical positioning and the reduced likelihood of anisekonia.[4] Recent reports refute this notion, concluding that the flexible open-loop AC IOL has similar if not better outcomes than the sclera-fixated IOL.[5,6] However, in some instances, neither capsule nor iris support is available, making the scleral-fixated IOL the only option.

Because of their anatomic location, sclera-fixated PCIOLs have a theoretic advantage over other IOLs in regard to complications, especially in eyes after trauma and in young patients.[7-9] They provide better visual acuity and binocularity, lead to a lower incidence of strabismus than contact lenses, and avoid the complications of ACIOLs, which are seen more with rigid closed loop IOLs than with open-loop and iris-claw IOLs. However, the surgical technique of sclera-fixated IOL is much more difficult than other IOL implantations, it results in sutures tracking into the eye, and there is surgical manipulation in the region of the ciliary body, which can cause hemorrhage.[10,11] Serious postoperative complications, such as knot and suture erosion,[12-14] IOL tilt, suture breakage, endophthalmitis, retinal detachment (RD),[15] choroidal hemorrhage,[13] elevated intraocular pressure (IOP),[16-19] and open-angle glaucoma, are well documented. Complication rates within 12 months of surgery are reported to below[18] and similar in children and adults.[20] However, over the long-term, unacceptably high rates of suture breakage and IOL dislocation in young patients have been recorded.[7]

Sutures

The Ethicon TG-160-2, Ethicon CIF-4 (Ethicon, New Jersey) can be used for *ab interno* methods. The Ethicon STC-6 straight needle is used in both methods. In general, 10-0 polypropylene has been the suture material of choice.[21]

PLACEMENT OF SCLERAL SUTURES

Originally, suturing techniques involved passing the needle from inside to outside (*ab interno*) the eye. Although this method may be quicker and is easier when penetrating keratoplasty is performed concomitantly, it is a blind procedure.[22]

As its name suggests, the outside to inside (*ab externo*) technique involves passing the needle from outside to inside, and was described by Lewis.[23] This is also undertaken blindly in that the intraocular exit-point of the needle is unseen, but by knowing the entry point sulcus positioning of the suture is more predictable.[24,25] With the *ab externo* technique, the anterior chamber can remain closed during needle passes. This avoids collapse of the ciliary sulcus in the hypotonic eye, thus facilitating accurate suture placement.[26]

SCLERAL SUTURE FIXATION TECHNIQUES

Simple Knotting Over the Sclera

In this technique, IOLs are attached to the sclera with two points of fixation. Formed polypropylene suture knot and suture ends over the sclera are covered by conjunctiva and the Tenon's capsule. However, despite its simplicity with regard to suture technique, conjunctival erosion is very common after this procedure.[27] Serious complications, such as endophthalmitis may also be seen.

Corneal Autografts for External Knots

The knots are covered with autologous lamellar corneal patches during the combined keratoplasty and scleral fixation. The patch is then covered with conjunctiva.[2] This method is safer with regard to sutural erosion but a corneal autograft protuberance is made over the sclera, which is seen as a disadvantage.

Covering with Fascia Lata or Dura Mater

Autologous fascia lata or lyophilized dura mater is used to cover the external knots. These patches are then covered with conjunctiva, which provides very good protection against suture exposure. However, removing fascia lata or supplying dura mater allografts could increase difficulty and cost. Moreover, during the postoperative period, externally recognizable patches on the eye may lead to physiological and cosmetic disturbances.[29,30]

Covering with Scleral Flaps

Covering with scleral flaps appears to be a favorable technique for scleral fixation. First, triangular limbal-based scleral flaps (3 × 1 mm) are fashioned. A previously formed knot on the sclera is placed under a triangular flap then this flap is closed and remains sutureless at the end of surgery. With this technique the maintenance of knot security within the sclera has benefits with regard to suture exposure, but if the flap is too thin it can easily be dehisced, macerated, or punctured. In addition, the knot may reposition through the scleral bed into the eye.[31]

Continuous-loop Fixation Technique

In this technique, the needle is passed through the haptic's eyelet/s and punctures the sclera in two places. One end of the suture is tied to the other end of the suture. The suture knot is then rotated in through the incision and out through the sclera. The knots are then rotated into the eye.[23] Therefore, with this type of arrangement a few knot-related problems are expected to arise. On the other hand, as each haptic requires two points of scleral fixation, a total of four needle punctures need to be made in the sclera, and thus there is a relatively higher risk of developing complications compared with the conventional two-needle punctures. In addition, suture knot rotation may cause IOL torque and tilt.

Four Points of Fixation Underneath the Superficial Scleral Flap

Herein, the suture knot is rotated in the same manner as during the previously mentioned procedure. The difference between the two procedures is in the fashioning of an L-shaped scleral flap for covering the suture.[32]This technique minimizes the possibility of conjunctival erosion, suture exposure and thinning of sclera, but the longer surgical time is considered to be a disadvantage.

Limbal-groove Incision and Double-suture Fixation

The limbal-groove incision and double-suture fixation method allows for a two-point fixation.[33] Two 3 mm scleral grooves are created horizontally at 3 and 9 o'clock, 0.5–0.75 mm from the limbus. The suture knot is trimmed and rotated into the scleral groove. This method allows the suture knot to be buried in the eye without the use of scleral flaps. There is a risk of suture knot protrusion.

Trans-scleral Fixation of Intraocular Lenses through Sclerotomy

In vitrectomy surgery, after the haptic is pulled close to the sclerotomy site, a suture is tied to the haptic of IOL from outside through the sclerotomy site. The remaining suture material is buried within the sclerotomy lips. Therefore, the risk of suture exposure is minimized. In this procedure of IOL fixation, the haptics should be situated symmetrically opposite each other. In addition, scleral suturing may cause damage to the retina.[34]

SCLERAL INCISION TECHNIQUE

During this procedure, a radial scleral incision is made and sutured with the knot buried within the incision. Problems associated with depth of incision and suture exposure are sometimes seen.[35]

SCLERAL FIXATION WITHOUT CONJUNCTIVAL DISSECTION

This technique is a variation of the traditional triangular scleral flap for scleral fixation and involves performing a conjunctival peritomy and dissecting a scleral flap anteriorly from a position 2–3 mm posterior to the limbus. Surgery begins in clear cornea and dissects a scleral pocket posteriorly, avoiding the need for scleral cautery. Conjunctival dissection is also avoided and sutured wound closure is unnecessary. A larger surface area can be created for suture passes than with triangular sclera flaps or scleral grooves.[36]However, scleral dissection and suture management are incredibly intricate.

SCLERAL TUNNEL TECHNIQUE

This is also a modified scleral flap technique. After dissecting conjunctiva, a conventional scleral tunnel is fashioned with a crescent blade. Passage of a double-armed suture through the roof of the scleral tunnel with subsequent retrieval of the suture ends through the external incision for tying facilitates scleral fixation[37] However, the technique seems to be logical for preventing suture exposure, as a thin flap can easily be dehisced, macerated or punctured with suture knot.

KNOTLESS SCLERAL FIXATION

Knotless scleral fixation describes the technique for implanting an IOL by scleral fixation sutures. This has the advantages of knotless fixation of the haptics and an out-in approach for passing the needle through the sclera.[38] Probably, the worst complication with this procedure is suture loosening, which could result in IOL decentration and tilt.

KNOT AND SUTURE BURYING INTO THE SCLERA WITHOUT FLAP, TUNNEL, INCISION OR GROOVE

The needle is passed through the sclera in a lamellar fashion next to where the suture protrudes from the sclera. Afterwards, the free end with the needle and the other end are tied using a classic suture-tying method. As the suture is being tied, a free end with the needle and a second piece in the form of a loop appear. A very small loop is required for the burial technique. Thus, when the suture is being tied, the suture attached to the IOL should be gripped at the point closest to the scleral entry and knotted. Thus, the suture loop becomes smaller. For the burial procedure, the free-stranded needle is passed through the loop and passed again in the same direction so a secondary loop is made over the first one. The free end is passed through the recently formed loop once more. Thus, the free needle grips the loop bound to the sclera. The needle is inserted into the sclera at the point closest to the preformed knot, and advanced in a lamellar fashion. The needle is retrieved after it is advanced more than the length of the loop onto which the sutures are held. The loop tied to the pulled suture is rotated and buried in the sclera. The suture mounted on the needle is seen at the scleral wound. If the suture is cut at the exit site, its end is retained in the sclera, providing entire burial of the loop and the end mounted on the needle (Fig. 6.1).[39] Author evaluated the sclera-sutured free 150 suture ends after a minimum 24 months of follow-up in 75 eyes of 75 patients and observed no intraoperative or postoperative complications related to the suture burial technique itself.[40]

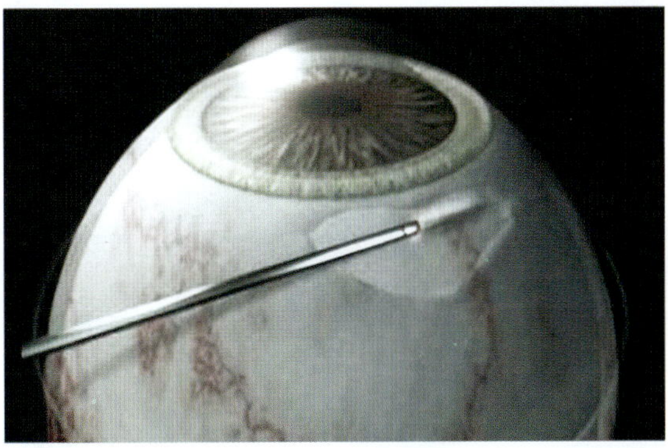

Fig. 6.1: Scleral pocket made with 23 G MVR blade

FIXATION OF THE HAPTICS IN A LIMBUS-PARALLEL SCLERA TUNNEL T_2 NO GLUE NO SUTURES TECHNIQUE (FIGS 6.2 TO 6.5)

This is our preferred technique. A 270 degrees conjunctival peritomy is done.Two partial thickness scleral grooves of 4 mm are fashioned 1.5 mm from the limbus, parallel to it at 10-8 o' clock and 4-2 o' clock using 25 G trocar. Two sclerotomies are made at the edges of the grooves using 23 G syringe. Three 23 G sclerotomy ports are made at 3 mm from limbus in inferotemporal, superotemporal and superonasal quadrants, respectively. Anterior vitrectomy is done routinely. Using a clear corneal incision a foldable lens is introduced into the anterior chamber. Using a

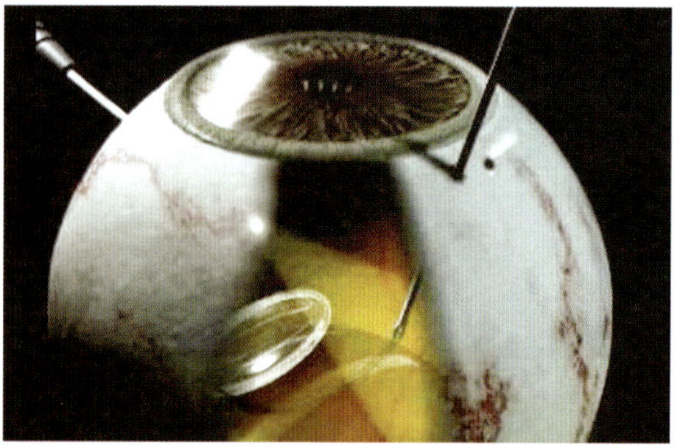

Fig. 6.2: Externalization of the haptic

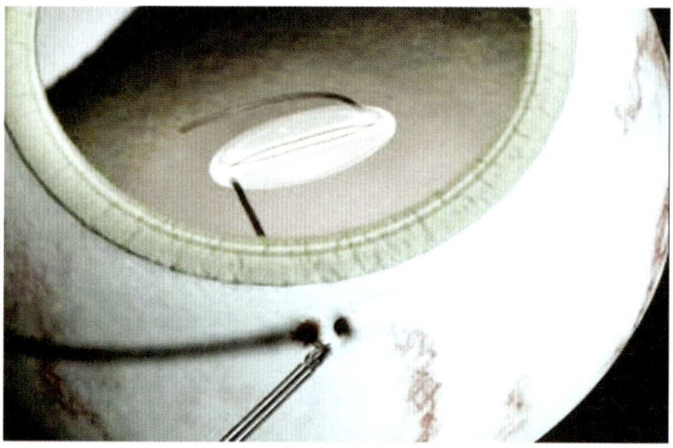

Fig. 6.3: Tucking of haptic into the scleral pocket

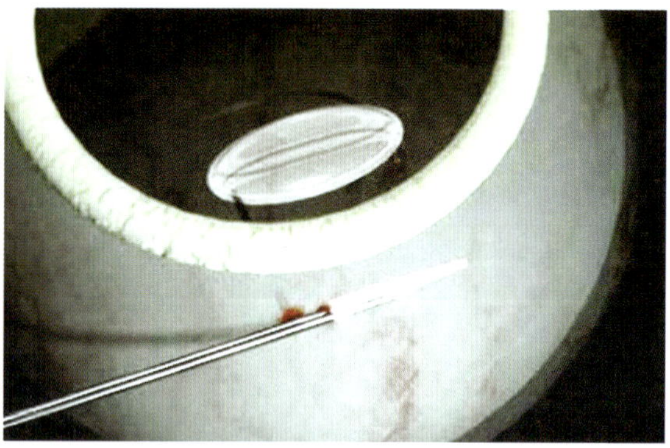

Fig. 6.4: Tucking of the other haptic

25 G vitrectomy forceps, inserted through the sclerotomies at the edges of the grooves the haptics are taken out and put into their respective grooves at 10-8 o' clock and 4-2 o' clock. In this procedure no suture is required, no blind procedure for passing the needle. This technique can be modified to make a corneoscleral tunnel and insert a nonfoldable 3-piece IOL also.

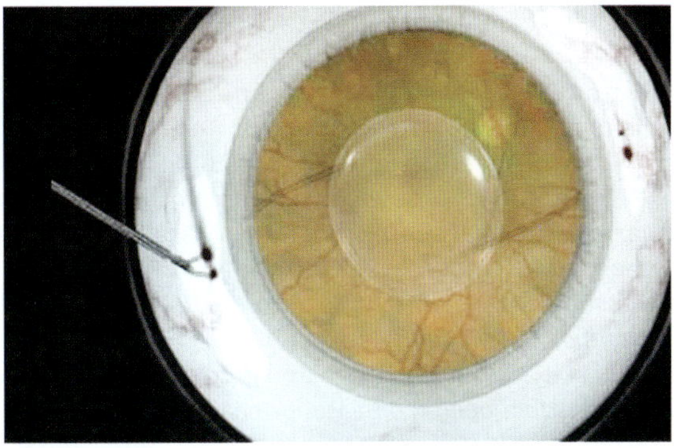

Fig. 6.5: Well centered IOL after the procedure

Many methods have been described to allow scleral fixation. Experienced surgeons have achieved excellent results with trans-sclerally sutured PCIOLs. Common to all scleral fixation technique is the need to cover, bury or rotate suture knots to prevent overlying conjunctival erosion and subsequent endophthalmitis. Each of these is different with regard to technical difficulty, potential postoperative problems and complications. For example, the sutures may erode through the scleral flaps and cause irritation. They may also loosen or break and cause either tilting or dislocation of the optic. In addition, a persistent suture extending between intraocular and extraocular environments may provide a track for bacteria to enter the eye and establish endophthalmitis.

A choroidal hemorrhage and detachment can occur from inadvertent injury to the ciliary body. The incidence of suprachoroidal hemorrhage is a function of procedure duration and intraoperative manipulation. Factors that increase the risk of hemorrhage include older age, history of hypertension, peripheral vascular disease, glaucoma, aortic stenosis, emphysema, eye surgery (risk increases with more procedures), and a need for excessive intraoperative manipulation (e.g., if concomitant procedures, such as removal of residual lens material, extensive vitrectomy, repair of large iris defects or iridoplasty are needed). Moreover, traction on the peripheral retina or vitreous during suture placement in the sulcus may increase the risk of retinal detachment. Numerous suggestions have been made to improve the accuracy of sulcus penetration, move away from *ab interno* suture techniques and move towards the *ab externo* approach, mirror systems, transillumination and endoscopy.[41]

In conclusion, surgeons should be experienced in their particular scleral fixation technique and receive continual training in all of the techniques. This represents great savings in terms of time, supply costs, and improved patient and surgeon satisfaction in both the short- and long-term.

References

1. Misra A,BurtonRL. Incidence of intraoperative complications during phacoemulsification in vitrectomized and nonvitrectomized eyes: prospective study. *J Cataract Refract Surg* 2005;31:1011-14.
2. Bhagat N, Nissirios N, Potdevin L, Chung J, Lama P, Zarbin MA, et al. Resident-performed phacoemulsification cataract surgery at New Jersey Medical School. *Br J Ophthalmol.* 2007; 91:1315-7.
3. Dick HB, Augustin AJ. Lens implant selection with absence of capsular support. *Curr Opin Ophthalmol.* 2001;12:47-57.
4. Evereklioglu C, Er H, Bekir NA, Borazan M, Zorlu F. Comparison of secondary implantation of flexible open-loop anterior chamber and scleral-fixated posterior chamber intraocular lenses. *J Cataract Refract Surg.* 2003;29:301-8.
5. Kwong YYY, Yuen HKL, Lam RF, Lee VYW, Rao SK, Lam DSC.Comparison of outcomes of primary scleral-fixated versus primary anterior chamber intraocular lens implantation in complicated cataract surgeries. *Ophthalmology.* 2007;114:80-5.
6. Donaldson KE, Gorscak JJ, Budenz DL, Feuer WJ, Benz MS, Forster RK. Anterior chamber and sutured posterior chamber intraocular lenses in eyes with poor capsular support. *J Cataract Refract Surg.* 2005;31:903-9.
7. Vote BJ, Tranos P, Bunce C, Charteris DG, Da Cruz L. Longterm outcome of combined pars plana vitrectomy and scleral fixated sutured posterior chamber intraocular lens implantation. *Am J Ophthalmol.* 2006;141:308-12.
8. Wagoner MD, Cox TA, Ariyasu RG, Jacobs DS, Karp CL. Intraocular lens implantation in the absence of capsular support; a report by the American Academy of Ophthalmology (Ophthalmic Technology Assessment). *Ophthalmology.* 2003; 110:840-59.
9. Epley KD, Shainberg M, Lueder GT, Tychsen L. Pediatric secondary lens implantation in the absence of capsular support. *J AAPOS.* 2001;5:301-6.
10. Hannush SB. Sutured posterior chamber intraocular lenses: Indications and procedure. *Curr Opin Ophthalmol.* 2000;11:233-40.
11. Kwong YYY, Yuen HKL, Lam RF, Lee VYW, Rao SK, Lam DSC. Comparison of outcomes of primary scleral-fixated versus primary anterior chamber intraocular lens implantation in complicated cataract surgeries. *Ophthalmology.* 2007;114:80-5.
12. Holland EJ, Daya SM, Evangelista A, Ketcham JM, Lubniewski AJ, Doughman DJ, Lane SS. Penetrating keratoplasty and transscleral fixation of posterior chamber lens. *Am J Ophthalmol.* 1992;114:182-7.
13. Solomon K, Gussler JR, Gussler C, Van Meter WS. Incidence and management of complications of transsclerally sutured posterior chamber lenses. *J Cataract Refract Surg.* 1993;19:488-93.
14. Uthoff D, Teichmann KD. Secondary implantation of scleralfixated intraocular lenses. *J Cataract Refract Surg.* 1998;24:945-50.
15. Asadi R, Kheirkhah A. Long-term results of scleral fixation of posterior chamber intraocular lenses in children. *Ophthalmology.* 2008;115:67-72.
16. Krause L, Bechrakis NE, Heimann H, Salditt S, Foerster MH. Implantation of scleral fixated sutured posterior chamber lenses: a retrospective analysis of 119 cases. *Int Ophthalmol.* 2009;29:207-12.
17. Heidemann DG, Dunn SP. Transsclerally sutured intraocular lenses in penetrating keratoplasty. *Am J Ophthalmol.* 1992;113:619-25.
18. Johnston RL, Charteris DG, Horgan SE, Cooling RJ. Combined pars plana vitrectomy and sutured posterior chamber implant. Arch Ophthalmol 2000;118:905-10. Available at: http://archopht. ama-assn.org/cgi/reprint/118/7/905.pdf. Accessed March 15, 2011.

19. Heidemann DG, Dunn SP. Visual results and complications of transsclerally sutured intraocular lenses in penetrating keratoplasty. *Ophthalmic Surg.* 1990;21:609-14.
20. Furuta M, Tsukahara S, Tsuchiya T. Pupillary elongation after anterior chamber lens implantation. *J Cataract Refract Surg.* 1986;12:273-5.
21. Pannu JS. A new suturing technique for ciliary sulcus fixation in the absence of posterior capsule. *Ophthalmic Surg.* 1997;19:751-4.
22. Apple DJ, Price FW, Gwin T, et al. Sutured retropupillary posterior chamber intraocular lenses for exchange of secondary implantation. The 12th annual binkhorst lecture, 1988. *Ophthalmology.* 1989;96:1241-7.
23. Lewis JS. Ab externo sulcus fixation. *Ophthalmic Surg.* 1991;22:692-5.
24. Arkin MS, Steinert RF. Sutured posterior chamber intraocular lenses. *Int Ophthalmol Clin.* 1994,34:67-85.
25. Duffrey RJ, Holland EJ, Agapitos PJ, et al. Anatomic study of transsclerally sutured intraocular lens implantation. *Am J Ophthalmol.* 1989;108:300-9.
26. Althaus C, Sundmacher R. Intraoperative intraocular endoscopy in transscleral suture fixation of posterior chamber lenses: consequences for suture technique, implantation procedure, and choice of PCL design. *Refract Corneal Surg.* 1993;9:333-9.
27. Özmen AT, Dogru M, Ertürk H, Özçetin H, Transsclerally fixated intraocular lenses in children. *Ophthalmic Surg Lasers.* 2002;33(5):394-9.
28. Bucci FA Jr, Holland EJ, Lindstrom RL. Corneal autografts for external knots in transsclerally sutured posterior chamber lenses. *Am J Ophthalmol.* 1991;112:353-4.
29. Bashshur Z, Ma'luf R, Najjar D, Noureddin B. Scleral fixation of posterior chamber intraocular lenses using fascia lata to cover the knots. *Ophthalmic Surg Lasers.* 2002;33:445-9.
30. Anand R, Bowman RW. Simplified technique for suturing dislocated posterior chamber intraocular lens to the ciliary sulcus. *Arch Ophthalmol.* 1990;108:1205-6.
31. Holland EJ, Daya SM, Evangelista A, et al. Penetrating keratoplasty and transscleral fixation of posterior chamber lens. *Am J Ophthalmol.* 1992;114: 182-7.
32. Rao SK, Gopal L, Fogla R, et al. Ab externo 4-point scleral fixation. *J Cataract Refract Surg.* 2000;26(1):9-10.
33. Bergren RL. Four-point fixation technique for sutured posterior chamber intraocular lenses. *Arch Ophthalmol.* 1994;112:1485-7.
34. Youn-Seok In, Joon-Hyun K, Byung-Joo S. Transscleral fixation of a dislocated IOL through sclerotomy. *J Cataract Refract Surg.* 2004;30:1163-6.
35. Monteiro M, Marinho A, Borges S, et al. Evaluation of a new IOL scleral fixation technique without capsular support. *J Fr Ophthalmol.* 2006;29(10): 1110-7.
36. Hoffman RS, Fine IH, Packer M. Scleral fixation without conjunctival dissection. *J Cataract Refract Surg.* 2006;32(11):1907-12.
37. Han Q, Chu Y. Combined suture-in-needle and scleral tunnel technique for scleral fixation of intraocular lens. *J Cataract Refract Surg.* 2007;33(8):1362-5.
38. Szurman P, Petermier K. et al. Z-suture: a new knotless technique for transscleral suture fixation of intraocular implants. *Br J Ophthalmol.* 2010; 94(2):167-9
39. Baykara M. Suture burial technique in scleral fixation. *J Cataract Refract Surg.* 2004;30:957-9.
40. Baykara M. Long-term results of a suture burial technique. *Eur J Ophthalmol.* 2008;18(3):368-70.
41. Hannush SB. Sutured posterior chamber intraocular lenses: indications and procedure. *Curr Opin Ophthalmol.* 2000;11(4):233-40.

7

chapter

Pukhraj Rishi
Tarun Sharma
Aditi Gupta

Advances in Retinopathy of Prematurity

ABSTRACT

Retinopathy of prematurity (ROP) is a proliferative retinopathy that develops in premature infants due to incomplete vasculogenesis of the retina at the time of birth. It remains a major cause of visual impairment despite ongoing continuous improvements in neonatal care. Several advances have been made in diagnosis and management of ROP over the past decade; however, many challenges still remain. More-severe ROP (prethreshold ROP and zone I ROP) has become more common in recent years, mainly due to increased survival of infants with very low birth weights and low gestational ages. According to American guidelines, screening is needed for all premature babies below 30-weeks gestational age and/or less than 1500 g at birth. Selected infants with a birth weight of 1500–2000 g or a gestational age of more than 30 weeks with an unstable clinical course, including those requiring cardiorespiratory support and who are believed by pediatrician to be at high risk, should also be screened for ROP. The first evaluation should be done by 31-weeks postconceptional age or by 4-weeks chronological age (whichever is later). In Indian scenario, it is recommended to start screening between 20 and 30 days of life, and that one screening session must be completed before day 30 of life. Screening must be done for babies born before 34-35 weeks of gestational age at birth and/or birth weight of 2000 gm or less. Earlier screening (before day 20 of life) is strongly recommended for babies under 30 weeks, and/or those with birth weight of 1500 gm or less. ROP-telescreening is an emerging aspect of neonatal care. Despite promising results from early treatment of ROP in the ETROP study, recalcitrant cases of ROP that are relatively unresponsive to all treatments still exist. The role for anti-VEGF agents in the management of such difficult cases will need to be evaluated fully. Future research focusing on genetic polymorphism influencing the outcome of ROP may provide useful information about the pathogenesis of the disease. Screening of genetic polymorphisms may also help identify and treat high-risk infants in a timely manner.

Introduction

Retinopathy of prematurity (ROP), previously known as retrolental fibroplasia (RLF) is a proliferative retinopathy that develops in premature infants due to incomplete vasculogenesis of the retina at the time of birth (Fig. 7.1). First described in 1942, it remains a major cause of visual impairment despite ongoing continuous improvements in neonatal care. World Health Organization's "Vision 2020 program"[1] has identified ROP as an important cause of blindness in both high and middle income countries.

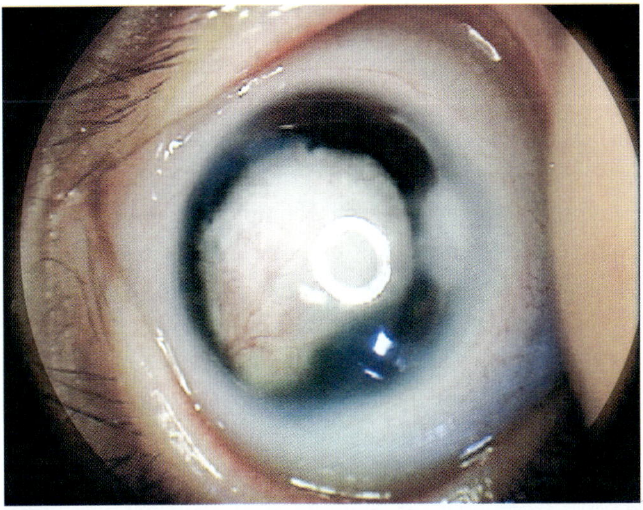

Fig. 7.1: External color photo of an eye showing retrolental fibroplasia—a feature typical of advanced ROP.

Color fundus photograph of the right eye reveals ROP sequelae over the posterior pole. Disk drag, falciform retinal fold involving the macula and macular heterotopia can be made out

Incidence

The overall incidence of ROP is estimated to be about 68% among infants having birth weight less than 1251 g and 98% among those having birth weight less than 750 grams.[2] A report from a national registry of children in USA indicated that ROP was the earliest cause of visual impairment.[2] More-severe ROP (prethreshold ROP and zone I ROP) has become more common in recent years, mainly due to increased survival of infants with very low birth weights and low gestational ages.[3]

Pathogenesis

The retinal vasculature begins in the 14–15th weeks postmenstrual age. The first stage is **vasculogenesis** characterized by *de novo* formation of retinal vessels, growing out of the optic disk into the inner retina as a wave of mesenchymal spindle cells.[4] These spindle cells migrate along the course of future major retinal blood vessels, forming primitive vascular tubes. Tissue-hypoxia-driven vascular development mediated by VEGF is not necessary for this stage. In the second stage of **angiogenesis**, endothelial proliferation, and capillary formation follow from the existing blood vessels. These new capillaries form peripheral parts of inner retinal vasculature, total outer retinal vasculature, and the perifoveal vasculature. VEGF secreted in response to retinal tissue hypoxia is needed to drive this stage of angiogenesis. The choroidal vessels (that are vascularized by the 6th week of gestation) supply the rest of the retina. The nasal portion of the retina is completely vascularized to the ora serrata by the 36th week of gestation. The larger temporal area usually is completed at 40–42 weeks (term).

Retinopathy of prematurity is a biphasic disease consisting of an initial vascular attenuation phase followed by a second fibrovascular proliferative phase.[5-7] Premature babies have incompletely vascularized retinas. Normally in utero, the development of the neural retina occurs anterior to the growing vasculature and the subsequent localized hypoxia stimulates the production of VEGF, drawing the vessels in the anterior hypoxic retina. Premature birth interrupts this normal process of retinal vascularization. First phase of ROP occurs from birth of baby to postmenstrual age approximately 30–32 weeks. It is characterized by retardation of normal retinal vascularization due to physiologically increased tissue oxygen tension postnatally (aggravated by supplemental oxygen). This relatively hyperoxic environment suppresses the VEGF mRNA expression and the normal VEGF-driven vascular growth, and it promotes apoptosis of vascular endothelial cells and vaso-obliteration.[8] VEGF activity in phase 1 is also inhibited by the low levels of IGF-1 that normally exerts a permissive role in VEGF-induced vascularization.[9] The second phase of ROP begins around 32–34 weeks postmenstrual age. As the baby matures, the nonvascularized retina becomes increasingly metabolically active due to continued programmed development of retinal neural cells, leading to tissue hypoxia. Hypoxia stimulates upregulation of proangiogenic growth, factors, such as VEGF and erythropoietin. This overproduction of VEGF, at a determined postmenstrual age (30–32 weeks) when IGF-1 increases and reaches normal levels, induces an uncontrolled neovascularization. In severe cases, this can lead to uncontrolled vascular growth into the vitreous that may lead

BOX 7.1: VASCULOGENESIS AND ANGIOGENESIS

Vasculogenesis: *De novo* formation of retinal vessels, growing out of the optic disk into the inner retina as a wave of mesenchymal spindle cells along the course of future major retinal blood vessels. VEGF plays no role.

Angiogenesis: Endothelial proliferation and capillary formation following from the existing blood vessels. Driven by VEGF secreted in response to tissue hypoxia.

to retinal detachment. The important role played by VEGF in this second phase of ROP, is the reason behind positive effects of anti-VEGF drugs in controlling neovascularization in ROP. Both the phases are summarized in Box 7.1.

The most important question that still remains unanswered regarding the pathogenesis of ROP is why it progresses in some premature infants despite timely and aggressive intervention, whereas it spontaneously regresses in other infants with similar clinical characteristics. Many causal risk factors have been proposed, to explain the same. Current research is focused upon identifying the genetic susceptibility of ROP. Based on a retrospective analysis in monozygotic and dizygotic twins, a 70% variance in the susceptibility of ROP was found to be from genetic factors.[10]

Risk Factors

Prematurity is the main causal factor for ROP. The birth weight, though also correlated to gestational age, is an independent risk factor for developing ROP.[11] Another important cause for ROP is the excessive retinal oxygenation.[12] STOP-ROP (Supplemental Therapeutic Oxygen for Prethreshold Retinopathy Of Prematurity) study was conducted to determine the efficacy and safety of supplemental oxygen administered to premature infants to reduce the progression to threshold ROP.[13] It was found that no benefit was achieved by keeping the oxygen saturation above 95%. However, higher oxygen saturation levels were not found to worsen the disease in prethreshold babies. Controlled oxygen supplementation, with lower oxygen targets at early gestational age and higher oxygen targets at older gestational age decreases the severity and incidence of ROP while inducing normal retinal development.[14]

Other reported risk factors for ROP are those associated with prematurity and low birth weight: hyperglycemia, frequent blood transfusions, bacterial and fungal late-onset sepsis, and light exposure. The Light-ROP study evaluated the role of light in stimulating the development of ROP. Patients were either exposed to normal light conditions in the nursery or shielded from ambient light conditions. There was no difference in the number of patients developing ROP in either group. Recently, the role of the ethnic and/or genetic predisposition to ROP is being studied in detail.[15] The incidence of ROP is noted to be more frequent in whites and in male gender. Genetic polymorphism altering the function of gene regulating VEGF has been proposed in the pathogenesis of ROP.[16]

The risk factors for ROP are enumerated in Box 7.2.

BOX 7.2: RISK FACTORS FOR ROP

- Prematurity
- Low birth weight
- Excessive retinal oxygenation
- Concurrent illnesses
- Anemia
- Hyperglycemia
- Frequent blood transfusions
- Bacterial and fungal late-onset sepsis
- Mechanical ventilation
- Seizures
- Apnea
- Bradycardia
- Intraventricular hemorrhage
- Light exposure
- Ethnic and/or genetic predisposition

Pathology

Histologically, stage I ROP is characterized by hyperplasia of the primitive spindle cells of the vanguard mesenchymal tissue at the demarcation line.[17] The ridge of stage II consists of further hyperplasia of the spindle cells, along with proliferation of the endothelial cells of the rear guard mesenchymal tissue. In stage III, extraretinal neovascular tissue emanates from the ridge, characterized by proliferation of endothelial cells and small, thin-walled vessels. There is condensation of vitreous into sheets and strands oriented anteriorly toward the equator of the lens. Such tractional forces of the vitreous draw the retina anteriorly (Fig. 7.2) and may lead to retinal detachment in stage 4 (Figs 7.3 and 7.4) and stage 5.

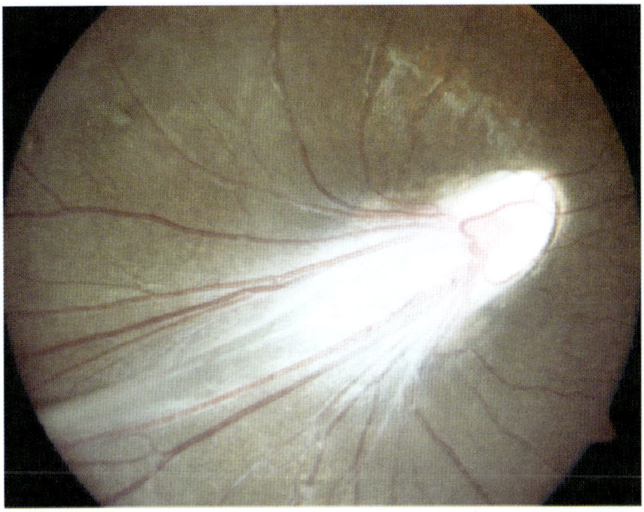

Fig. 7.2: Color fundus photograph of the right eye reveals ROP sequelae over the posterior pole. Disk drag, falciform retinal fold involving the macula and macular heterotopia can be made out.

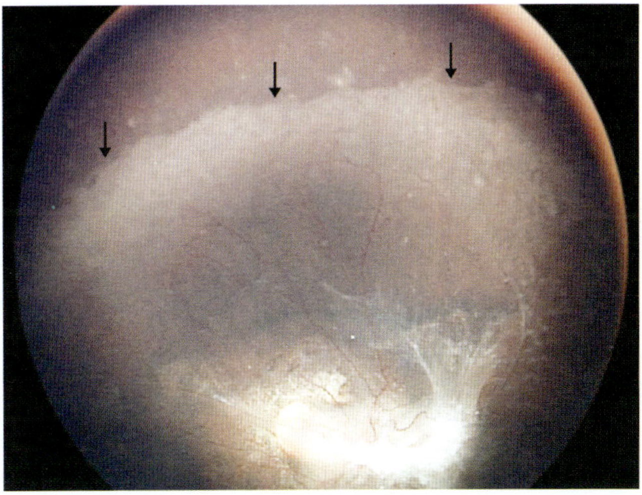

Fig. 7.3: Color fundus (Retcam) photo showing tractional retinal detachment involving the macula. Note the distinct demarcation between the vascular and avascular retina (arrows).

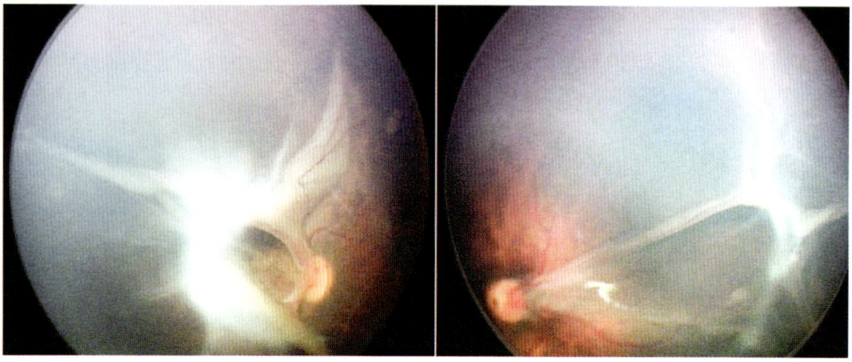

Fig. 7.4: Color fundus (Retcam) photo showing tractional retinal detachment—ROP stage 4b.

Classification

The prevalent classification for ROP is International Classification of Retinopathy of Prematurity Revisited. The International Classification of Retinopathy of Prematurity (ICROP) published the consensus classification in 2 parts, the first in 1984 and later expanded in 1987. It included zone, stage, and the presence or absence of plus disease.[18] Zone refers to the location of disease, stage refers to severity, and the extent is described by clock hours. Each zone is centered on the optic disk rather than the macula, in contrast to standard retinal drawings. Zone I is a circle with optic nerve as its center point and radius equal to twice the disk-fovea distance. Zone II extends centrifugally from the edge of Zone I to the nasal ora serrata. Zone III is the temporal crescent remnant. Figure 7.5 depicts the zones I–III. Box 7.3 provides the definitions of ROP in corresponding zones. Regarding the staging, immature blood vessels ending without any demarcation are classified as no ROP or stage 0. Stage 1 consists of a flat demarcation line between vascular and avascular retina.

BOX 7.3: ICROP DEFINITION OF LOCATION AND SEVERITY OF ROP

Zone I ROP: When ≥1 clock hour (sector) of ROP is seen within zone I.

Zone II ROP: When retinal vessel maturation has not occurred to within 1 disk diameter of the nasal ora serrata in nasal most 2 contiguous clock hours (sectors) and ≥1 clock hour of ROP is seen within zone II, with no ROP in zone I.

Zone III ROP: When retinal vessel maturation has occurred to within 1 disk diameter of the nasal ora serrata in those 2 contiguous clock hours (sectors) and ≥1 clock hour of ROP is present elsewhere in the eye.

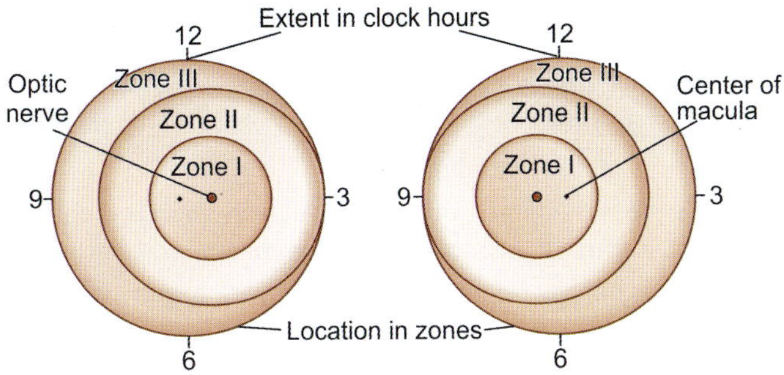

Fig. 7.5: Schematic diagram showing classification of ROP based on location and extent of disease. Severity of disease is another important criteria to be factored-in while assessing the disease.

Stage 2 is an elevated ridge. Stage 3 is extraretinal neovascular tissue along the ridge extending into the vitreous. Stage 4A refers to a partial retinal detachment not involving the fovea, and stage 4B is a partial retinal detachment involving the fovea. Stage 5 is a total retinal detachment, that can again be classified into subtypes according to the configuration of the funnel of retinal detachment.

The Committee to Revisit ICROP in 2005 provided three major additions to ICROP—aggressive posterior ROP (AP-ROP), preplus disease, and a clinical pearl for clarification of the extent of zone I.[19] AP-ROP is ill defined ROP with plus disease in zone I or sometimes posterior zone II. Stage 3 of AP-ROP is often intraretinal and can be deceptively featureless. AP-ROP may not pass through the typical stages of disease and progresses rapidly to stage 4 or 5. AP-ROP may appear as only a flat network of neovascularization at the deceptively featureless junction between vascularized and nonvascularized retina and may be easily overlooked by a less experienced observer. It is observed in the smallest premature infants, and requires prompt laser treatment. Such aggressive disease was previously called as 'Rush disease'. The salient features of AP-ROP are enumerated in Box 7.4.

Preplus disease refers to an intermediate level of plus disease between normal and plus disease.[20] Preplus disease is defined as vascular abnormalities of the posterior pole, consisting of more arterial tortuosity and more venous dilatation than normal that are insufficient for the diagnosis of plus disease. Signs of preplus disease early in the course of ROP have been shown to be strongly associated with development of severe ROP that require laser treatment. The diagnosis of preplus disease, thus, has prognostic value.[21] Whereas, conventional 'plus disease' refers only to eyes with at

BOX 7.4: CHARACTERISTICS OF AGGRESSIVE POSTERIOR ROP (AP-ROP)

- Posterior location (zone 1 or sometimes, posterior zone II)
- Prominent plus disease
- Ill-defined nature of the retinopathy
- Posterior pole vessels show increased dilation and tortuosity in all 4 quadrants that is out of proportion to the peripheral retinopathy
- Shunting occurs from vessel to vessel within retina and not solely at the junction between vascular and avascular retina
- Usually, it does not progress through the classic stages 1 to 3
- Typically extends circumferentially and is often accompanied by a circumferential vessel
- Performing indirect ophthalmoscopy with a 20 D condensing lens instead of a 25 or 28 D lens may help distinguish the deceptively featureless neovascularization of AP-ROP.

least two quadrants of dilation as well as tortuosity meeting or exceeding that in the standard photograph of plus disease.[22] Other signs of plus disease include iris vascular engorgement, pupillary rigidity, and vitreous haze. Plus disease occurs when the peripheral vascular shunting of blood is so overwhelming that it results in marked venous dilation and arterial tortuosity in the posterior pole. Plus disease is the hallmark of rapidly progressive ROP and is notated by adding a plus sign after the number of the ROP stage.

Finally, the Committee to Revisit ICROP provided the clarification of the extent of zone I. When a 25 or 28 D indirect ophthalmoscopy condensing lens is used to view the posterior pole, zone 1 is the area viewed by placing the nasal edge of the optic nerve at one edge of the field of view. Thus, if any ROP is evident in the entire field of view of that lens, the ROP must be in zone I. Two other terms associated with ROP include 'popcorn lesions' and 'hot dog'. 'Popcorn lesions' refer to small isolated tufts of neovascular tissue lying on the surface of the retina, and may be seen posterior to the ridge. Such lesions do not constitute the degree of fibrovascular growth that is a necessary condition for stage 3. They usually regress completely over several weeks. 'Hot dog' refers to a red hot active ridge, probably the site of increasing vascular channels. If noted on zone 1 or 2, it has a poor prognostic sign. This area may regress with cicatrix floating in the vitreous cavity and nonpatent ghost vessels still visibly attached to the retina (a second ridge would clearly be identified anterior to this cicatrix). In less fortunate eyes, this area may be the site of a true retinal detachment (no advancing ridge would be visible and the vessels would not be ghostly but engorged).

Screening Guidelines

ROP screening is done via a dilated examination by indirect ophthalmoscopy using 20 D or 28 D condensing lens with scleral depression. In a joint statement from the American Academy of Pediatrics, American Academy of Ophthalmology, and American Associations for Pediatric Ophthalmology and Strabismus,[3] screening guidelines were recommended based on the results of CRYO-ROP and ETROP. According to American guidelines, screening is needed for all premature babies below 30-weeks gestational age and/or less than 1500 g at birth. Selected infants with a birth weight of 1500-2000 g or a gestational age of more than 30 weeks with an unstable clinical course, including those requiring cardiorespiratory support and who are believed by pediatrician to be at high risk, should also be screened for ROP.[23] The first evaluation should be done by 31-weeks postconceptional age or by 4-weeks chronological age (whichever is later). Examinations thereafter should be performed on a 1 week, 2-week, or 3-week basis (depending on findings) until there is evidence of vascularization into zone III without any previous zone I or II disease, full retinal vascularization, postmenstrual age of 45 weeks with no prethreshold ROP or complete regression of treated ROP. In most cases, at least two examinations should be carried. One examination may be sufficient if it is shown unequivocally that retinal vascularization is complete bilaterally.

The British Association for Perinatal Medicine and the College of Ophthalmologists recommend screening all infants <1,500 g at birth.[24] However, these Western guidelines may not be suitable for developing countries like India.[25] In a series from south India, 26.1% of infants with threshold ROP were found to have a birth weight of >l,500 g, and that there was one infant with 1,950 g birth weight that developed threshold disease.[26] It was suggested that developing countries likely need to modify western screening guidelines and in India, there may be need for routine screening of premature infants with a birth weight of up to 2000 g.[26] Further, Jalali et al recently defined ROP screening criteria for India.[27] They recommended to start screening between 20 and 30 days of life, and that one screening session must be completed before day 30 of life. Screening must be done for babies born before 34–35 weeks of gestational age at birth and/or birth weight of 2000 g or less. Earlier screening (before day 20 of life) is strongly recommended for babies under 30 weeks, and/or those with birth weight of 1500 g or less.

Differential Diagnosis

Stage 5 of ROP can present like a white retrolental fibrous mass, causing leukocoria. At this stage, it is important to exclude other causes of leukocoria in infants. The causes of leukocoria in an infant include retinoblastoma, cataract, Coats' disease (usually unilateral and more common in boys) or diffuse choroidal hemangioma, persistent fetal vasculature syndrome, formerly called persistence of primary hyperplastic vitreous (usually unilateral and associated with microphthalmia and prominent ciliary processes); chronic vitreous hemorrhage, infectious causes, such as endogenous endophthalmitis and toxocariasis, Norrie's disease, incontinentia pigmenti, retinochoroidal coloboma, and congenital retinoschisis (Box 7.5). Spotaneously regressed ROP and ROP sequelae should be differentiated from familial exudative vitreoretinopathy (FEVR). The differential diagnoses for ROP are enumerated in Box 7.5.

BOX 7.5: DIFFERENTIAL DIAGNOSIS OF LEUKOCORIA

- Retinoblastoma
- Cataract
- Coats' disease
- Persistent fetal vasculature syndrome (persistent hyperplastic primary vitreous)
- Chronic vitreous hemorrhage
- Toxocariasis
- Endogenous endophthalmitis
- Norrie's disease
- Incontinentia pigmenti
- Retinochoroidal coloboma
- Congenital retinoschisis

Management

Treatment guidelines of ROP are summarized in Table 7.1.

CRYO-ROP study recommended treatment for threshold ROP, defined as 5 contiguous or 8 cumulative clock hours of stage 3 ROP in zone I or II in the presence of "plus" disease. Of threshold eyes left untreated, 50% developed adverse structural outcomes (e.g. retinal detachment) 12 months after randomization.[22]

The ETROP study tested the hypothesis that earlier treatment of high-risk infants would result in a better visual outcome than conventional treatment at threshold.[28,29] Prethreshold ROP is divided into highrisk or type 1 and lowrisk or type 2, based on eyes that have a risk of 15% or more of

TABLE 7.1: Management algorithm for ROP

		Zone 1	Zone 2	Zone 3
Stage 1	Plus	Retinal ablation	Close observation	Observation*
	No Plus	Close observation	Observation	Observation
Stage 2	Plus	Retinal ablation	Seriously consider retinal ablation	Observation
	No Plus	Close observation**	Observation	Observation
Stage 3	Plus	Retinal ablation†	Retinal ablation	Observation
	No Plus	Retinal ablation	Close observation	Observation
Stage 4 and Stage 5 ROP need surgery				

These are approximate guidelines. Exact management may differ according to clinical judgment of treating ophthalmologist
*Observation refers to 2 weekly follow-up
**Close observation refers to 1 weekly follow-up
†Retinal ablation is done to avascular retina with or without involving the ridge

BOX 7.6: DEFINITION OF THRESHOLD (DEFINED BY CRYO-ROP STUDY) AND PRETHRESHOLD ROP (DEFINED BY ETROP STUDY)

Threshold ROP:

Zone I or II, 5 contiguous or 8 composite hours of stage 3 ROP, with plus disease

Prethreshold ROP:

Type 1/ high risk

1. Zone I ROP, any stage with plus disease,
2. Zone I ROP, Stage III without plus disease, and
3. Zone II ROP, Stage II or III with plus disease

Type 2/ Low risk

1. zone I, stage 1 or 2 without plus disease
2. zone II, stage 3 without plus disease

adverse outcomes in the ETROP study. Revised treatment guidelines based on results of ETROP are that 'type 1' ROP should be treated promptly within 72 hours of diagnosis. These eyes include:

1. Zone I ROP, any stage with plus disease.
2. Zone I ROP, stage III without plus disease, and
3. Zone II ROP, stage II or III with plus disease.

These new guidelines effectively include all babies with threshold ROP defined in the original CRYO-ROP study.[22] The number of clock hours of disease is no longer the determining factor in recommending ablative treatment.

Box 7.6 summarizes the features of threshold and prethreshold disease. It is also recommended that 'type 2' ROP should be observed closely. These eyes include:

1. Zone I, stage 1 or 2 without plus disease
2. Zone II, stage 3 without plus disease.[29]

Several studies have been conducted on ROP, important ones are listed in Box 7.7

BOX 7.7: CLINICAL STUDIES ON ROP

- CRYO-ROP: Cryotherapy for Retinopathy of Prematurity Study
- ETROP: Early Treatment for Retinopathy of Prematurity Study
- STOP-ROP: Supplemental Oxygen for the Treatment of Prethreshold Retinopathy of Prematurity Trial
- PHOTO-ROP: Photographic Screening for Retinopathy of Prematurity Study
- LIGHT-ROP: Effects of Light Reduction on Retinopathy of Prematurity Study
- BEAT-ROP: Bevacizumab Eliminates the Angiogenic Threat of Retinopathy of Prematurity Study
- HOPE: High Oxygen Percentage in Retinopathy of Prematurity Study
- MIC: Microplasmin in children (for stage 4 ROP)

Treatment Modality

Conventional treatment for acute phase ROP has evolved from cryotherapy in the 1980s to the current gold standard LASER therapy beginning in the 1990s (Fig. 7.6). Cryotherapy can be performed either transsclerally (for posterior disease) or transconjunctivally after topical, local or general anesthesia. It involves ocular complications like intraocular hemorrhage, conjunctival hematoma, conjunctival laceration, and systemic side effects like bradycardia.

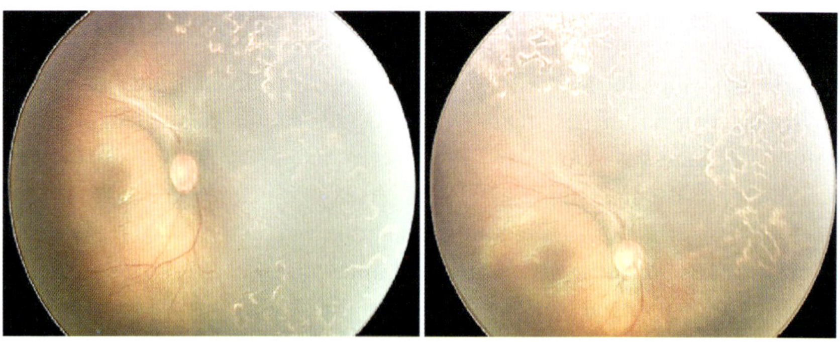

Fig. 7.6: Color fundus (Retcam) photos showing laser photocoagulation scars in fundii with regressed ROP.

Currently, laser photocoagulation is the standard of care for ROP. Cryotherapy is no longer preferred for routine avascular retinal ablation in premature babies, due to the various side effects. Few indications of cryotherapy over laser treatment include poor fundus visibility and lack of availability of laser. The side effects of laser are significantly less than cryotherapy, the ocular tissues are less traumatized, posterior zone 1 disease is easily treated, and general anesthesia is not necessary. The aim of treatment is near-confluent ablation of avascular retina, with burns spaced one-half burn width apart, from the ora serrata up to the ridge for 360 degrees. Signs of regression of ROP are listed in Box 7.8. Complications of laser include corneal haze, burns of the iris, cataracts, and burns of tunica vasculosa lentis causing intraocular hemorrhages. During subsequent examinations, laser is done to the skip areas, if any. Persistent plus disease or fibrovascular proliferation is other indication for additional treatment.

BOX 7.8: SIGNS OF REGRESSION OF ROP AFTER RETINAL ABLATION

- Lack of increase in severity/ lack of progression to next stage
- Regression of all signs of plus disease including return of vessels to normal caliber and resolution of vessel tortuosity
- Change in color in the ridge from salmon pink to white
- Transgression of vessels through the demarcation line
- Commencement of the process of replacement of active ROP lesions by scar tissue
- Improvement in media clarity
- Improvement in pupillary dilatation
- Clearing of retinal and preretinal hemorrhages.

Advancement of ROP after retinal ablation may need further treatment. Signs are:

1. Focal areas of active neovascularization.
2. Persistent plus disease.
3. Lack of regression.

Scleral buckling surgery and/or lens sparing vitrectomy are the treatment options for eyes that have progressed to Stage 4 despite adequate laser photocoagulation. Stage 4 ROP was earlier managed with scleral buckling; however, this procedure had certain limitations. It did not restore normal retinal anatomy and was unsuitable for cases with very posterior disease, though it was satisfactory for relieving peripheral traction. Although the lens is spared during scleral buckling procedure, anisometropia can still occur and be a cause of amblyopia. Lens-sparing vitrectomy is more capable of relieving the posterior traction and the results have been satisfactory for selected cases of stage 4 ROP (Figs 7.7 and 7.8).[30]

The surgical management of stage 5 ROP has been unsatisfactory. Lens-sacrificing vitrectomy is the standard approach to manage stage 5 ROP. However, the surgical risk is high and outcomes of stage 5 eyes remain poor despite surgical intervention.

Antivascular endothelial growth factor (VEGF) therapy is currently being tried with success in ROP. Bevacizumab is an anti-VEGF monoclonal antibody. Bevacizumab Eliminates the Angiogenic Threat of Retinopathy of Prematurity (BEAT-ROP) study is currently underway to determine the efficacy of intravitreal bevacizumab in the treatment of ROP compared to a control group receiving conventional laser therapy, in neonates with acute stage 3 ROP in zone I or posterior zone II with plus disease.[31] Other studies have also reported bevacizumab to be beneficial for ROP.[32,33]

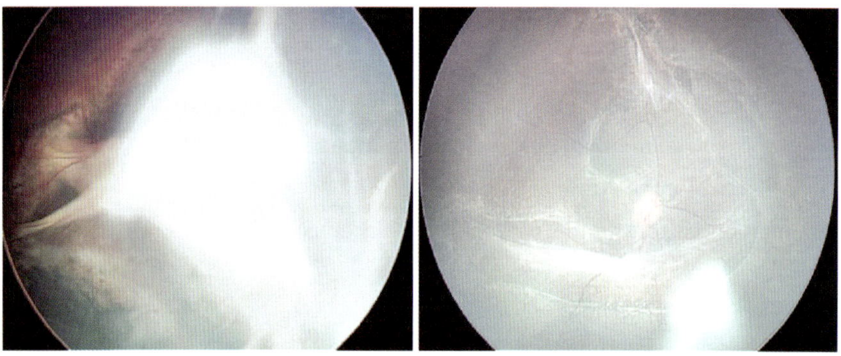

Fig. 7.7: Color fundus (RetCam) photos showing stage 4b ROP, before (left) and after (right) surgery. Note the attached posterior pole despite the distorted pathoanatomy.

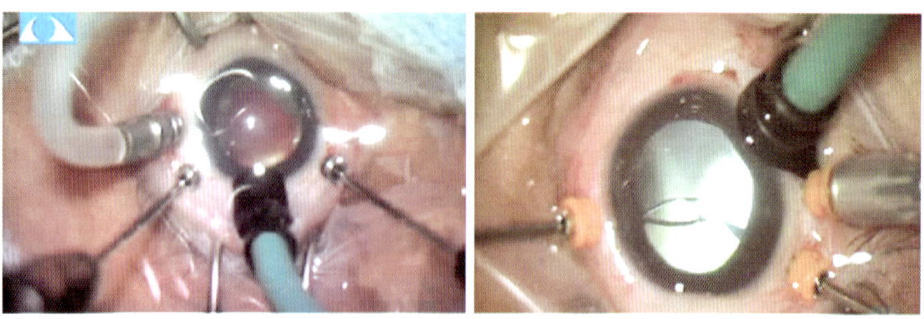

Fig. 7.8: 25 G Chandelier illumination (green cable) through 4th port gives excellent illumination to facilitate true bimanual dissection in these technically challenging eyes.

Recombinant human erythropoietin (rhEPO) has also been tried as treatment for ROP. However, no significant difference has been noted between the administration of rhEPO and the incidence and severity of ROP.[34] Presently, the data are inconclusive regarding role of rhEPO in ROP and its further clinical utility is yet to be determined.

Consequences

There are potentially visually significant consequences to ROP that require lifetime follow-up in these babies. Such complications, though more prevalent in babies who have been treated, can still occur in those who had less severe stages of ROP. Patients with ROP are at greater risk for refractive errors, strabismus, glaucoma, cataracts and retinal detachment later in life. Approximately 70% of infants with significant ROP became myopic in the first year of life. Eyes with macular heterotopia (temporal macular drag) and straightened blood vessels show increased prevalence of myopia and high myopia.[35] Myopia in adults who were born full-term is typically axial, due to an increase in axial length. Myopia in adult eyes of previously premature infants with a history of ROP is found to be because of higher corneal curvatures rather than axial myopia.[36] Astigmatism greater than 2 diopters, well within the amblyogenic range if uncorrected is present in up to 20% of eyes with a history of significant ROP at 3 years of age.[37] The incidence of strabismus in infants with a history of ROP ranges up to 20.3%. It has been reported that many infants with strabismus at 6 months no longer had strabismus 3 months later. Hence, conservative management of strabismus in infants with a history of ROP is clinically indicated.[38] Retinal detachment is found in 25.6%, and cataract in 83.7%. Other complications include decreased visual acuity, retinal pigmentary changes, thin areas in the periphery, macular heterotopia, macular dragging, and retinal tears,[39] glaucoma (angle closure, open-angle, and neovascular[40] and exudative retinopathy.[41]

Advances

IMAGING

The development of contact wide-field digital retinal imaging (RetCam) has proved very useful for documentation and follow-up of the babies having ROP.

COMPUTER-ASSISTED QUANTIFICATION OF PLUS DISEASE

Much progress has been made in last few years in automated assessment of plus disease. The assessment of plus disease is hampered by subjectivity. The diagnosis of plus disease is based on comparison with the standard photograph that was first used for the CRYO-ROP study.[22] Hence, there is large interobserver variation in the diagnosis of plus disease since different examiners interpret this photograph in different ways. Freedman et al found that three principal investigators in the CRYO-ROP study disagreed on the presence of plus disease in 40% images.[42] Chiang found that out of 22 experts, all agreed on the presence or absence of plus disease in only 12% of images.[43]

A computer program, called 'ROPtool,' has been developed to automatically trace retinal blood vessels and measure their tortuosity.[44] It expresses tortuosity as 'tortuosity index,' and a tortuosity index greater than 10 has more tortuosity than the average of all vessels in the standard photograph of plus disease.

TELESCREENING

Several studies have shown that remote screening for ROP is feasible.[45-47] Telescreening for ROP can play an important role, especially in areas with limited access to ophthalmic care. Studies have shown that single-image and multiple-image telemedicine examinations perform comparably in the determination of a recommended follow-up interval and in the detection of plus disease.[48]

Conclusion

Several advances have been made in diagnosis and management of ROP over the past decade; however, many challenges still remain. Despite promising results from early treatment of ROP in the ETROP study, recalcitrant cases of ROP that are relatively unresponsive to all treatments still exist. The role for anti-VEGF agents in the management of such difficult cases will need to be evaluated fully.[49] It is also unknown whether curtailing supplemental oxygen will have a beneficial effect on ROP without causing other morbidities.[50,51] Future research focusing on genetic polymorphism influencing the outcome of ROP may provide useful information about the pathogenesis of the disease. Screening of genetic polymorphisms may also help identify and treat high risk infants in a timely manner.[15,16]

References

1. Gilbert C, Foster A. Childhood blindness in the context of Vision 2020—the right to sight. *Bull World Health Organ.* 2001;79:227-32.
2. Hatton DD, Schwietz E, Boyer B, et al. Babies count: the national registry for children with visual impairments, birth to 3 years. *J Am Assoc Pediatr Ophthalmol. Strabismus* 2007;11:351-5.
3. Good WV, Hardy RJ, Dobson V, Palmer EA, Phelps DL, Quintos M, Tung B; Early Treatment for Retinopathy of Prematurity Cooperative Group. The incidence and course of retinopathy of prematurity: findings from the early treatment for retinopathy of prematurity study. *Pediatrics.* 2005;116(1):15-23.
4. Hughes S, Yang H, Chan-Ling T. Vascularisation of the human fetal retina: roles of vasculogenesis and angiogenesis. *Invest Ophthalmol Vis Sci.* 2000;41: 1217-28.
5. Shastry BS. Genetic susceptibility to advanced retinopathy of prematurity (ROP). *J Biomed Sci.* 2010;17:69.
6. Chen J, Stahl A, Hellstrom A, Smith LE. Current update on retinopathy of prematurity: screening and treatment. *Curr Opin Pediatr.* 2011;23(2):173-8.
7. Smith LEH. Pathogenesis of retinopathy of prematurity. *Semin Neonatol.* 2003;8:469-73.
8. Fleck BW, McIntosh N. Pathogenesis of retinopathy of prematurity and possible preventive strategies. *Early Hum Dev.* 2008;84(2):83-8.
9. Romagnoli C. Risk factors and growth factors in ROP. *Early Hum Dev.* 2009,85(10 Suppl):S79-82. Epub 2009 Oct 14.
10. Bizzarro MJ, Hussain N, Jonsson B, et al: Genetic susceptibility to retinopathy of prematurity. *Pediatrics.* 2006; 118:1858-1863.
11. Darlow BA, Hutchinson JL, Henderson-Smart DJ, Donohue DA, Simpson JM, Evans NJ. Prenatal risk factors for severe retinopathy of prematurity among very preterm infants of the Australian and New Zealand Neonatal Network. *Pediatrics.* 2005;115:990-6.
12. Flynn JT, Bancalari E, Snyder ES, Goldberg RN, Feuer W, Cassady J, et al. A cohort study of transcutaneous oxygen tension and the incidence and severity of retinopathy of prematurity. *N Engl J Med.* 1992;326:1050-4.
13. The STOP-ROP Multicenter Study Group. Supplemental therapeutic oxygen for prethreshold retinopathy of prematurity (STOP-ROP), a randomized, controlled trial. I: Primary outcomes. *Pediatrics.* 2000;105:295-310.
14. Sears JE, Pietz J, Sonnie C, Dolcini D, Hoppe G. A change in oxygen supplementation can decrease the incidence of retinopathy of prematurity. *Ophthalmology.* 2009;116(3):513-8.
15. Holmström G, van Wijngaarden P, Coster DJ, Williams KA. Genetic susceptibility to retinopathy of prematurity: the evidence from clinical and experimental animal studies. *Br J Ophthalmol.* 2007;91(12):1704-8.
16. Shastry BS. Genetic susceptibility to advanced retinopathy of prematurity (ROP). *J Biomed Sci.* 2010;25;17:69.
17. Foos RY. Pathologic features of clinical stages of retinopathy of prematurity. In: Flynn JT, Tasman WS, eds. Retinopathy of prematurity. New York: Springer-Verlag; 1992:23-36.
18. The Committee for the Classification of Retinopathy of Prematurity. An international classification of retinopathy of prematurity. Arch Ophthalmol. 1984; 102:1130-34.

19. An International Committee for the Classification of Retinopathy of Prematurity. The International Classification of Retinopathy of Prematurity Revisited. *Arch Ophthalmol.* 2005;123:991-9.
20. Wallace DK, Kylstra JA, Chesnutt DA, Prognostic significance of vascular dilation and tortuosity insufficient for plus disease in retinopathy of prematurity. *J AAPOS.* 2000;4:224-9.
21. Wallace DK, Freedman SF, Hartnett ME, Quinn GE. Predictive Value of Pre-plus Disease in Retinopathy of Prematurity. *Arch Ophthalmol.* 2011;129(5):591-6
22. Cryotherapy for Retinopathy of Prematurity Cooperative Group. Multicenter trial of cryotherapy for retinopathy of prematurity: Preliminary results. Arch Ophthalmol. 1988;106:471-9.
23. Section on Ophthalmology, American Academy of Pediatrics, American Academy of Ophthalmology, American Association for Pediatric Ophthalmology and Strabismus. Screening Examination of Premature Infants for Retinopathy of Prematurity. *Pediatrics.* 2006:117;572-6.
24. Retinopathy of prematurity: Guidelines for screening and treatment. The report of a Joint Working Party of The Royal College of Ophthalmologists and the British Association of Perinatal Medicine. *Early Hum Dev.* 1996;46:239-58.
25. Gharaibeh A, Khassawneh M, Khriesat W, Alkhatib S, Migdadi Y. Adopting Western Retinopathy of Prematurity Screening Programs in Eastern Countries, are we Screening Properly? *Middle East Afr J Ophthalmol.* 2011;18(3):209-13.
26. Deshpande DA, Chaturvedi M, Gopal L, Ramachandran S, Shanmugasundaram R. Treatment of threshold retinopathy of prematurity. *Indian J Ophthalmol.* 1998;46(1):15-9.
27. Jalali S, Azad R, Trehan HS, Dogra MR, Gopal L, Narendran V. Technical aspects of laser treatment for acute retinopathy of prematurity under topical anesthesia. *Indian J Ophthalmol.* 2010;58(6):509-15.
28. Good WV, Hardy RJ, ETROP Multicenter Study Group. The multicenter study of early treatment for retinopathy of prematurity (ETROP) *Ophthalmology.* 2001;108:1013-14.
29. Early Treatment for Retinopathy of Prematurity Cooperative Group. Revised indications for the treatment of retinopathy of prematurity: Results of the early treatment of retinopathy of prematurity randomized trial. *Arch Ophthalmol.* 2003;121: 1684-94.
30. Bhende P, Gopal L, Sharma T, Verma A, Biswas RK. Functional and anatomical outcomes after primary lens-sparing pars plana vitrectomy for Stage 4 retinopathy of prematurity. *Indian J Ophthalmol.* 2009;57(4):267-71.
31. Mintz-Hittner H. BEAT-ROP study. http://www.clinicaltrials.gov. [Accessed 19 March 2010].
32. Wu WC, Yeh PT, Chen SN, Yang CM, Lai CC, Kuo HK. Effects and complications of bevacizumab use in patients with retinopathy of prematurity: a multicenter study in taiwan. *Ophthalmology.* 2011;118(1):176-83.
33. Mintz-Hittner HA, Kennedy KA, Chuang AZ. Efficacy of intravitreal bevacizumab for stage 3+ retinopathy of prematurity. *N Engl J Med.* 2011;364(7):603-15.
34. Shah N, Jadav P, et al. The effect of recombinant human erythropoietin on the development of retinopathy of prematurity. *Am J Perinatol.* 2010; 27:67-71.

35. Quinn GE, Dobson V, Davitt BV, et al. Progression of myopia and high myopia in early treatment for retinopathy of prematurity study: findings to 3 years of age. *Ophthalmology*. 2008; 115:1058-1064.
36. Baker PS, Tasman W. Myopia in adults with retinopathy of prematurity. *Am J Ophthalmol*. 2008; 145:1090-1094.
37. Davitt BV, Dobson V, Quinn GE, et al. Astigmatism in the early treatment for retinopathy of prematurity study. *Ophthalmology*. 2009; 116:332-339.
38. Vanderveen DK, Coats DK, Dobson V, et al. Prevalence and course of strabismus in the first year of life for infants with prethreshold retinopathy of prematurity. *Arch Ophthalmol*. 2006;124:766-773.
39. Kaiser RS, Trese MT, Williams GA, Cox Jr. MS. Adult retinopathy of prematurity. Outcomes of rhegmatogenous retinal detachments and retinal tears. *Ophthalmology*. 2001; 108:1647-1653.
40. Gallo J.E., Holmstrom G., Kugelberg U et al. Regressed retinopathy of prematurity and its sequelae in children aged 5-10 years. *Br J Ophthalmol*. 1991;75:527-531.
41. Brown MM, Brown GC, Duker JS, et al. Exudative retinopathy of adults: a late sequela of retinopathy of prematurity. *Int Ophthalmol*. 1994; 95(18):281-285.
42. Freedman SF, Kylstra JA, Hall JG, Capowski JJ, Plus disease in retinopathy of prematurity - photographic evaluation by an expert panel (abstract). *Invest Ophthalmol Vis Sci*. 1995;36: 76.
43. Chiang MF, Jiang L, Gelman R, et al. Interexpert agreement of plus disease diagnosis in retinopathy of prematurity. *Arch Ophthalmol*. 2007;125:875-80.
44. Wallace DK, Zhao Z, Freedman SF. A pilot study using 'ROPtool' to quantify plus disease in retinopathy of prematurity, J AAPOS, 2007;11:381-7.
45. Ells AL, Holmes JM, Astle WF, Williams G, et al. Telemedicine approach to screening for severe retinopathy of prematurity: a pilot study. *Ophthalmology*, 2003; 110:2113-17.
46. Schwartz SD, Harrison SA, Ferrone PJ, Trese MT, Telemedical of Prematurity Planning Study Group. Resolving our uncertainty about oxygen therapy. *Pediatrics*. 2003;112:1415-19.
47. Chiang MF, Keenan JD, Starren J, et al. Accuracy and reliability of remote retinopathy of prematurity diagnosis, *Arch Ophthalmol*. 2006;124:322-7.
48. Lajoie A, Koreen S, Wang L, et al. Retinopathy of prematurity management using single-image vs multiple-image telemedicine examinations. *Am J Ophthalmol*. 2008;146(2):298-309.
49. Lutty GA, Chan-Ling T, Phelps DL, et al. Proceedings of the Third International Symposium on Retinopathy of Prematurity: an update on ROP from the lab to the nursery. *Mol Vis*. 2006;12:532-80.
50. Cole CH, Wright KW, Tarnow-Mordi W, Phelps DL, Pulse Oximetry Saturation Trial for prevention of Retinopathy of Prematurity Planning Study Group, Resolving our uncertainty about oxygen therapy. *Pediatrics*. 2003;112:1415-19.
51. Wallace DK, Oxygen Saturations and Retinopathy of Prematurity - Are We On Target? *J AAPOS*. 2006;10:382-3.
52. Flynn JT, Chan-Ling T. Retinopathy of prematurity: two distinct mechanisms that underlie zone 1 and zone 2 disease. *Am J Ophthalmol*. 2006; 142(1):46 59.

53. Azad RV, Pal N, Chandra P. Enhanced mydriasis during indirect diode laser therapy for threshold retinopathy of prematurity. *J Pediatr Ophthalmol. Strabismus*. 2006; 43:54-5.
54. Boyle EM, Freer Y, KhanOrakzai Z, Watkinson M, Wright E, Ainsworth JR, McIntosh N. Sucrose and nonnutritive sucking for the relief of pain in screening for retinopathy of prematurity: a randomised controlled trial. *Arch Dis Child Fetal Neonatal* 2006;91(3):F166-F168.
55. Engle WA; American Academy of Pediatrics Committee on Fetus and Newborn, "Age Terminology During the Perinatal Period", *Pediatrics*. 2004, 114(5):1362

8
chapter

Neha Sinha
Sandeep Saxena

Current Concepts in Central Serous Chorioretinopathy

ABSTRACT

Central serous chorioretinopathy (CSCR) is characterized by serous detachment of the neurosensory retina. Elevated circulating cortisol and epinephrine levels have been implicated in the pathogenesis of CSCR. The disease can be classified into acute and chronic types with good and poor visual recovery, respectively. Indocyanine green (ICG) angiography has highlighted the importance of the choroidal circulation in the pathogenesis of CSCR. With the help of OCT, it is now possible to identify subtle or even subclinical CSCR and progression of disease. Recent advances in the diagnostics and treatment help in better understanding of the disease.

Introduction

Central serous chorioretinopathy (CSCR) is a disease in which a serous detachment of the neurosensory retina occurs over an area of leakage from the choriocapillaris through the retinal pigment epithelium (RPE). It may be divided into 2 distinct clinical presentations.

ACUTE CSCR

The acute form is classically unilateral and characterized by one or more focal leaks at the level of RPE on fluorescein angiography. The neurosensory detatchment contains clear subretinal fluid but may be cloudy or have subretinal fibrin in some cases. This form is self-limiting and does not lead to gross visual deficit after resolution (Figs 8.1 and 8.2).

CHRONIC CSCR

The chronic form is believed to be due to diffuse RPE disease and is usually bilateral. It presents with diffuse RPE atrophic changes, varying

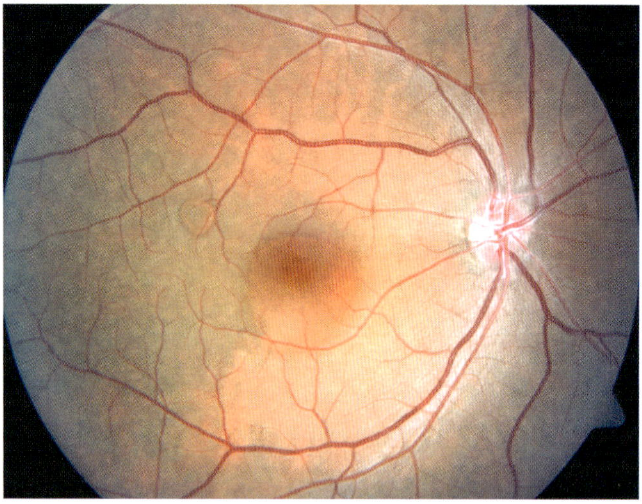

Fig. 8.1: Acute central serous chorioretinopathy: Color fundus photograph shows neurosensory detachment of the macula along with a pigment epithelial detachment

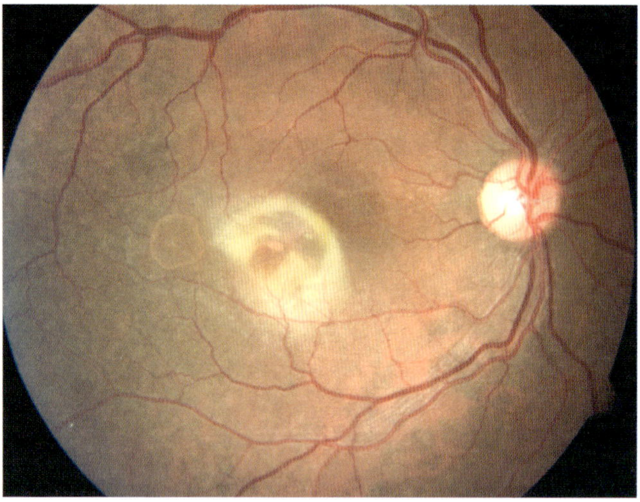

Fig. 8.2: Acute central serous chorioretinopathy: Color fundus photograph shows neurosensory detachment of the macula along with subretinal fibrin and a pigment epithelial detachment

degrees of subretinal fluid, RPE alterations, and RPE tracks (Fig. 8.3). It is characterized by diffuse areas of RPE leakage on fluorescein angiography. It has a relatively poor visual prognosis.

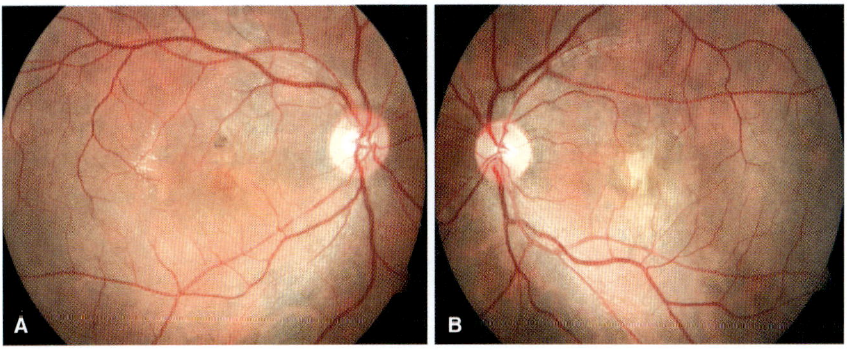

Figs 8.3A and B: Chronic central serous chorioretinopathy showing retinal pigment epithelial alterations and exudation **A.** RPE alterations; **B.** Exudation

Pathophysiology

Previously it was thought that CSCR occurs due to focal choroidal vasculopathy and abnormal ion transport across the RPE. The discovery of indocyanine green (ICG) angiography has highlighted the importance of the choroidal circulation in the pathogenesis of CSCR. ICG angiography has demonstrated both multifocal choroidal hyperpermeability and hypofluorescent areas suggestive of focal choroidal vascular compromise. Some investigators believe that initial choroidal vascular compromise subsequently leads to secondary dysfunction of the overlying RPE.[1,2]

Some studies using multifocal electroretinography have demonstrated bilateral diffuse retinal dysfunction even when CSCR was active only in one eye.[3]These studies support the belief of diffuse systemic effect on the choroidal vasculature.

Elevated circulating cortisol and epinephrine, which affect the autoregulation of the choroidal circulation are also involved in the pathogenesis of CSCR as seen in patients of systemic hypertension, obstructive sleep apnea and type A personalities.[4] Furthermore, Tewari et al[5] demonstrated impaired autonomic response with significantly decreased parasympathetic activity and significantly increased sympathetic activity in patients with CSCR. Corticosteroids have a direct influence on the expression of adrenergic receptor genes and thus contribute to the overall effect of catecholamines on the pathogenesis of CSCR. Consequently, multiple studies have conclusively implicated the effect of corticosteroids in the development of CSCR. Carvalho-Recchia et al[6] showed in a series that 52% of patients with CSCR had used exogenous steroids within 1 month of presentation as compared with 18% of control subjects.

Cotticelli et al[7] showed an association between *Helicobacter pylori* infection and CSCR. The prevalence of *H. pylori* infection was 78% in patients with CSCR compared with a prevalence of 43.5% in the control group. The authors proposed that *H. pylori* infection may represent a risk factor in CSCR, though no further studies have substantiated this claim.

Epidemiology

VISUAL MORBIDITY

Central serous chorioretinopathy typically resolve spontaneously in most of the patients (80–90%) with final visual acuity 20/25 or better vision. Even with return of good central visual acuity, many of these patients still notice dyschromatopsia, loss of contrast sensitivity, metamorphopsia, and rarely nyctalopia. Patients with classic CSCR have a 40–50% risk of recurrence in the same eye. Risk of choroidal neovascularization from previous CSCR is considered small (<5%) but has an increasing frequency in older patients.[8,9]

Approximately, 5–10% of patients may fail to recover 20/30 or better visual acuity. These patients often have recurrent or chronic serous retinal detachments, resulting in progressive RPE atrophy and permanent visual loss to 20/200 or worse. The final clinical picture represents diffuse retinal pigment epitheliopathy.

Otsuka et al[10] reviewed a subset of patients who presented with a severe variant of CSCR over a mean follow-up period of 10.6 years. These patients have had multifocal lesions and bullous retinal detachments with shifting fluid and fibrin deposition. During the follow-up period, 52% of patients experienced recurrences of CSCR ranging from 1–5 episodes. However, 80% of eyes regained a visual acuity of better than 20/40, and 52% returned to a visual acuity of 20/20 or better. Eventually, patients reached a state of quiescent disease.

RACE

Central serous chorioretinopathy is uncommon among African Americans but appears severely among Hispanics and Asians.

SEX

This condition affects men 6–10 times more often than women.

AGE

Central serous chorioretinopathy is most commonly seen in patients between the ages of 20 and 55 years. It may manifest in older age (more than 50 years). Spaide et al[11] reviewed 130 consecutive patients with CSCR and found that their age at the first diagnosis ranged from 22.2 to 82.9 years with a mean age of 49.8 years. Patients, who presented at 50 years or older were found to have bilateral disease with a decreased male predominance (2.6:1) and showed more diffuse RPE changes. Furthermore, the patients had systemic hypertension or a history of corticosteroid use.[12]

SIGNS AND SYMPTOMS

Patients with CSCR typically present with following signs and symptoms:

1. Central visual loss
2. Metamorphopsia (especially micropsia)
3. Positive scotoma
4. Loss of color saturation
5. Loss of contrast sensitivity
6. Delayed retinal recovery time (photostress test).

The decreased vision usually is improved by a small hyperopic correction.

Clinical examination shows a serous retinal detachment which may be very subtle, often requiring slit-lamp biomicroscopy examination for detection.[13] Pigment epithelial detachments, RPE mottling and atrophy, subretinal fibrin and rarely subretinal lipid or lipofuscinoid flecks may also be seen.[14]

Pathogenesis

The advent of ICG angiography has highlighted the importance of the choroidal circulation to the pathogenesis of central serous CSCR. Indocyanine green angiography has demonstrated both multifocal choroidal hyperpermeability and hypofluorescent areas suggestive of focal choroidal vascular compromise. Some investigators believe that initial choroidal vascular compromise subsequently leads to secondary dysfunction of the overlying RPE.[15]

Type A personality and systemic hypertension may be associated with CSCR.[16]

Allibhai et al[17] reported an association with a drug, sildenafil citrate and CSCR. Fraunfelder and Fraunfelder[18] further evaluated the association of

CSCR with sildenafil. After reviewing 1,500 cases of the ocular side effects of sildenafil, they have found 11 men had CSCR. The symptoms resolved following cessation of sildenafil in 8 of 11 patients but recurred in 3 of these patients upon restarting the drug. A causal relationship could not be determined due to the cyclic nature of CSCR but suggested that patients with refractory CSCR should consider cessation of sildenafil use.

Systemic associations of CSCR include organ transplantation, exogenous steroid use, Cushing syndrome, systemic hypertension, sleep apnea, systemic lupus erythematosus, pregnancy, gastroesophageal reflux disease, and use of psychopharmacologic medications.[4,17,19-22]

Haimovici et al[23] evaluated systemic risk factors for CSCR in 312 patients and 312 control subjects. They found that systemic steroid use and pregnancy were most strongly associated with CSCR. Other risk factors included antibiotic use, alcohol use, untreated hypertension and allergic respiratory disorders.

LABORATORY STUDIES

Laboratory tests are not very helpful in the diagnosis. An occasional elevated level of plasminogen activator inhibitor may be found in a patient with CSCR.

Fundus Fluorescein Angiography

Fundus fluorescein angiography (FA) of a classical case of CSCR shows one or more focal leaks at the level of the RPE (Figs 8.4 and 8.5). Usually, two types of pattern are seen. In the early stage, leakage is seen as a hyperfluorescent dot which later on expands into a large dot within the area of macular detachment called *inkblot* type. Sometimes, it rises under the neurosensory detachment as a *smoke stack*. The ink blot pattern is more common than smoke stack. The smoke stack pattern is thought to be related to the increased concentration of protein in the fluid. The classic *"smokestack"* appearance of the fluorescein leak is seen only in 10–15% of cases. In this pattern, a diffuse retinal pigment epitheliopathy demonstrates focal granular hyperfluorescence corresponding to window defects and blockage caused by RPE atrophy and clumping with one or more areas of subtle continued leakage.

Indocyanine Green Angiography

Indocyanine green angiography (ICG angiography) has shown hypofluorescent areas early in the angiogram followed by late hyperfluorescence and leakage

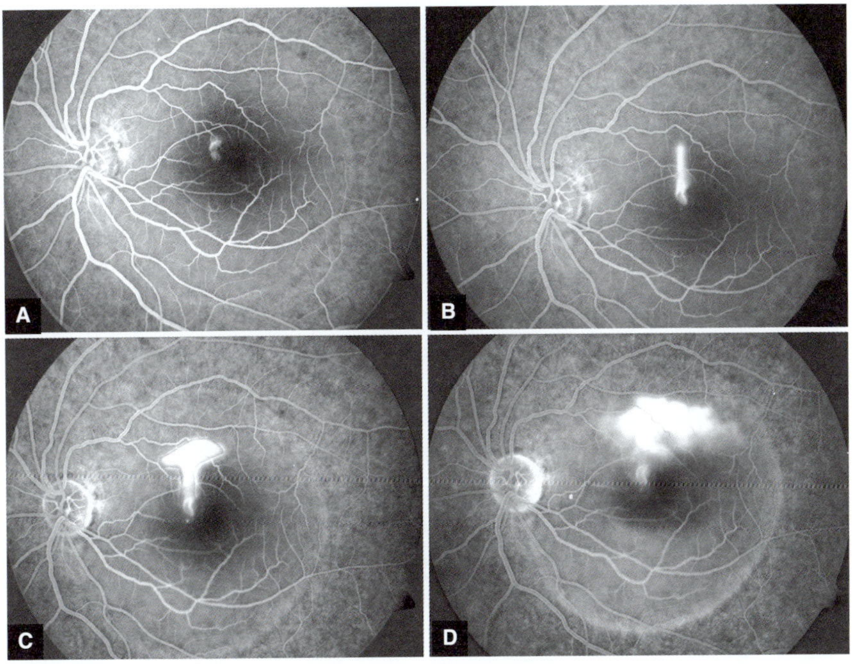

Figs 8.4A to D: Acute central serous chorioretinopathy: Fundus fluorescein angiography showing A: Hyperfluorecent dot, B: Linear expanded dot, C and D: increasing smoke stacks appearances (umbrella pattern)

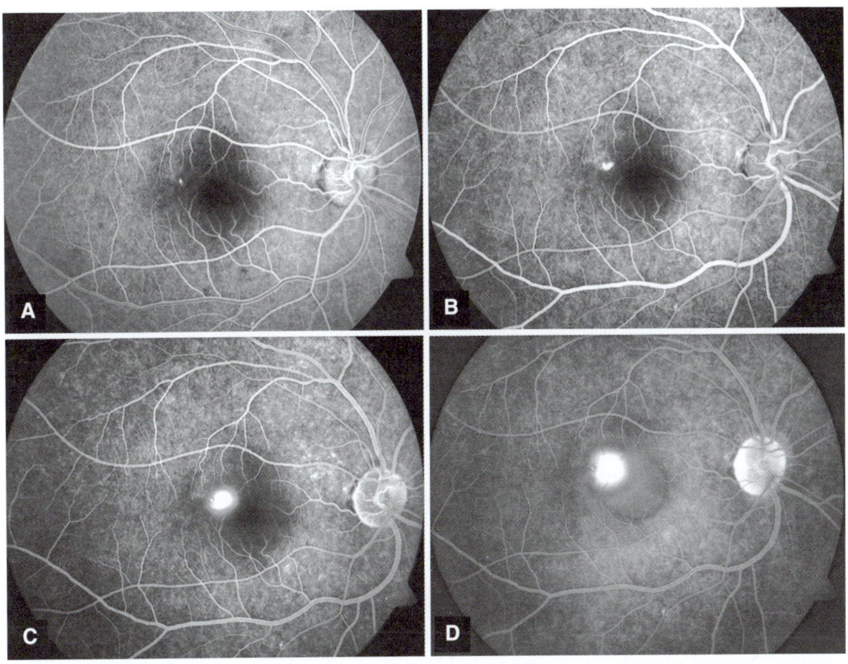

Figs 8.5 Ato D: Acute central serous chorioretinopathy: Fundus fluorescein angiography shows gradual expanding ink blot appearances

in choroidal vasculature. Often, multiple areas of leakage are seen on ICG angiography that are not evident clinically or on FA. According to some researchers, characteristic mid phase findings on ICG angiography allows differentiation from occult choroidal neovascularization in older individuals. Multiple patches of hyperfluorescence are presumably due to choroidal hyperpermeability, which in later phases, results in silhouetting or negative staining of larger choroidal vessels.

Scanning laser ophthalmoscopy is a newer technology to evaluate the retina. Ooto et al[24] showed that adaptive optics is useful in evaluating cone abnormalities associated with visual acuity loss in eyes with central serous chorioretinopathy.

Optical Coherence Tomography

Optical coherence tomography (OCT) can demonstrate subretinal fluid, pigment epithelial detachments, and retinal atrophy. It is especially helpful in identifying subtle or even subclinical, neurosensory macular detachments.

OCT features of acute and chronic CSCR are summarized below.[25]

ACUTE CSCR (FIGS 8.6 TO 8.8)

1. Thickening of the neurosensary retina with detachment
2. Retinal pigment epithelial detachment
3. Combination of both—1 and 2
4. Presence of moderately high reflective mass bridging the detached neurosensary retina and RPE with subretinal fibrin.

CHRONIC CSCR (FIG. 8.9)

1. Foveal atrophy and thinning
2. Cystoid changes at the fovea
3. Associated complications may show RPE rip and choroidal neovascularisation.

Three-dimensional Optical Coherence Tomography

Three-dimensional optical coherence tomography may be performed using an SD-OCT scanning protocol that achieves high sampling density in all 3 dimensions and acquires high density volumetric data of the macula. Volume rendering of the 3-dimensional data generates a 3-dimensional image. The data can be processed to provide comprehensive structural information. The unprecedented visualization provided by this technology enables determination of specific alterations in the characteristics of the retinal anatomy. Three-

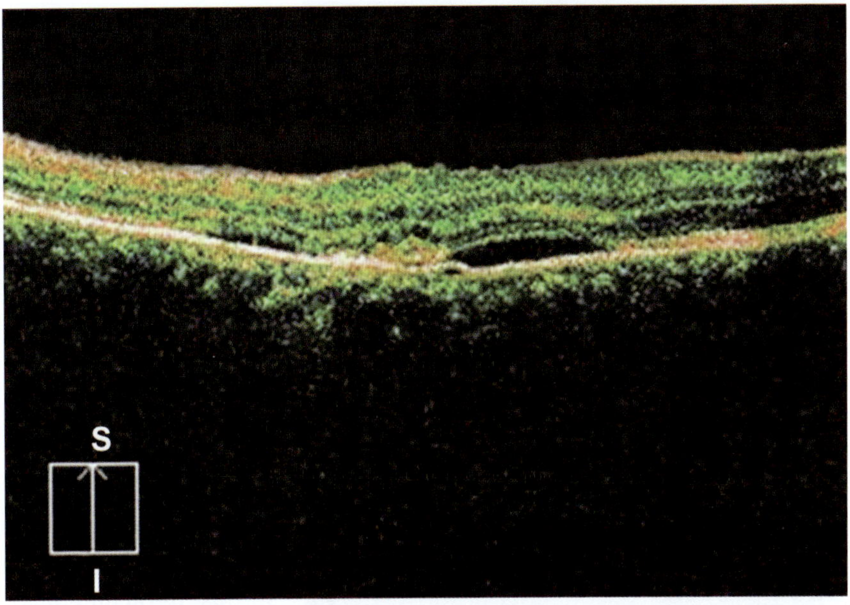

Fig. 8.6: Acute central serous chorioretinopathy: Spectral domain optical coherence tomography shows serous detachment of macula and pigment epithelial detachment

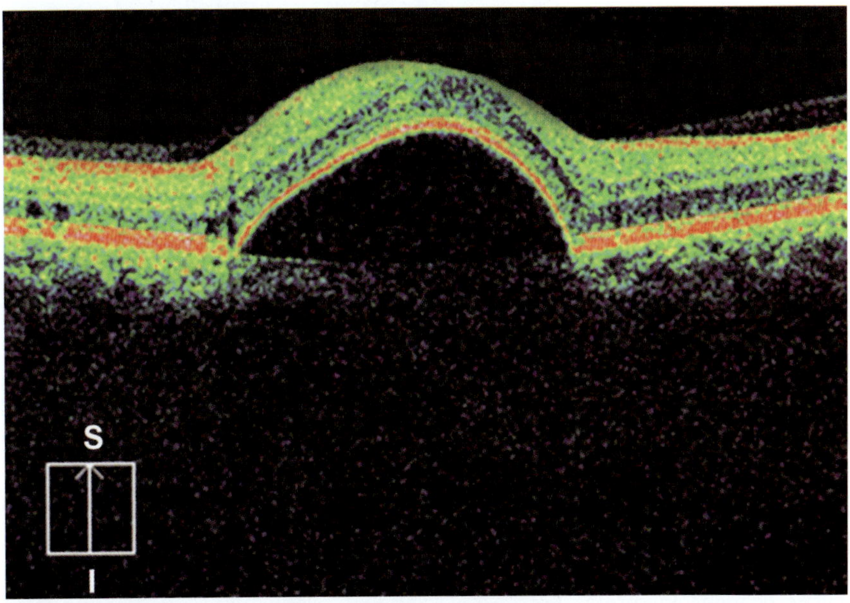

Fig. 8.7: Acute central serous chorioretinopathy: Spectral domain optical coherence tomography shows large pigment epithelial detachment

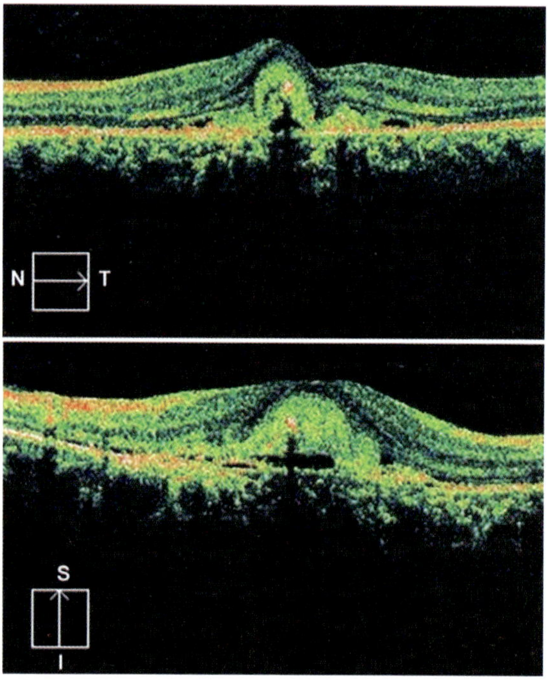

Fig. 8.8: Acute central serous chorioretinopathy: Spectral domain optical coherence tomography shows subretinal fibrin, serous detachment of macula and pigment epithelial detachment

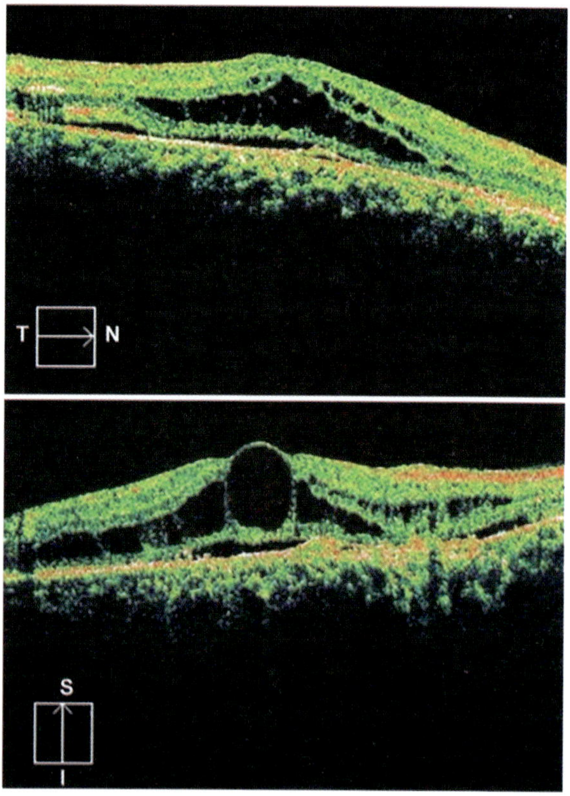

Fig. 8.9: Chronic central serous chorioretinopathy: Spectral domain optical coherence tomography shows serous detachment of macula, pigment epithelium detachment, cystic changes in retina, and proliferating cells on retinal pigment epithelium and back surface of neurosensory retina

dimensional OCT data can be used to segment measure, and map intraretinal layer thicknesses. Currently, the clinical applications of 3D retinal imaging are being evaluated for selective visualization of macular layers. SD-OCT shows morphologic alterations in the retinal pigment epithelium.

Quantitative and topographic assessment of pigment epithelium detachment (PEDs) on spectral domain single-layer retinal pigment epithelium (SD-OCT SL-RPE) map compares well with fluorescein angiography. SD-OCT SL-RPE map is indeed a noninvasive advanced tool for documentation of quantitative and topographic distribution of PEDs and obviates the need for fluorescein angiography for monitoring the progress of PEDs in eyes with CSCR (Fig. 8.10).

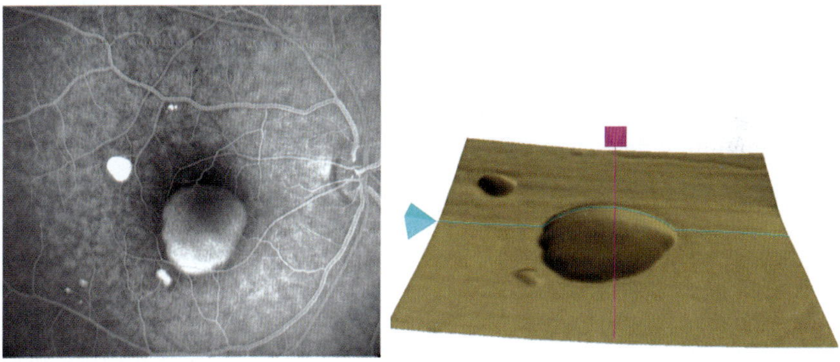

Fig. 8.10: Central serous chorioretinopathy: Three-dimensional spectral domain optical coherence tomography retinal pigment epithelium map shows topographic and quantitative distribution of pigment epithelial detachments in 512 x 128 macular cube when compared to fundus fluorescein angiography

Multifocal Electroretinography

Multifocal electroretinography is a technique which allows simultaneous recording of the focal electroretinographic responses from multiple retinal locations.[26] Due to impairment of the central macular function in CSCR, first-order mfERG responses will demonstrate reduced response amplitude especially in the rings arising from the central macula. Delayed implicit times may also be observed in the area of serous macular detachment, but in some it might be seen in areas without retinal detachment and even in unaffected fellow eyes suggesting more widespread retinal dysfunction in CSCR. Chappelow and Marmor [27] first described the persistently reduced focal electrical responses on multifocal electroretinography in eyes with resolved CSCR. Furthermore, investigators including Lai et al[28] are using multifocal electroretinography as a means of assessing the efficacy and safety of new treatment modalities for CSCR (Fig. 8.11).

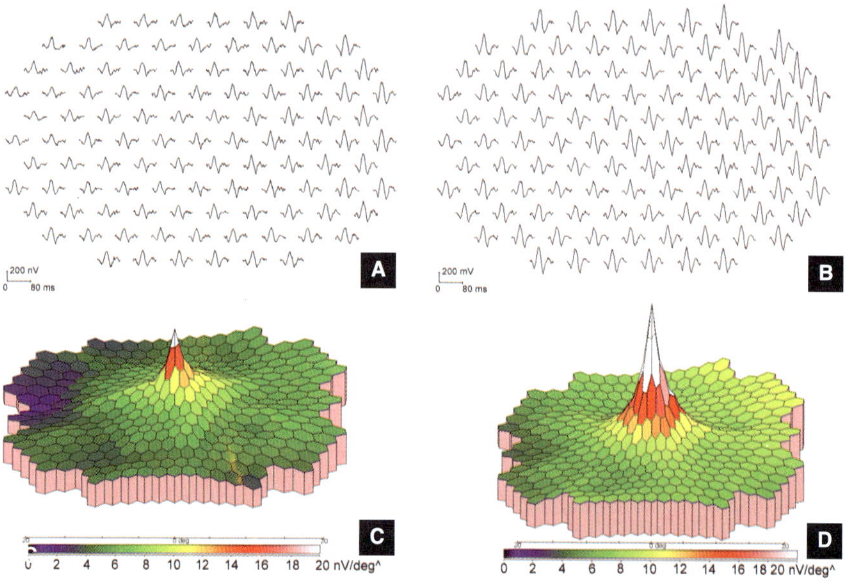

Figs 8.11A to D. Serial first-order kernel multifocal electroretinography assessment of central serous chorioretinopathy: **A:** Trace array and **B:** Three-dimensional response density plot at the initial presentation showing reduced response amplitude at the central macula. **C:** Trace array and **D:** Three-dimensional response density plot after resolution of exudative macular detachment showing recovery of the multifocal electroretinography responses indicating recovery of macular function *(Courtesy:* Dr. Timothy Y Y Lai, Hong Kong)

Fundus Autofluorescence

Fundus flurorescein is a noninvasive imaging technique, which evaluates the structural and metabolic condition of the RPE cells at macula. In acute CSCR, a localized spot of reduced autofluorescence may be observed corresponding to area of focal RPE defect. Mild diffuse increase in autofluorescence might be observed due to increase metabolic activity of RPE cells (Figs 8.12 and 8.13).[29-31] In chronic CSCR, irregularity in the level of autofluorescence might be seen with both areas of reduced and increased autofluorescence. Reduced activity is due generalized RPE atrophy or loss of photoreceptors.[29-31]

Microperimetry

Micrometry (using the Nidek MP-1 microperimeter) has shown lower retinal sensitivity in the macula even once visual acuity returned to 20/20. Ojima et al[32,33] showed that areas of reduced sensitivity were typically focal and localized to clinically apparent regions of irregular RPE.

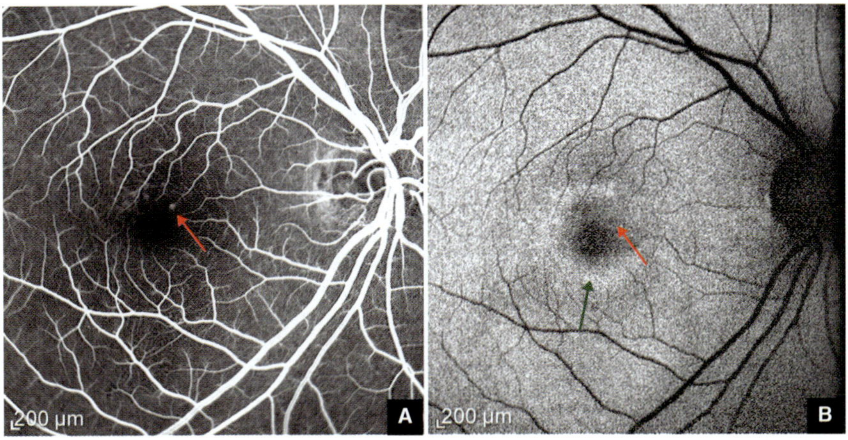

Figs 8.12A and B: A: Early phase fluorescein angiography showing a focal point of leakage (red arrow) in acute central serous chorioretinopathy. B: Fundus autofluorescence image of the same eye showing a localized spot of hypofluorescence due to focal loss of RPE corresponding to the leakage site on FA (red arrow). An area of increased autofluorescence (green arrow) can also be seen surrounding the macula due to increased metabolic activity of RPE cells (*Courtesy:* Dr. Timothy Y Y Lai, Hong Kong)

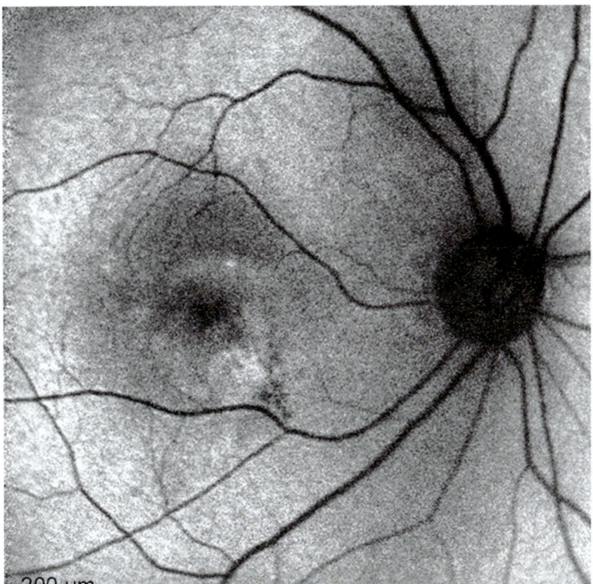

Fig. 8.13: Fundus autofluorescence image of a chronic central serous chorioretinopathy showing irregular level of autofluorescence signals. Areas of reduced autofluorescence are suggestive of retinal pigment epithelial atrophy, whereas areas of increased autofluorescence are suggested of increased RPE activity (*Courtesy:* Dr. Timothy Y Y Lai, Hong Kong)

TREATMENT

Medical

- Efficacy of tranquilizers or beta-blockers is unknown. Furthermore, an evaluation of 230 consecutive patients with central serous chorioretinopathy found that use of psychopharmacologic agents (e.g., anxiolytics, antidepressants) was a risk factor for CSCR. Use of corticosteroids in the treatment of CSCR should be avoided because it may result in exacerbation of serous detachments
- Tatham and Macfarlane [34] described a case series of patients who were treated with propranolol for CSCR. They suggested that beta-blockade had a hypothetical mechanism in treating CSCR. Further evidence is needed to substantiate this potential treatment
- Mifepristone was used in the treatment of chronic CSCR by Nielsen et al.[35]
- Bevacizumab (Avastin) is a humanized monoclonal antibody that inhibits all active isoforms of VEGF and is approved by USFDA since 2004 for treatment of metastatic colorectal cancer. It has been used to successfully treat the rare complication of choroidal neovascularization following CSCR.[36-38] Variable reports are available in literature about the efficacy of intravitreal therapy (Figs 8.14 and 8.15).

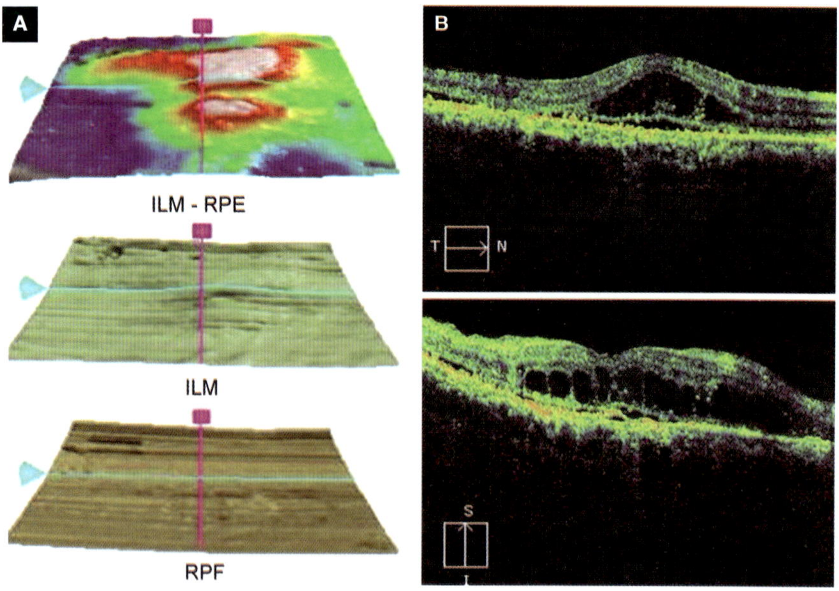

Figs 8.14A and B: Intravitreal bevacizumab in chronic central serous chrioretinopathy: Pre treatment: A: Macular topography in ILM-RPE, ILM and RPE maps and B: Neurosensory detachment and cystic changes in macula

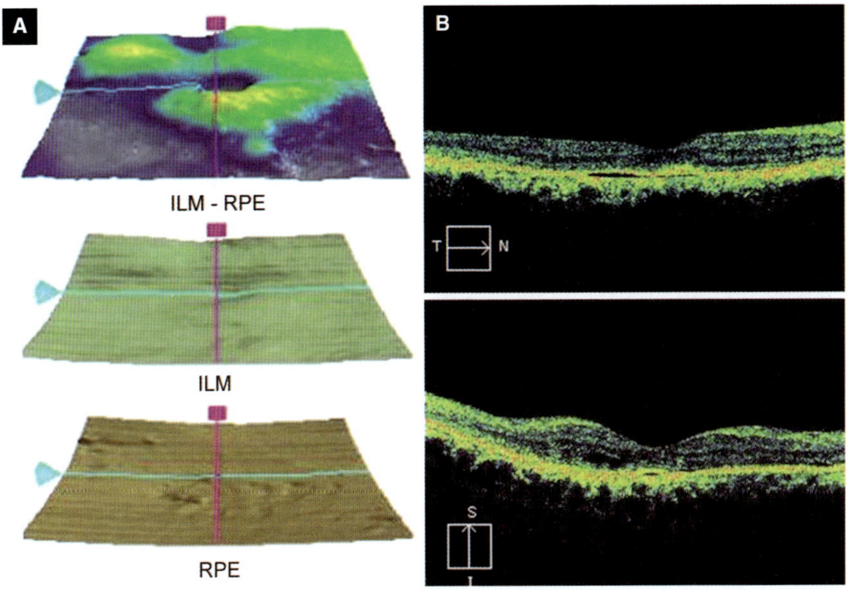

Figs 8.15A and B: Intravitreal bevacizumab in chronic central serous chrioretinopathy: Post-treatment: A: Macular topography in ILM-RPE, ILM and RPE maps and B: Residual neurosensory detachment, resolution of cystic changes in macula and reappearance of foveal contour

- Finasteride (phosphodiesterase inhibitor) may represent a novel medical treatment for chronic central serous chorioretinopathy.[39]

Laser Photocoagulation

Laser photocoagulation should be considered under the following circumstances:

1. Persistence of a serous retinal detachment for more than 4 months.
2. Recurrence in an eye with visual deficit from previous CSCR.
3. Presence of visual deficits in opposite eye from previous episodes of CSCR.
4. Occupational or other patient's need requiring prompt recovery of vision.

Laser treatment also may be considered in patients with recurrent episodes of serous detachment with a leak located more than 300 μm from the center of the fovea.[40,41] Laser treatment does not appear to improve the final visual prognosis, but it shortens the course of the disease and decreases the risk of recurrence for CSCR.[42,43] It affect the final contrast sensitivity, which was found to be lesser in patients treated with early laser as compare to patients kept on the conservative management. Some evidence suggests that patients with chronic CSCR (diffuse retinal pigment epitheliopathy) may have better prognosis with laser treatment.

Photodynamic Therapy

Photodynamic therapy (PDT) has growing support in the literature as a treatment of chronic CSCR and recently in acute phases of this condition. PDT is known to have a direct effect on the choroidal circulation but was limited by potential adverse effects, such as macular ischemia. Lai et al[28] has described half dose verteporfin with significantly decreased the rates of adverse events with these modifications. They proposed 3 mg/m^2 of verteporfin infused over 8 minutes, followed 2 minutes later with ICG guided PDT. Of the eyes treated, 85% showed complete resolution of the neurosensory retinal detachment and/or pigment epithelial detachment by 1 month after treatment. Use of verteporfin and PDT was first reported in 2003 in the setting of CSCR. Yannuzzi et al[44] described using ICG angiography to first identify areas of choroidal hyperpermeability that were then targeted with PDT. Subsequent studies using PDT protocols established by the Treatment of Age-Related Macular Degeneration with Photodynamic Therapy (TAP) study have reported case series that support the use of PDT, especially in the setting of chronic CSCR with neurosensory detachments. PDT is believed to hasten both fluid resorption and visual recovery.

Reibaldi et al[45] evaluated the treatment efficacy of standard-fluence PDT versus low-fluence PDT using microperimetry. The study found improvement of macular sensitivity following treatment along with greater efficacy in treatment overall using low-fluence PDT. Multiple authors have also begun to use PDT as a first-line therapy for acute focal leaks from CSCR with reported success. Most papers describe resolution of subretinal fluid within 1 month of treatment.

Chan et al[46] demonstrated that there is evidence of choroidal vascular changes on ICG with regard to choroidal permeability and vascular remodelling. ICG mediated photothrombosis is a technique using a low-intensity laser combined with ICG dye infusion to treat focal areas of hyperpermeability in the choroid. Like PDT, it addresses treatment to the level of the choroidal vasculature.[47] An 810 nm laser is applied after infusion of ICG dye.

Transpupillary Thermotherapy

Without prior ICG dye, investigators have also used the 810 nm laser as transpupillary thermotherapy (TTT) with moderate anecdotal success.[48,49] However, Penha et al[50] described severe retinal thermal injury in a 31-year-old man following this treatment modality and recommended caution for this adverse event following ICG mediated TTT treatment.

Micropulse Yellow Laser Therapy

Micropulse yellow laser therapy is one of the newer treatment modality which resolves leakage and retinal detachment without scarring or retinal damage. The IQ 577 (Iridex Corporation, Mountain View, CA, U.S.A.) laser is a solid-state, multimode laser. In micropulse mode, the laser energy is delivered in short pulses. The laser stays on only 10 to 15% of the time (depending on duty cycle selected) generating less heat and producing less damage to the retina than continuous-wave photocoagulation. The 577 nm yellow wavelength is ideal for CSR and other retinal applications because it is highly selective for the RPE. Oxyhemoglobin in the RPE absorbs yellow light better than any other wavelength, while xanthophylls have negligible uptake of yellow light, localizing the effects to the RPE and further protecting the fovea.[51] The results from a small series of patients with central serous retinopathy treated with the yellow laser have been very encouraging.

FOLLOW-UP

Most patients with central serous chorioretinopathy receive follow-up care for 3 months to determine whether the fluid resolves spontaneously.

COMPLICATIONS

- Retinal pigment epithelial decompensation from recurrent attacks leads to RPE atrophy and subsequent retinal atrophy. RPE decompensation is a manifestation of CSCR but may also be considered as a long-term complication[52]
- A minority of patients develops choroidal neovascularization at the site of leakage and laser treatments. A retrospective review of cases shows that one-half of these patients may have had signs of occult choroidal neovascularization at the time of treatment. In the other patients, the risk of choroidal neovascularization may have been increased by the laser treatment[9]
- Acute bullous retinal detachment may occur in otherwise healthy patients with CSCR. This appearance may mimic Vogt-Koyanagi-Harada disease, rhegmatogenous retinal detachment or uveal effusion. A case report also has implicated the use of corticosteroids in CSCR as a factor increasing the likelihood of subretinal fibrin formation. Reducing the corticosteroid dose frequently will lead to resolution of the serous retinal detachment.[53]

PROGNOSIS

- Serous retinal detachments typically resolve spontaneously in most patients with patients (80–90%) returning to 20/25 or better vision[54,55]
- Patients with classic CSCR (characterized by focal leaks) have a 40–50% risk of recurrence in the same eye[13,54,55]
- In spite of return of good central visual acuity, many of these patients still notice dyschromatopsia, loss of contrast sensitivity, metamorphopsia, or nyctalopia[54]
- These patients often have recurrent or chronic serous retinal detachments, resulting in progressive RPE atrophy and permanent visual loss to 20/200 or worse. The final clinical picture represents diffuse retinal pigment epitheliopathy
- Risk of choroidal neovascularization from previous CSCR is considered small (<5%) but has an increasing frequency in older patients diagnosed with CSCR.[8,13]

References

1. Okushiba U, Takeda M. Study of choroidal vascular lesions in central serous chorioretinopathy using indocyanine green angiography. *Nippon Ganka Gakkai Zasshi*. 1997;101:74-82.
2. Iijima H, Iida T, Murayama K, Imai M, Gohdo T. Plasminogen activator inhibitor 1 in central serous chorioretinopathy. *Am J Ophthalmol.* 1999;127:477-8.
3. Marmor MF, Tan F. Central serous chorioretinopathy: bilateral multifocal electroretinographic abnormalities. *Arch Ophthalmol.* 1999;117:184-8.
4. Leveque TK, Yu L, Musch DC, Chervin RD, Zacks DN. Central serous chorioretinopathy and risk for obstructive sleep apnea. *Sleep Breath.* 2007;11:253-7.
5. Tewari HK, Gadia R, Kumar D, Venkatesh P, Garg SP. Sympathetic-parasympathetic activity and reactivity in central serous chorioretinopathy: a case-control study. *Invest Ophthalmol Vis Sci.* 2006;47:3474-8.
6. Carvalho-Recchia CA, Yannuzzi LA, Negrao S, Spaide RF, Freund KB, Rodriguez-Coleman H. Corticosteroids and central serous chorioretinopathy. *Ophthalmology.* 2002;109:1834-7.
7. Cotticelli L, Borrelli M, D'Alessio AC, Menzione M, Villani A, Piccolo G. Central serous chorioretinopathy and Helicobacter pylori. *Eur J Ophthalmol* 2006; 16:274-8.
8. Gomolin JE. Choroidal neovascularization and central serous chorioretinopathy. *Can J Ophthalmol.* 1989;24:20-3.
9. Matsunaga H, Nangoh K, Uyama M, Nanbu H, Fujiseki Y, Takahashi K. [Occurrence of choroidal neovascularization following photocoagulation treatment for central serous retinopathy]. *Nippon Ganka Gakkai Zasshi.* 1995;99(4):460-8.
10. Otsuka S, Ohba N, Nakao KA. Long-term follow-up study of severe variant of central serus chorioretinopathy. *Retina.* 2002;22:25-32.
11. Spaide RF, Campeas L, Haas A, Yannuzzi LA, Fisher YL, Guyer DR. Central serous chorioretinopathy in younger and older adults. *Ophthalmology.* 1996;103:2070-9; discussion 2079-80.
12. Polak BC, Baarsma GS, Snyers B. Diffuse retinal pigment epitheliopathy complicating systemic corticosteroid treatment. *Br J Ophthalmol.* 1995;79:922-5.

13. Gass JD. Central serous chorioretinopathy and white subretinal exudation during pregnancy. *Arch Ophthalmol.* 1991;109:677-81.
14. Piccolino FC, Borgia L. Central serous chorioretinopathy and indocyanine green angiography. *Retina.* 1994; 14:231-42.
15. Yannuzzi LA. Type-A behavior and central serous chorioretinopathy. *Retina.* 1987; 7:111-31.
16. Jampol LM, Weinreb R, Yannuzzi L. Involvement of corticosteroids and catecholamines in the pathogenesis of central serous chorioretinopathy: a rationale for new treatment strategies. *Ophthalmology.* 2002; 109:1765-6.
17. Allibhai ZA, Gale JS, Sheidow TS. Central serous chorioretinopathy in a patient taking sildenafil citrate. *Ophthalmic Surg Lasers Imaging.* 2004;35:165-7.
18. Fraunfelder FW, Franufelder FT. Central serous chorioretinopathy associated with sildenafil. *Retina.* 2008; 28:606-9.
19. Cunningham ET Jr, Alfred PR, Irvine AR. Central serous chorioretinopathy in patients with systemic lupus erythematosus.*Ophthalmology.* 1996;103:2081-90.
20. Bouzas EA, Scott MH, Mastorakos G, Chrousos GP, Kaiser-Kupfer MI. Central serous chorioretinopathy in endogenous hypercortisolism. *Arch Ophthalmol.* 1993;111:1229-33.
21. Mansuetta CC, Mason JO 3rd, Swanner J, Feist RM, White MF Jr, Thomley ML. An association between central serous chorioretinopathy and gastroesophageal reflux disease. *Am J Ophthalmol.* 2004;137:1096-100.
22. Tittl MK, Spaide RF, Wong D, Pilotto E, Yannuzzi LA, Fisher YL. Systemic findings associated with central serous chorioretinopathy.*Am J Ophthalmol.* 1999;128: 63-8.
23. Haimovici R, Koh S, Gagnon DR, Lehrfeld T, Wellik S. Risk factors for central serous chorioretinopathy: a case-control study.*Ophthalmology.* 2004;111:244-9.
24. Ooto S, Hangai M, Sakamoto A, Tsujikawa A, Yamashiro K, Ojima Y, et al. High-resolution imaging of resolved central serous chorioretinopathy using adaptive optics scanning laser ophthalmoscopy. *Ophthalmology.* 2010;117:1800-9,
25. Bhende M, Nair BK (2006) Central serous chorioretinopathy. In: Saxena S, Meredith Ta (eds) Optical coherence tomography in retinal diseases. Jaypee, New Delhi, pp137-144
26. Sutter EE, Tran D. The field topography of ERG components in man-I. The photopic luminance response. *Vision Res.* 1992;32:433-46.
27. Chappelow AV, Marmor MF. Multifocal electroretinogram abnormalities persist following resolution of central serous chorioretinopathy.*Arch Ophthalmol* 2000;118:1211-5.
28. Lai TY, Chan WM, Li H, Lai RY, Liu DT, Lam DS. Safety enhanced photodynamic therapy with half dose verteporfin for chronic central serous chorioretinopathy: a short term pilot study. *Br J Ophthalmol.* 2006;90:869-74.
29. Eandi CM, Ober M, Iranmanesh R, et al. Acute central serous chorioretinopathy and fundus autofluorescence. *Retina.* 2005;25:989-93.
30. Ruckmann A, Fitzke FW , Fan J et al. Abnormalities of fundus autofluorescence in central serous retinopathy. *Am J Ophthalmol.* 2002;133:780-86.
31. Spaid RF, Klancnik JM Jr. Fundus autofluorescence and central serous chorioretinopathy. Ophthalmology.
32. Ozdemir H, Karacorlu SA, Senturk F, Karacorlu M, Uysal O. Assessment of macular function by microperimetry in unilateral resolved central serous chorioretinopathy. *Eye (Lond).* 2008;22:204-8.
33. Ojima Y, Tsujikawa A, Hangai M, et al. Retinal sensitivity measured with microperimeter 1 after resolution of central serous chorioretinopathy. *Am J Ophthalmol.* 2008;146:77-84.

34. Tatham A, Macfarlane A. The use of propranolol to treat central serous chorioretinopathy: an evaluation by serial OCT. *J Ocul Pharmacol Ther.* 2006;22:145-9.
35. Nielsen JS, Weinreb RN, Yannuzzi L, Jampol LM. Mifepristone treatment of chronic central serous chorioretinopathy. *Retina.* 2007;27:119-22.
36. Huang WC, Chen WL, Tsai YY, Chiang CC, Lin JM. Intravitreal bevacizumab for treatment of chronic central serous chorioretinopathy. *Eye (Lond).* 2009;23:488-9.
37. Torres-Soriano ME, Garcia-Aguirre G, Kon-Jara V, Ustariz-Gonzales O, Abraham-Marin M, Ober MD. A pilot study of intravitreal bevacizumab for the treatment of central serous chorioretinopathy (case reports). *Graefes Arch Clin Exp Ophthalmol.* Sep 2008;246:1235-9.
38. Chan WM, Lai TY, Liu DT, Lam DS. Intravitreal bevacizumab (avastin) for choroidal neovascularization secondary to central serous chorioretinopathy, secondary to punctate inner choroidopathy, or of idiopathic origin. *Am J Ophthalmol.* 2007;143:977-983.
39. Forooghian, Farzin ; Meleth, Annal D ; Cukras, Catherine ; Chew, Emily Y ; Wong, Wai T, Meyerle, Catherine B .Finasteride for chronic central serous chorioretinopathy; Retina 2011 Volume 31, 766-771
40. Watzke RC, Burton TC, Woolson RF. Direct and indirect laser photocoagulation of central serous choroidopathy. *Am J Ophthalmol* 1979; 88:914-8.
41. Robertson DM, Ilstrup D. Direct, indirect, and sham laser photocoagulation in the management of central serous chorioretinopathy. *Am J Ophthalmol.* 1983;95:457-66.
42. Burumcek E, Mudun A, Karacorlu S, Arslan MO. Laser photocoagulation for persistent central serous retinopathy: results of long-term follow-up. *Ophthalmology.* 1997; 104:616-22.
43. Taban M, Boyer DS, Thomas EL, Taban M. Chronic central serous chorioretinopathy: photodynamic therapy. *Am J Ophthalmol.* 2004;137:1073-80.
44. Yannuzzi LA, Slakter JS, Gross NE, Spaide RF, Costa DL, Huang SJ. Indocyanine green angiography-guided photodynamic therapy for treatment of chronic central serous chorioretinopathy: a pilot study. *Retina.* 2003;23:288-98.
45. Reibaldi M, Boscia F, Avitabile T, et al. Functional Retinal Changes Measured by Microperimetry in Standard-Fluence vs Low-Fluence Photodynamic Therapy in Chronic Central Serous Chorioretinopathy. *Am J Ophthalmol.* 2011;151:953-960.e2.
46. Chan WM, Lam DS, Lai TY, Tam BS, Liu DT, Chan CK. Choroidai vascular remodelling in central serous chorioretinopathy after indocyanine green guided photodynamic therapy with verteporfin: a novel treatment at the primary disease level. *Br J Ophthalmol.* 2003;87:1453-8.
47. Costa RA, Scapucin L, Moraes NS, Calucci D, Melo LA Jr, Cardillo JA. Indocyanine green-mediated photothrombosis as a new technique of treatment for persistent central serous chorioretinopathy. *Curr Eye Res.* 2002;25:287-97.
48. Hussain N, Khanna R, Hussain A, Das T. Transpupillary thermotherapy for chronic central serous chorioretinopathy. *Graefes Arch Clin Exp Ophthalmol.* 2006;244: 1045-51.
49. Shukla D, Kolluru C, Vignesh TP, Karthikprakash S, Kim R. Transpupillary thermotherapy for subfoveal leaks in central serous chorioretinopathy. *Eye (Lond).* 2008;22:100-6.
50. Penha FM, Aggio FB, Bonomo PP. Severe retinal thermal injury after indocyanine green-mediated photothrombosis for central serous chorioretinopathy. *Am J Ophthalmol.* 2007;143:887-9.

51. Chen SN, Hwang JF, Tseng LF, Lin CJ. Subthreshold diode micropulse photocoagulation for the treatment of chronic central serous chorioretinopathy with juxtafoveal leakage Ophthalmology. 2008 ;115:2229-34.
52. Yap EY, Robertson DM. The long-term outcome of central serous chorioretinopathy. *Arch Ophthalmol.* 1996;114:689-92.
53. Gass JD, Little H. Bilateral bullous exudative retinal detachment complicating idiopathic central serous chorioretinopathy during systemic corticosteroid therapy. *Ophthalmology.* 1995;102:737-47.
54. Hooymans JM. Fibrotic scar formation in central serous chorioretinopathy developed during systemic treatment with corticosteroids.*Graefes Arch Clin Exp Ophthalmol.* 1998; 236:876-9.
55. Cardillo Piccolino F, Eandi CM, Ventre L, Rigault de la Longrais RC, Grignolo FM. Photodynamic therapy for chronic central serous chorioretinopathy. *Retina.* 2003; 23:752-63.
56. Ober MD, Yannuzzi LA, Do DV, Spaide RF, Bressler NM, Jampol LM. Photodynamic therapy for focal retinal pigment epithelial leaks secondary to central serous chorioretinopathy. *Ophthalmology.* 2005;112:2088-94

9

chapter

Dananjay Shukla

Idiopathic Macular Telangiectasia

ABSTRACT

Idiopathic macular telangiectasia (IMT) is a common but underdiagnosed macular disease. The condition manifests itself in two discrete presentations: one which resembles mild Coats' disease and causes visual loss by macular edema is labeled type 1 IMT; the more subtle but more common variant, which causes visual loss by foveal atrophy, pigment migration and subretinal neovascularization, is called type 2 IMT. While type 1 can be diagnosed clinically, type 2 IMT needs to be differentiated from microvascular diseases like diabetic macular edema as well as heredomacular degenerations. Fluorescein angiography and optical coherence tomography aid diagnosis for both types of IMT; fundus autofluorescence helps in early diagnosis of IMT2. Photocoagulation is the treatment of choice for IMT1. IMT2 is slowly progressive, but most patients maintain good vision in at least one eye. Treatment is, therefore, not required till the proliferative stage is reached. Although no treatment has an established value. Inhibitors of vascular endothelial growth factor, especially bevacizumab, probably provides best visual outcomes at proliferative stage of IMT2. Transpupillary thermotherapy and photodynamic therapy have modest but more stable outcomes. Macular telangiectasia study may soon provide the final answers to the lingering questions about the cause, pathology, natural history and management of this enigmatic disease.

History and Evolution of Terminology

The term "retinal telangiectasia" refers to an irregular dilation, incompetence and leakage of the retinal capillaries, which may occur anywhere in the fundus from posterior pole to the periphery. This term was first used by Reese to refer to a spectrum of capillary anomalies from *Leber's miliary aneurysms* to Coats' disease as part of a continuum.[1] When only the capillaries of foveal avascular zone are involved, the term *parafoveal telangiectasia* has been used. This rather vague nomenclature was firmed up by Gass and Oyakawa as *idiopathic juxtafoveolar retinal telangiectasis (IJFRT)*, to exclude the more common telangiectasia secondary to retinal vascular diseases.[2] Gass and Blodi revisited this classification a decade later to present a detailed and comprehensive system, still used and respected by peers.[3] Yannuzzi and colleagues simplified this complex classification and called the condition *idiopathic macular telangiectasia* (IMT).[4] The Macular Telangiectasia (MacTel) study, a large 5-year multicenter study, has given a still simpler name to the condition: *macular telangiectasia* or *MacTel*.[5] Till the MacTel terminology gains currency, we prefer to call this disease IMT, in deference to the fact that this is, till date, an idiopathic condition by definition.

Classification of Idiopathic Macular Telangiectasia

Gass and Blodi divided IJFRT into three clinical categories: Type 1 was unilateral with features suggestive of a forme fruste of Coats' disease. Type 2 was bilateral, and the most common type. However, the telangiectasias were barely visible or *occult* in most cases. Type 3 was rare, was characterized by perifoveal capillary occlusion and associated with cardiovascular or central nervous system diseases. Each type had two subtypes A and B. The subtype B was generally less common, had less defined clinical features, and systemic associations. They also provided a 5-stage grading for the most common subtype, 2A in this study, which was also the largest study of natural history of the condition.[3] Yannuzzi et al have removed the rare type 3, which they called occlusive telangiectasia, as well as all the B-subtypes, retaining only two types.[4] Type 1 or aneurysmal telangiectasia is similar to type 1A of Gass and Blodi, a milder variant of Coats' disease, with similar demographics, clinical features and response to treatment (Fig. 9.1). Type 2 or perifoveal telangiectasia is similar to Gass type 2A, with occult telangiectasia and minimal exudation (Table 9.1). Type 2 IMT typically appears as a gray opacification of macula, with or without intraretinal crystalline deposits, right-angled venules and stellate plaques of migrating retinal pigment, which Gass and Blodi believed to be the precursor of intra- and subretinal neovascularization (Figs 9.2 and 9.3). Yannuzzi et al reduced the 5-stage grading of type 2A IJFRT into only two stages of type 2 IMT: a non-proliferative stage, and a later stage of neovascular proliferation, almost invariably associated with significant visual loss.

Epidemiology and Natural History

IMT was so far believed to be a rare retinal disease, mainly due to low awareness. One of the purposes of the MacTel study is to present evidence

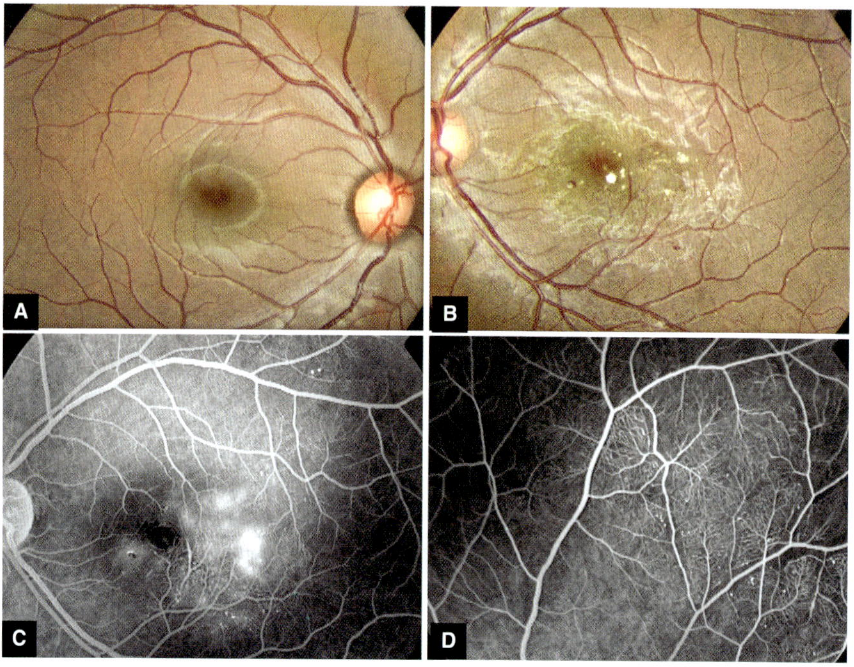

Figs 9.1A to D: Type 1 idiopathic macular telangiectasia (IMT1). **A and B:** In this patient is characterized by unilateral presence of obvious telangiectasia, hard exudates and macular edema in the left eye (LE); right eye (RE) is normal. **C and D:** In the late arteriovenous phase of fluorescein angiography, telangiectasia are more prominent on the temporal aspect of foveal avascular zone (FAZ), with prominent leakage of dye. Note the extramacular extension of the telangiectasia, which are also observed in the superotemporal midperiphery

TABLE 9.1: Differences between type1 and type 2 IMT

Feature	IMT Type 1	IMT Type 2
Mean age (years)	40	50–60
Sex	Males	No gender bias
Laterality	Unilateral	Bilateral
Clinical visibility	Obvious telangiectasia; exudates	Occult; graying of macula
Thickening (OCT)	Significant; common	Rare; atrophy common
Visual prognosis	Most lose vision if untreated	Most retain vision within 1–2 Snellen lines; unless neovascularization occurs
Leakage (FFA)	Significant; extra-macular also	Subtle; parafoveal
Treatability	Responds to Laser	Refractory to treatment

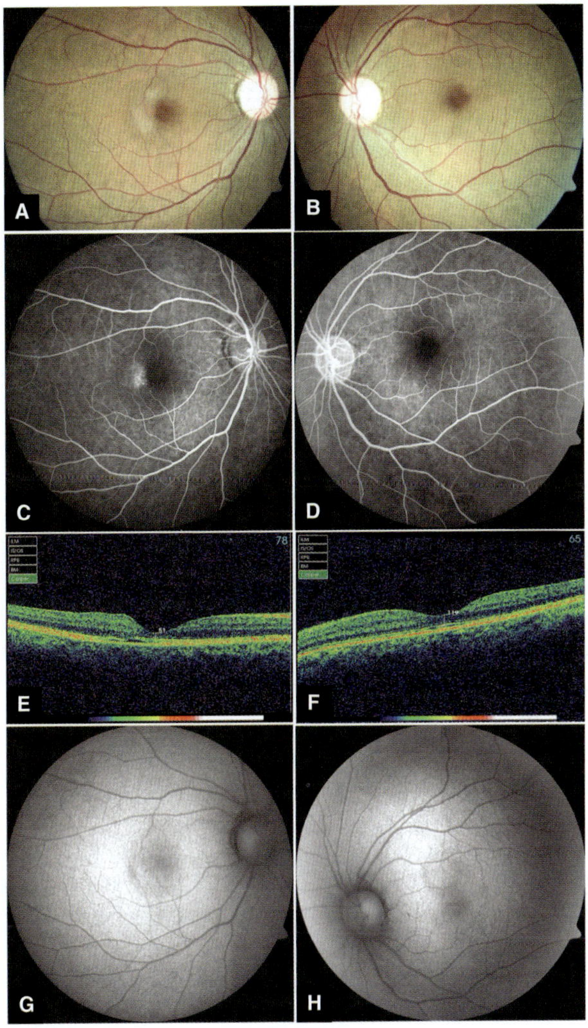

Figs 9.2A to H: Early stage of type 2 idiopathic macular telangiectasia (IMT2). **A:** RE shows gray opacification of central macula temporally. The visible microaneurysms and two dot hemorrhages temporal to gray area are secondary to background diabetic retinopathy. **B:** LE shows no evidence of IMT; only a few scattered drusen are visible. **C:** Late arteriovenous phase of FA clearly shows the temporal telangiectasia in RE, which are beginning to leak. **D:** Late phase FA shows no IMT in LE. **E:** Spectral domain OCT (SD-OCT, Topcon) shows foveal thinning (central thickness: 51μm) in RE and shallow subfoveal fluid (normal foveal thickness in Indian eyes is approximately 120-170μm). F: SD-OCT LE shows nearly normal foveal thickness and contours. **G and H:** Fundus autofluorescence study reveals increased signal (reduced masking of autofluorescence) from central macula (which is very dark in healthy eyes) in both the eyes, thus, confirming the presence of early IMT2 in LE, before it was detectable with either FA or OCT in LE

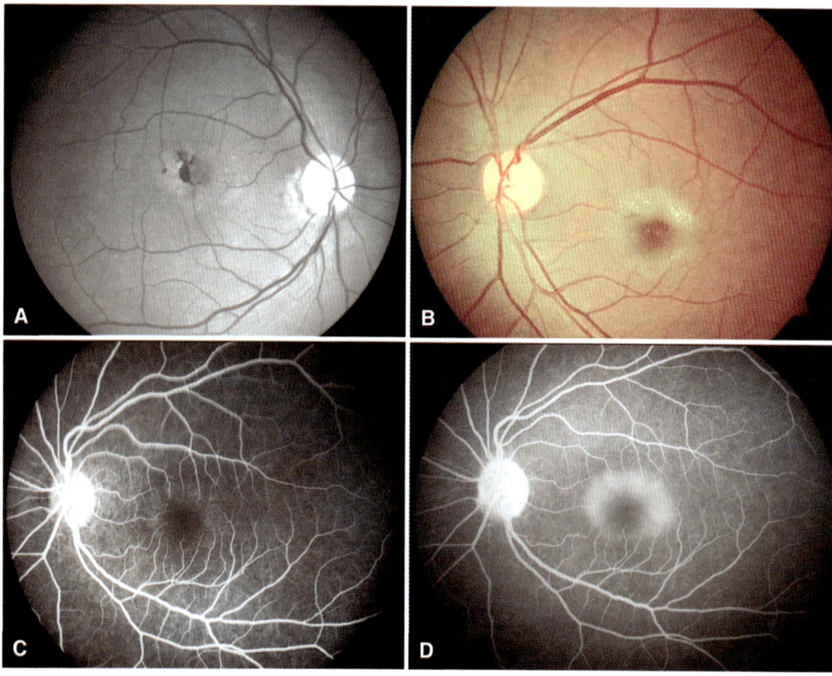

Figs 9.3A to D: Nonproliferative type 2 IMT: Showing other salient clinical features. **A and B:** RE shows a prominent stellate plaque of pigment migration at the temporal aspect of the gray ring. Temporal to the pigment plaque, a right-angled venule is seen descending from the superotemporal arcade. The venule dips backwards into deeper capillary plexus at right angle, hence the name. The vertical dip into retina appears as an abrupt termination of the venule, sometimes marked by a faint pigment, as seen here. A few crystalline deposits are also visible, more prominently in LE **C and D:** FA in midphase shows the telangiectasia, which are present 360^0 around FAZ in this eye. Late phase shows a soft leak from the telangiectasia, which is much fainter, compared to the leakage from type 1 IMT

and eliminate this misconception.[5] IMT, particularly type 2, is now widely known to be more common than previously believed; [6-8] Klein and colleagues recently estimated the prevalence of type 2 IMT to be 1 in 1000 in the large population-based Beaver Dam Study;[8] though according to MacTel study managers, this figure might also be an underestimation.[6]

Type 1 IMT was reported in less than a third of the cases series by Gass and Blodi.[2] It frequently results in a moderate visual loss due to cystoid macular edema, which, if untreated, generally results in progressive visual loss.[9] Type 2 IMT is more of an enigma: visual loss is almost invariable with onset of subretinal neovascularization (SRNV);[2,3,9] but the natural course of nonproliferative IMT is not clear. While Gass and Blodi averred that a gradual visual loss occurred due to foveal atrophy, it was not documented longitudinally in their case series. The later authors disagree on the extent and frequency of visual loss in IMT2.[10,11] We retrospectively analyzed 104 patients (203 eyes) with type 2 IMT, and found that the visual prognosis is not black-and-white.[12] While a gradual visual decline does occur in most patients, a majority (85%) maintain vision within 2 Snellen lines of the presentation. Most patients presenting with good vision (6/12 or better), retain it at least in one eye, irrespective of the development of SRNV, which occurs in only a minority (5%) of the eyes. The major cause for visual loss in our series was subfoveal pigment migration. But decline in visual acuity is not necessarily the only cause for patient's symptoms in type 2 IMT. Charbel Issa and colleagues have suggested that measurements of visual scotoma, metamorphopsia and near vision may be more sensitive parameters of visual dysfunction than visual acuity in these patients.[13,14]

Diagnostic Investigations

Gass and Blodi described fluorescein angiography (FA) as the key investigation,[2,3] and it remains the gold standard for diagnosis till date.[9] In type 1 IMT, FA reveals leakage from the clinically obvious telangiectasia, and also capillary dropouts and peripheral telangiectasia occasionally (Figs 9.1C and D). FA is more useful in type 2 IMT where it confirms the diagnosis in early or doubtful cases. In the earliest stage of IJFRT 2A described by Gass and Blodi, no visible lesion is seen in the macula while FA shows a characteristic though faint late leakage from the telangiectasia, most prominently at the temporal aspect of foveal avascular zone (FAZ); the telangiectasia themselves are not visible in the mid-arteriovenous phase.[3] In the later stages, the macula develops a gray opacification, sometimes in a bull'seye pattern. By this time, both the telangiectasia and their leakage are obvious (Figs 9.3C and D). When SRNV is present, its intense leakage is super-imposed over the faint leakage of the telangiectasia (Fig.9.4).[2,3,9-12]

Optical coherence tomography (OCT) has become the second most favored tool for diagnosis of IMT after FA. In type 1 IMT, OCT only shows what is obvious on biomicroscopy and angiography: macular thickening.[9]In type 2 IMT, however, OCT reveals tell-tale features, which though not pathognomonic, are very helpful in clinching the diagnosis. The most dramatic OCT feature of IMT 2 is foveal atrophy, which is completely in contrast to the angiographic leakage, and the expected macular thickening (Figs 9.2E and 9.4C).[9,12,15] The second most common feature is foveal outer lamellar splitting (Fig. 9.4C), which like foveal atrophy, can also be observed in several other conditions, but helps in diagnosis in combination with other clinical features and FA.[9,15]

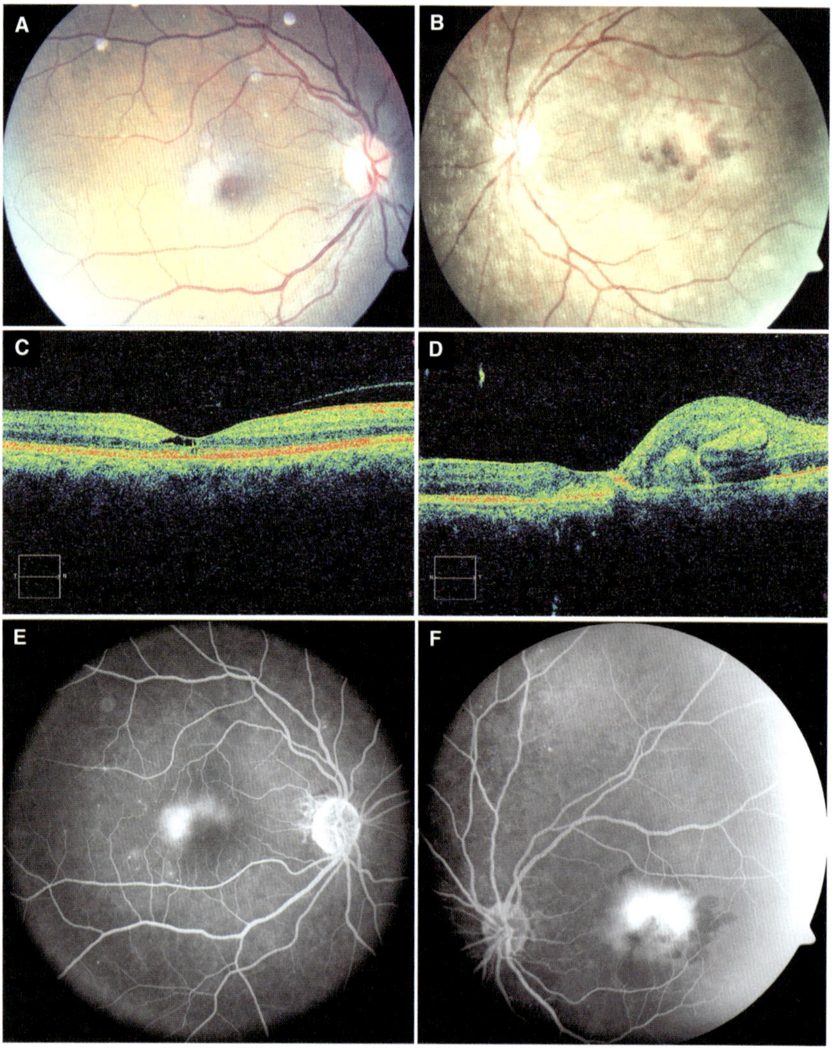

Figs 9.4A to F: Proliferative type 2 IMT. **A:** This diabetic patient shows a gray sheen in RE due to nonproliferative IMT with diabetic retinopathy manifesting as numerous microaneurysms. It is critical but easy to differentiate IMT from diabetic macular edema, as no thickening or hard exudates are visible clinically or on OCT (see Fig. 9.4C). **B:** LE shows asteroid hyalosis, which clouds the view of a large subretinal neovascularization above and temporal to the central macula. **C:** SD-OCT (Cirrus) dramatically differentiates IMT2 from diabetic macular edema, by revealing foveal atrophy (thinning) rather than thickening. Also note the lamellar splitting in inner and outer fovea, characteristic of IMT2. **D:** Horizontal OCT in LE reveals a large intra- and subretinal neovascular membrane with parafoveal edema encroaching temporal fovea. **E and F:** Late phase FA reveals background microaneurysms and soft leakage from telangiectasia in both eyes. Note the intense leak from superotemporal SRNV superimposed over the faint capillary leak in LE. The extravasated blood blocks fluorescence.

Fundus autofluorescence (FAF) is a well-known phenomenon, but has recently re-emerged as a diagnostic tool with the use of Confocal Scanning Laser Ophthalmoscopy (CSLO) to optimize the low intensity autofluorescence image of the fundus. FAF measures the accumulation of lipofuscin (a metabolic residue of relentless phagocytosis and aging of the retinal pigment epithelium) in the fundus, a common sequel of several degenerative diseases of the outer retina and retinal pigment epithelium.[16] Increased FAF signal from fovea, apparently due to loss of luteal pigment, is now considered one of the earliest (earlier than the subclinical late FA leakage as mentioned above) and most sensitive and specific sign of IMT2 (Figs 9.2B,D,F, and H).[6]

Fundus microperimetry has already been used to plot central scotomas in IMT2;[14] adaptive optics imaging was recently super-imposed on SLO to measure cone density,[17] and another CSLO based tool; confocal blue-reflectance imaging has been suggested as a possible noninvasive alternative to FA in type 2 IMT.[18] As technology continues to improve, imaging for IMT2 is likely to become completely noninvasive, and yet more diagnostic and predictive of the disease outcome.

Differential Diagnosis

Many common retinal conditions mimic IMT1, which include branch retinal vein occlusion, retinal arterial macroaneurysm, and radiation retinopathy. The patient demographics, systemic evaluation and history, and Coats' like clinical features generally exclude secondary causes of retinal telangiectasia. The differential diagnosis of IMT2 is more interesting; it includes not only vascular but degenerative conditions also. Diabetic maculopathy needs to be frequently differentiated from IMT2 in a diabetic patient (Figs 9.4A, C, and E). In our experience, the most common conditions which mimic IMT2 include heredomacular degenerations causing bull's eye appearance and central serous chorioretinopathy in young patients, and age-related macular degeneration in the older age group, particularly when associated with SRNV. Less common conditions are those causing crystal deposition in the posterior pole, including Tamoxifen retinopathy and Bietti's crystalline dystrophy. In such scenarios, FA and OCT, along with clinical evaluation, are sufficient to arrive at the diagnosis without subjecting the patient to electrophysiological tests and perimetry.

Pathophysiology and Systemic Associations

Type 1 and 2 IMT appear to be different diseases. While IMT1 is characterized by a vascular pathology driving the disease course, IMT2 now appears to be essentially a degenerative disease, primarily affecting the neural retina; vascular pathology merely adding to the disease manifestations. Though IMT2 was initially described by Gass and Blodi as a perifoveal capillary disease,[3] Gass, with his keen understanding and foresight, subsequently pointed out that IMT2 was not a disease of dilated leaky blood vessels. The central visual loss due to photoreceptor atrophy (which he diagnosed without the benefit of OCT) and the absence of cystoid macular edema suggested that the primary pathology lay in perifoveal neural cells or Muller cells.[19] Gass explained the disease progression by suggesting that the dilatation, remodeling and proliferation of the outer retinal capillary plexus were associated with capillary invasion of the outer retina, resulting in photoreceptor atrophy. This was followed by pigment migration into the inner retina, and finally, development of the intraretinal neovascularization into subretinal space.[19] Thus, Gass suggested that in IMT2 (as in retinal angiomatous proliferation), the neovascularization originated from the retina rather than from choroid (Figs 9.4B,D, and F). This pattern of neovascularization was later called as type 3 neovascularization by Yannuzzi,[20]and is the reason why the classification of SRNV in IMT 2 as classic and occult may be futile.[12]

Gass' suspicion of Muller cell dysfunction plays a major role in pathogenesis was supported by a recent report on the immunohistochemistry of IMT2.[21] This report also confirmed the loss of macular pigment in IMT2, which was already demonstrated by noninvasive investigations like FAF (Figs 9.2G, and H) and confocal blue-reflectance imaging, supporting the concept of IMT2 as a degenerative disease of the outer retina and RPE.

Another pathogenetic aspect of IMT2 was highlighted by the early histopathological report of Eliassi-Rad and Green, who demonstrated changes similar to diabetes in perifoveal capillaries: basement membrane thickening, loss of pericytes and capillary endothelial degeneration.[22] Though systemic vascular diseases like diabetes and hypertension are not causally related to IMT 2, we and other investigators, including MacTel study, found these systemic associations in more than half of the patients.[7,12] Other systemic associations of IMT 2 include genetic susceptibility (mainly ATM gene dysfunction) which was observed in 26–57% European subjects. It is suggested that ATM gene causes impaired tolerance to oxidative stress and compromises DNA repair, leading to retinal telangiectasia.[23]

Treatment of IMT

Type 1 IMT results in visual loss due to cystoid macular edema, and treatment, therefore, consists of laser photocoagulation to the obvious capillary abnormalities. However, spontaneous improvement has also been described.[2,3,9,10] Intravitreal injection of triamcinolone acetonide is also an option; but macular edema can rebound, and therefore not as useful.[9] Anti-vascular endothelial growth factor (VEGF) antibodies, mainly bevacizumab, have been reported to produce no visual or anatomical benefit in IMT1.[24]

Most interventional studies have focused on type 2 IMT. Since over 80% of eyes which develop SRNV in IMT2 end up with a vision of 6/60 or less,[25]therefore, the proliferative stage should always be treated. However, treatment of nonproliferative IMT2 has also been attempted by several authors, mostly without success; no treatment has been shown to prevent disease progression.[6] While intravitreal triamcinolone is not helpful,[26] laser photocoagulation may actually harm by inducing subretinal neovascularization.[9] Anti-VEGF treatments have also failed almost universally,[27-29] though a recent small case series showed visual and anatomical improvement in presence of subfoveal neural detachment.[30] A role of antioxidant supplementation has also been suggested.[9]

SRNV in IMT2 has been treated with transpupillary thermotherapy (TTT), photodynamic therapy (PDT) and anti-VEGF agents, either alone or in combination. Since the neovascularization starts intraretinally (type 3), surgical removal is contraindicated.[9] We have reported stabilization of vision and regression of neovascularization in over 90% of our 13 patients (14 eyes) with SRNV in IMT2 with TTT; achieved with a single treatment session in 85% eyes.[31] Similar results have been reported in a smaller series (7 eyes) and with more sessions (2.4) with PDT: 5 stabilized, one improved and one declined with SRNV regression in all eyes.[32] The advantage of anti-VEGF agents lies in their ability to improve vision in some cases. In the largest and most recent case series of 9 eyes, vision improved in 3 eyes, and was stable in 4 eyes with 2.2 injections of bevacizumab: a definite improvement over the results with TTT or PDT. SRNV was found to be regressed in 8 eyes out of 9.[28]

It may be concluded that IMT1 typically requires treatment with conventional photocoagulation, particularly when progressive visual loss due to macular edema is observed. IMT2 is usually refractory to treatment at nonproliferative stage. SRNV definitely requires treatment: though definite conclusions about choice of treatment cannot be drawn based on current evidence; anti-VEGF agents, particularly bevacizumab, appear to obtain the best outcomes, PDT or TTT may be added in cases refractory to standalone anti-VEGF treatment.

Summary

IMT is a subtle yet not uncommon condition, which closely resembles several other common vascular and degenerative macular diseases. The complexity and urgency of diagnosis are increased by the coincidence of diabetes, and the subsequent confusion with diabetic macular edema. While photocoagulation remains the gold standard for the treatment of diabetic macular edema, it is actually harmful in IMT2. Similarly, familiarity with IMT can avoid unnecessary investigations for heredomacular degenerations as well. We now have a working knowledge of visual prognosis of IMT2, the most common, but ironically the most underdiagnosed and misdiagnosed type of IMT. One can reassure most patients that they are likely to retain good vision in at least one eye for 2–3 years, and neovascular complications develop only in a minority of the patients. Final and long-term answers about the natural history, prognosis, histopathology, genetics and potential treatments of IMT will hopefully soon be available from the MacTel study, which comprises more than 30 centers in Europe, USA, Israel and Australia, with 400 participants enrolled since 2005, and which has just about begun to publish its findings.[5-7]

References

1. Reese AB. Telangiectasis of the retina and Coats' disease. *Am J Ophthalmol.* 1956;42:1-8.
2. Gass JD, Oyakawa RT. Idiopathic juxtafoveolar retinal telangiectasis. *Arch Ophthalmol.* 1982;100:769-80.
3. Gass JDM, Blodi BA. Idiopathic juxtafoveolar retinal telangiectasis: update of classification and follow-up study. *Ophthalmology.* 1993;1536-46.
4. Yannuzi JA, Bardal AMC, Freund KB, et al. Idiopathic macular telangiectasia. *Arch Ophthalmol.* 2006;124:450-460.
5. MacTel website https://secure.emmes.com/emmesweb/projects/mactel-0 (Accessed 16 Jul 2010)
6. Gillies MC. Progress report: the MacTel project. *Retina Today.* 2010;5: 35-37.
7. Clemons TE, Gillies MC, Chew EY, et al. Baseline characteristics of participants in the natural history study of macular telangiectasia (MacTel): MacTel Project Report No. 2. *Ophthalmic Epidemiol.* 2010;17:66-73.
8. Klein R, Blodi BA, Meuer SM, et al. The prevalence of macular telangiectasia type 2 in the Beaver Dam eye study. *Am J Ophthalmol.* 2010;150:55-62.
9. Charbel Issa P, Scholl HPN, Helb HM, et al. Macular telangiectasia. In: Holz FG, Spaide RF (eds) Medical retina. Springer: Heidelberg 2007:183-97.
10. Chew EY. Parafoveal telangiectasis. In: Ryan SJ, Hinton DR, Schachat AP, Wilkinson CP, eds. Retina. 4th ed. vol 2. Philadelphia: Elsevier; 2006:1409-15.
11. Watzke RC, Klein ML, Folk JC, et al. Long term juxtafoveal retinal telangiectasia. *Retina.* 2005;25:727-35.
12. Shukla D, Gupta SR, Neelakantan N, et al. Type 2 Idiopathic Macular telangiectasia: long term visual prognosis and incidence of subretinal neovascularization. Retina (in press).
13. Charbel Issa P, Holz FG, Scholl HP. Metamorphopsia in patients with macular telangiectasia type 2. *Doc Ophthalmol.* 2009;119:133-40.

14. Charbel Issa P, Helb HM, Rohrschneider K, et al. Microperimetric assessment of patients with type 2 idiopathic macular telangiectasia. *Invest Ophthalmol Vis Sci*. 2007;48:3788-95.
15. Cohen SM, Cohen ML, El-Jabali F, et al. Optical coherence tomography findings in nonproliferative group 2A idiopathic juxtafoveal retinal telangiectasis. *Retina*. 2007;27:59-66.
16. Schmitz-Valckenberg S, Holz FG, Bird AC, et al. Fundus autofluorescence imaging: review and perspectives. *Retina*. 2008;28:385-409.
17. Ooto S, Hangai M, Takayama K, et al. High-resolution photoreceptor imaging in idiopathic macular telangiectasia type 2 using adaptive optics scanning laser ophthalmoscopy. *Invest Ophthalmol Vis Sci*. 2011;52:5541-50.
18. Charbel Issa P, Berendschot TT, Staurenghi G, et al. Confocal blue reflectance imaging in type 2 idiopathic macular telangiectasia. *Invest Ophthalmol Vis Sci*. 2008;49:1172-77.
19. Gass JD. Histopathologic study of presumed parafoveal telangiectasis. *Retina*. 2000;20:226-27.
20. Yannuzzi LA, Freund KB, Takahashi BS. Review of retinal angiomatous proliferation or type 3 neovascularization. *Retina*. 2008;28:375-84.
21. Powner MB, Gillies MC, Tretiach M, et al. Perifoveal müller cell depletion in a case of macular telangiectasia type 2. *Ophthalmology*. 2010;117:2407-16.
22. Eliassi-Rad B, Green WR. Histopathologic study of presumed parafoveal telangiectasis. *Retina*. 1999;19:332-35.
23. Barbazetto IA, Room M, Yannuzzi NA, et al. ATM gene variants in patients with idiopathic perifoveal telangiectasia. *Invest Ophthalmol Vis Sci*. 2008;49: 3806-11.
24. Takayama K, Ooto S, Tamura H, et al. Intravitreal bevacizumab for type 1 idiopathic macular telangiectasia. Eye 2010;24:1492-97.
25. Engelbrecht NE, Aaberg TM Jr., Sung J, et al. Neovascular membranes associated with idiopathic juxtafoveolar telangiectasis. *Arch Ophthalmol*. 2002;120: 320-24.
26. Wu L, Evans T, Arévalo JF, Berrocal MH, Rodríguez FJ, Hsu M, Sánchez JG. Long-term effect of intravitreal triamcinolone in the nonproliferative stage of type II idiopathic parafoveal telangiectasia. *Retina*. 2008; 28:314-19.
27. Charbel Issa P, Finger RP, Kruse K, Baumüller S, Scholl HP, Holz FG. Monthly ranibizumab for nonproliferative macular telangiectasia type 2: a 12-month prospective study. *Am J Ophthalmol*. 2011;151:876-86.
28. Roller AB, Folk JC, Patel NM, et al. Intravitreal bevacizumab for treatment of proliferative and nonproliferative type 2 idiopathic macular telangiectasia. *Retina*. 2011 May 21. [Epub ahead of print]
29. Matt G, Sacu S, Ahlers C,et al. Thirty-month follow-up after intravitreal bevacizumab in progressive idiopathic macular telangiectasia type 2. *Eye*. 2010;24: 1535-41.
30. Lira RP, Silva VB, Cavalcanti TM, de Souza AC, Pinto AP. Intravitreous ranibizumab as treatment for macular telangiectasia type 2. *Arch Ophthalmol*. 2010;128:75-1078.
31. Shukla D, Singh J, Kolluru CM, et al. Transpupillary thermotherapy for subfoveal neovascularization secondary to group 2A idiopathic juxtafoveolar telangiectasis. *Am J Ophthalmol*. 2004;138:147-49.
32. Potter MJ, Szabo SM, Sarraf D, et al. Photodynamic therapy for subretinal neovascularization in type 2A idiopathic juxtafoveolar telangiectasis. *Can J Ophthalmol*. 2006;41:34-37.

10

chapter

Deependra Vikram Singh
Yog Raj Sharma

Recent Advances in Management of Retinal Vascular Occlusions

ABSTRACT

Retinal vein occlusion (RVO) is second most common medical retinal disorder seen by ophthalmologists in clinical practice. Vast advancements have been made in the field of diagnosis, management and understanding pathogenesis of RVO over last decade. The major advancements have been the availability of OCT for macular assessment and anti-VEGF therapies. Also the newer modalities like laser anasmosis, arteriovenous sheathotomy, radial optic neurotomy, and isovolemic hemodilution have been introduced and tested. The chapter intends to provide a brief synopsis of such advancements for both residents and retina experts.

Introduction

Retinal vein occlusion (RVO) is one of the most common causes of acquired retinal vascular abnormality in adults and a frequent cause of visual loss. There are few data on the prevalence of RVO in the general population, with current estimates derived largely from studies in white populations.[1-3] However, a recently published pooled analysis from 11 major studies from United States, Europe, Asia, and Australia has found the incidence of branch retinal vascular occlusion (BRVO) to be 4.4 per 1000 persons and 0.8 per 1000 persons for central retinal vein occlusion (CRVO) in general population.[4] The prevalence of RVO was similar between men and women, and increased with age. The prevalence of BRVO was highest in Asians and Hispanics and lowest in whites.

This chapter will focus on recent advances in management of RVO observed over last decade. Such discussion can be initiated only after

TABLE 11.1: Objectives, eligibility and visual results of BVOS and CVOS

BVOS study[5,6]	CVOS study[7-9]
Evaluated Argon Laser photocoagulation for treatment of BRVO patients having BCVA from 20/40 to 20/200. 139 eyes studied. • To determine whether scatter argon laser photocoagulation can prevent the development of neovascularization • To determine whether peripheral scatter argon laser photocoagulation can prevent vitreous hemorrhage • To determine whether macular argon laser photocoagulation can improve visual acuity in eyes with macular oedema reducing vision to 20/40 or worse.	Multi-center, randomized, controlled clinical trial designed to answer the following three questions: • To determine whether photocoagulation therapy can help prevent iris neovascularization in eyes with central vein occlusion (CVO) and evidence of ischemic retina • To assess whether grid-pattern photocoagulation therapy will reduce loss of central visual acuity due to macular edema secondary to CVO • To develop new data base describing the course and prognosis for eyes with CVO.

understanding pathogenesis of RVO and a brief reference to two major studies (Table 10.1) for BRVO and CRVO.[5-9]

Pathogenesis

Despite being grouped together, BRVO and CRVO differ significantly in the etiology, pathogenesis, natural course and management.

BRANCH RETINAL VEIN OCCLUSION

The BRVO is considered to be the result of age-related arteriosclerosis of retinal arteriole compressing the retinal venule at A-V crossing where they share a common sheath. Once the occlusion occurs, increased vascular pressure behind the occlusion may lead to leakage of fluid and small molecules across the vascular wall and into the surrounding retinal tissue, resulting in local edema. Vitreous traction may facilitate the development of cystoid macular edema (CME). In addition, vascular endothelial damage to the affected vein may induce low-grade, chronic inflammation of the retinal microvasculature and up regulation of inflammatory mediators. These mediators include prostaglandins, leukotrienes, intercellular adhesion molecule-1 (ICAM-1), integrins, tumor necrosis factor-α and vascular endothelial growth factor (VEGF).[10] Many of these cytokines weaken the blood-retina barrier and perpetuate CME. Late onset retinal ischemia leads to neovascularization and recurrent vitreous hemorrhage and tractional retinal detachments. Long-standing macular edema from BRVO can also lead to formation of large cysts and inner lamellar or full thickness macular hole.

CENTRAL RETINAL VEIN OCCLUSION

Pathogenesis of CRVO is poorly understood and is believed to be multifactorial. Most hypotheses revolve around the combination of factors causing external compression on optic nerve and/or central retinal vein along with hematological factors promoting venous stasis and increased coagulability resulting in obstruction of central retinal vein posterior to lamina cribrosa. Increased intravascular pressure proximal to the resultant central retinal venous occlusion contributes to fluid leakage into the retina, resulting in retinal edema. Vision loss from CRVO is usually due to CME, ischemic maculopathy, capillary nonperfusion, posterior segment neovascularization, vitreous hemorrhage, anterior segment neovascularization (iris or angle), and neovascular glaucoma (NVG). Chronic CME can lead to pigmentary degeneration and photoreceptor loss with a permanent central scotoma. The common site of neovascularization is the anterior segment but it can also occur in the posterior segment (e.g., optic nerve, retina). The risk of neovascularization increases with the degree of retinal ischemia. Anterior segment neovascularization and NVG is most likely to develop during the first few months after the occlusion (100 days glaucoma).

The argon laser treatment was evaluated in BVOS and CVOS with special reference to eligibility criteria, prevention of vascularization, and visual recovery (Table 10.1)

Recent Advances in the Management of RVO

The management of RVO has witnessed paradigm shifts after two major advancements in the field of medical retina. First is the availability of optical coherence tomography (OCT) and second is intravitreal injections. Table 11.3 summarizes the major advancements that will be discussed in this section.

Epidemiology

NATURAL COURSE OF CRVO

In evidence based analysis, McIntosh et al reviewed 53 studies with data from 3,271 eyes with CRVO and found that most eyes had visual acuity less than 20/40 at base line.[11] Although 6 studies reported an improvement in VA, none of these improvements resulted in VA better than 20/40. Up to 34% of eyes with nonischemic CRVO converted to ischemic CRVO over a 3-year period. In ischemic CRVO cases, neovascular glaucoma developed in at least 23% of eyes within 15 months. In nonischemic CRVO cases, macular edema resolved in approximately 30% of eyes over time, and subsequent neovascular glaucoma was rare. The most accepted definition of ischemic CRVO was presence of at least 10 disk areas of capillary nonperfusion on fundus fluorescein angiography. In his retrospective analysis of 66 eyes with CRVO Harey et al found that among the nonischemic eyes with initial visual acuity of 20/70 or worse, 59% improved, 27% showed no change, and 14% deteriorated on resolution of macular edema, whereas in ischemic CRVO, 41% improved, 41% did not change, and 18% deteriorated.[12] While the authors have highlighted the importance of differentiating ischemic from nonischemic CRVO, they have also stressed the limitation of FFA in indentifying all ischemic cases. Therefore, they have suggested use of functional tests like, relative afferent pupillary defect, electroretinography, visual acuity, and peripheral visual fields to assist categorization of CRVO cases.

NATURAL COURSE OF BRVO

Although the natural course of BRVO is much more favorable than CRVO, untreated BRVO patients can develop irreversible loss of vision from vitreous hemorrhage, traction retinal detachments and persisting macular edema and traction. Also the patients with BRVO are more likely to suffer from carotid artery obstruction and atherosclerosis. A large volume of data on natural course of BRVO is still missing from literature.

Diagnosis

OPTICAL COHERENCE TOMOGRAPHY

Availability of time domain and spectral domain OCTs has revolutionized the management of many retinal diseases including RVO. Because OCT imaging is a noncontact procedure and the infrared measurement beam is barely perceived by the test subject, testing is well tolerated by patients. The rapid acquisition time of OCT permits multiple images to be acquired simultaneously with different cross-sectional image planes, providing a comprehensive assessment of the macula. Optical coherence tomography provides information that complements information supplied by fundus photography and fluorescein angiography. By allowing direct visualization of retinal pathology on a morphologic level, OCT can be used for initial diagnosis and providing guidelines for management decisions. The advent of new pharmacologic therapies for the treatment of retinal diseases such as macular edema and choroidal neovascularization has enhanced the utility of OCT as a means of determining the therapeutic anatomic response.

Currently, most clinical trials that are evaluating retinal treatments use OCT response as a secondary outcome. Traditionally, BVOS recommended no intervention for macular edema in BRVO till BCVA is better than 20/60; however, a large number of macular BRVO patients are found to have significant macular edema and cystoid changes on OCT with BCVA better than 20/60. Such patients are now frequently offered treatments to prevent further visual loss and restore the macular function earlier rather than waiting for BCVA to drop below 20/60. Figure 10.1 shows a similar case where a macular BRVO patient was treated for macular edema and BCVA of 20/40. OCT has become an excellent non invasive tool for serial follow-up of such patients, especially when macular edema shows recurrences. OCT allows detection, evaluation and documentation of any vitreomacular traction associated with macular edema in BRVO patients. These patients can be counseled for possibility of vitreous surgery in future and also about the chances of worsening with laser photocoagulation. Although rare, a spontaneous posterior vitreous detachment can sometimes lead to improvement in such patients. The same can be confirmed with OCT. Figure 10.2 shows an example of such case. OCT can precisely outline the extent of involvement by macular edema. The cases showing no foveal involvement can be safely observed with serial OCTs and subjected to peripheral scatter photocoagulation on development of retinal ischemia. Figure 10.3 shows an example of such case.

In CRVO, OCT is again very helpful in detecting and quantifying macular edema. The resolution of macular edema and its recurrence is also nicely depicted on serial macular scans. Figure 10.4 shows OCT scans of an ischemic CRVO with macular edema before and after the anti-VEGF injections. Late cases show thinning of retina suggestive of loss of NFL and photoreceptors.

Systemic Work-up

ROLE OF ATHEROSCLEROSIS

A large number of studies have found a higher risk of atherosclerosis in RVO patients.[3,13] In a recent meta-analysis of 21 observational studies including 2,915 patients with RVO, O'Mahoney et al evaluated the role of 3 major risk factors of atherosclerosis in RVO patients.[13] They observed a more than 3.5-times higher risk of RVO in cases with systemic hypertension. About 2.5 times higher risk of RVO was associated with hyperlipidemia, but there was only a modest correlation between RVO and the presence of diabetes mellitus.

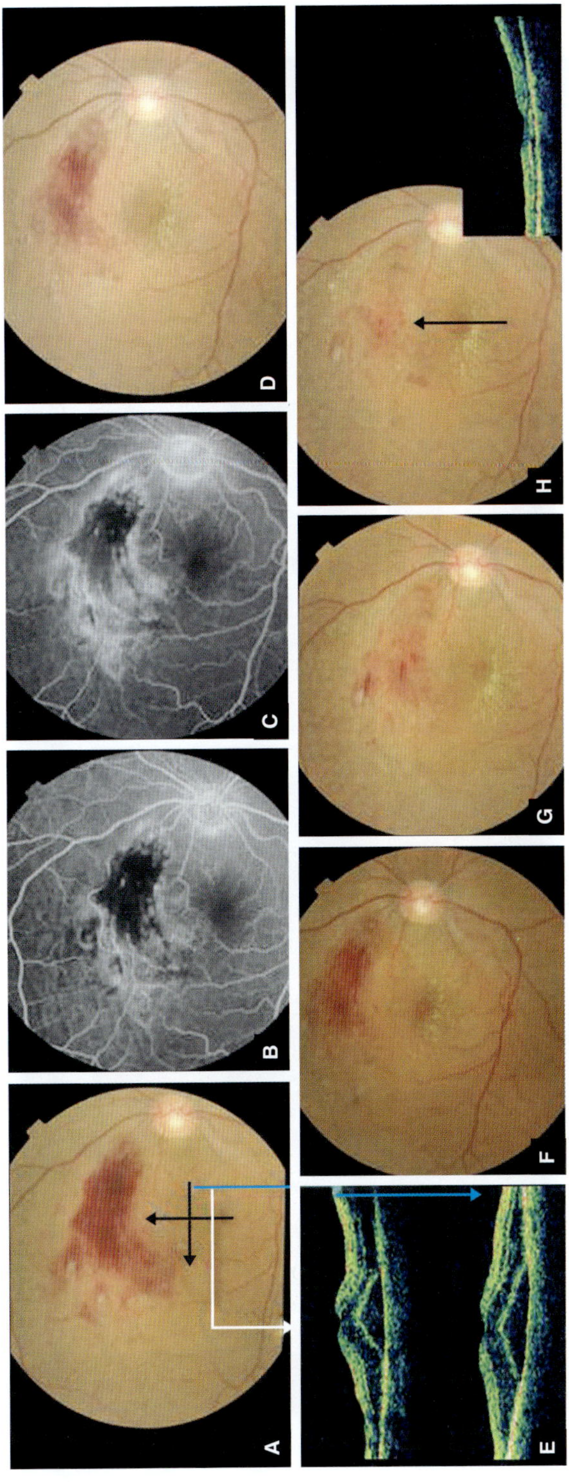

Figs 10.1A to H: Serial fundus photographs and OCT of a 60-year female with macular BRVO. Color and FFA photographs (A to C) are showing ischemia and retinal edema. OCT scans (D) showing foveal involvement by macular edema and subretinal fluid. Serial photographs (E to H) showing improvement after 2 intravitreal Ranibizumab injections at 1, 2, 3 and 6 months

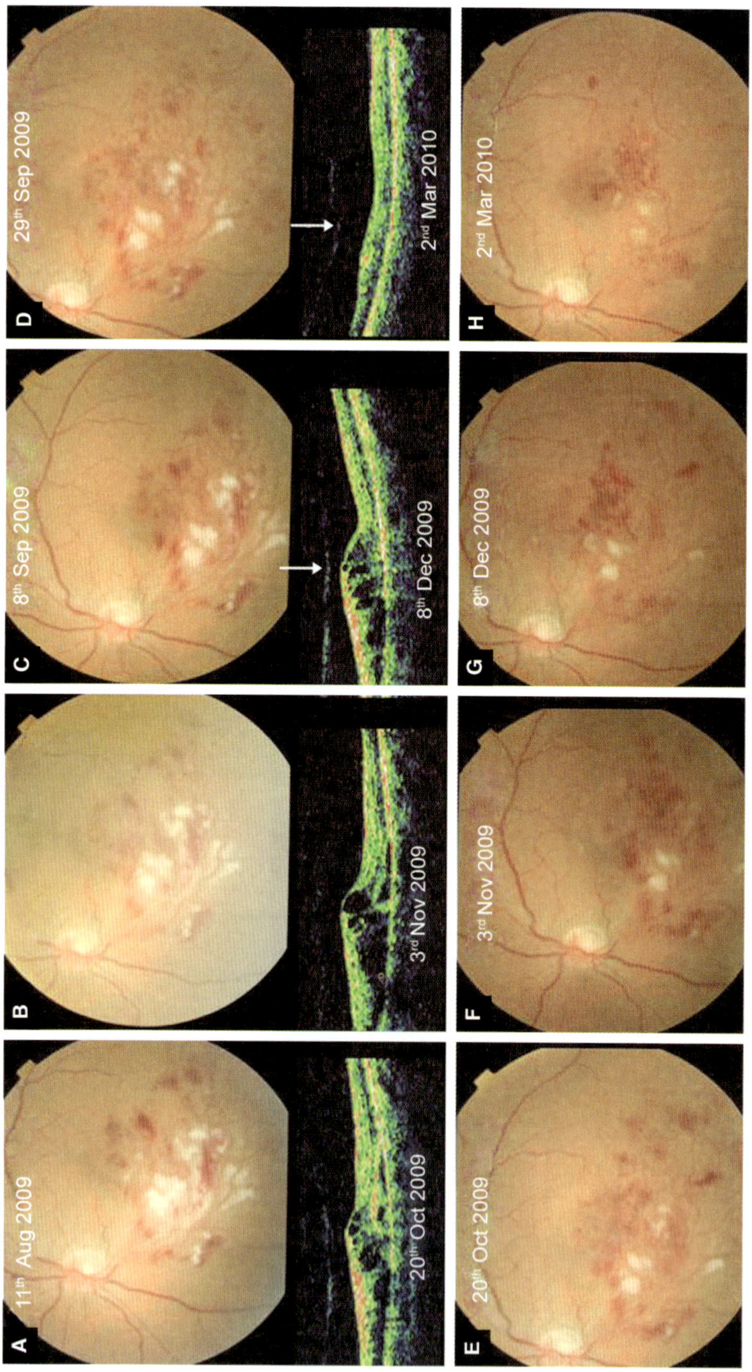

Figs 10.2A to H: Serial fundus photographs and OCT of a 45 year female with inferiotemporal BRVO, and showing resolution following 2 bevacizumab injections and spontaneous posterior vitreous detachment (white arrow)

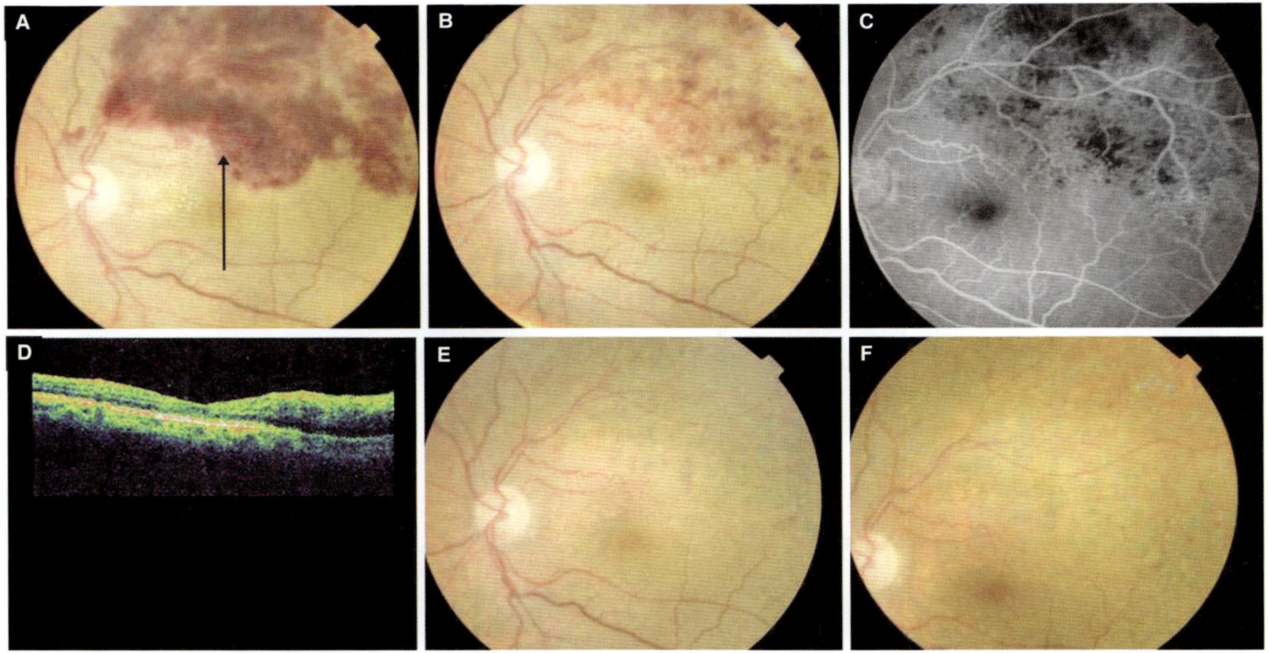

Figs 10.3A to F: Serial fundus photographs of an 80 years female with superotemporal BRVO. Fundus photographs (A and B) showing retinal edema not involving macula confirmed on OCT. Fundus fluorescein angiography photographs (C and D) done at 3 months after hemorrhages were resolved show ischemia and collaterals. Fundus photographs (E and F) showing resolved retinal edema and laser marks at 6 months follow-up (E) and 9 months follow-up (F)

ASSOCIATION WITH CAROTID ARTERY OBSTRUCTION

Carotid artery changes have been regarded as an important indicator of the extent of systemic atherosclerosis.[14,15] Brown et al[16] and Green et al[17] have demonstrated, some association between presence of carotid lesions and the pathogenesis of ischemic RVO, using digital subtraction angiography and histopathologic analysis, respectively. With recent advances and wide application of ultrasonographic examinations, carotid artery evaluation is being conducted as a simple and non-invasive procedure and is encountered more commonly even in routine clinical ophthalmology. In a recent study of patients with RVO, carotid artery evaluation was done on 58 eyes of 57 patients aged between 51 years and 88 years to investigate the relationship between RVO and carotid artery lesions.[18] Thirty-nine patients (40 eyes) had CRVO, and 18 patients (18 eyes) had BRVO. It is further demonstrated that the prevalence of plaques in the carotid artery was 49% among CRVO patients older than 50 years of age; the prevalence among those older than 70 years of age was significantly higher than that among individuals of similar age who attended the examination center (controls). Clinical characteristics of CRVO patients with carotid lesions in the present study included a significantly higher frequency (79%) of the ischemic type shown by fluorescein angiography. Compared with 49% of CRVO cases, only

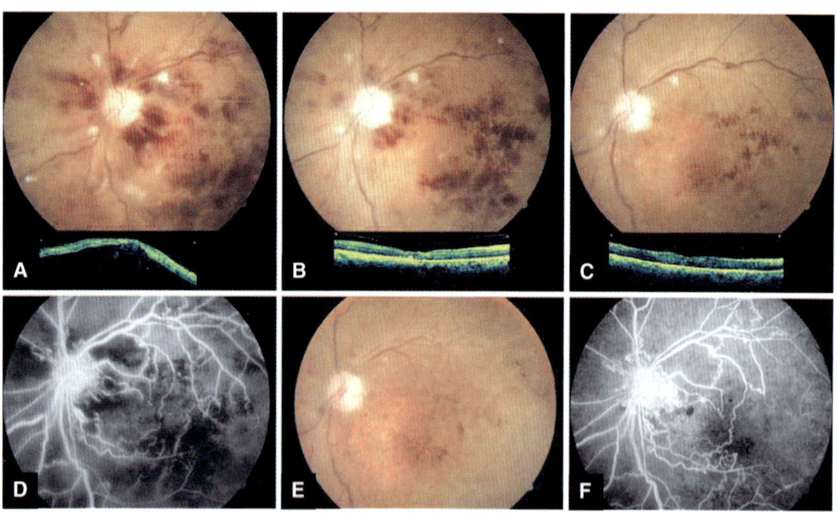

Figs 10.4A to F: Fundus, FFA photographs of 85 years old male with ischemic CRVO.

Serial pictures at 1month (B), 3 months (C) and 6 months (E) showing resolution of macular edema and hemorrhages but worsening retinal ischemia in spite of monthly bevacizumab injections.

22% of BRVO cases had a plaque in the carotid artery, showing a lower prevalence of carotid lesions in BRVO although there was no significant difference.

ROLE OF LABORATORY INVESTIGATIONS IN YOUNG PATIENTS

Changes in the blood vessel wall, changes in the blood flow, and changes in blood coagulability are known as *Virchow's triad*. These interrelated factors have been known to be responsible for the formation of thrombi in blood vessels as described by Virchow in the nineteenth century. Increased blood viscosity, Factor V Leiden, hyperhomocysteinemia, and protein C or S deficiency have been considered to play a role in the development of CRVO.[19-22] There are certain acquired hypercoagulable states also, including elevated antiphospholipid antibodies (AP-Abs; lupus anticoagulant [LA] and anticardiolipin antibodies [ACAs]). Lahey et al investigated whether hypercoagulability plays a role in thrombus formation in patients with central retinal vein occlusion (CRVO) who are less than 56 years of age.[23] Fifty-five patients with CRVO less than 56 years old (mean age, 44 years) underwent laboratory evaluation for homocysteine, activated protein C resistance, protein C activity, protein S activity, antithrombin III activity, antiphospholipid antibodies, and anticardiolipin antibodies. The results were compared with previously drawn age-matched control groups obtained by the same laboratory for statistical significance. Twenty-seven percent CRVO patients had one positive test result suggesting hypercoagulability. Compared with the control groups, these patients less than 56 years old with CRVO had a higher incidence of coagulation abnormalities by laboratory testing. Among the parameters tested, Hyperhomocysteinemia and circulating antiphospholipid antibodies were significantly more common in the CRVO patients ($P < 0.05$) compared with age-matched controls. Another useful data comes from a meta-analysis of thrombophilic risk factors that found only elevated homocysteine and anticardiolipin antibodies to be associated with CRVO.[24] A recent large case-control study, however, found no association between CRVO and thrombophilic risk factors, including homocysteine levels and anticardiolipin antibodies.[25] Recurrent CRVO has also been reported with elevated homocysteine in one study, but associations with anticardiolipin antibodies and factor V Leiden were not identified as risk factors in a multivariate study comparing patients with recurrent CRVO to those with one CRVO.[26] In view of contradictory results the need for further evaluation of the role of hypercoagulability states in RVO cannot be over emphasized.

Interventions for RVO

The conventional management of RVO as outline by BVOS and CVOS studies has been discussed elsewhere and a brief reference is provided in Table 10.1 and 10.2. While grid and sectoral scatter photocoagulation has been quite rewarding for BRVO, the CRVO continues to carry very poor visual prognosis and conventional management is far from satisfactory. The high incidence of severe vision loss associated with CRVO has prompted many researchers to explore a number of new strategies for its management. The focus of these interventions is on 2 major issues:

1. Treatment of recurrent macular edema and resulting photoreceptor loss.
2. Reversal of retinal ischemia by either promoting collaterals, or bypassing the occluding vein, or by suppressing the overactive thrombotic mechanisms.

INTRAVITREAL STEROIDS

Although the safety of intravitreal trimamcinolone acetonide (IVTA) is known since as early as 1981,[27] its wider clinical use for macular edema started only a decade back after more studies on safety and efficacy in patients with uveitis and diabetic macular edema became available.[28,29] Since TA was found to have antiangiogenic, antiproliferative and antiedematous effects its use for macular edema from CRVO started in 2002 with large number of reports describing treatment benefit from intravitreal triamcinolone in terms of visual acuity and macular edema.[30-34] IVTA was used in doses of 4 mg, 2mg and 1 mg. However, all studies found the visual benefits to be transient and lasting for 6 months maximum and a high incidence of side effects like rising intraocular pressure (IOP), cataract formation and endophthalmitis. The need to have larger studies on steroid use in macular edema was felt.[35] Finally to explore the role of IVTA in management of RVO, The Standard Care versus Corticosteroid for Retinal Vein Occlusion (SCORE) study, sponsored by the National Institutes of Health, National Eye Institute, was initiated. It consisted of 2 multicenter, randomized, Phase III clinical trials comparing the efficacy and safety of standard care with intravitreal injection(s) of triamcinolone acetonide (hereafter referred to as intravitreal triamcinolone) in either a 1 mg or a 4 mg dose for vision loss associated with macular edema secondary to CRVO and BRVO.[36-38] Figure 10.5 shows a CRVO patient managed with IVTA.

To summarize, while the IVTA was not found useful in patients with BRVO, it was found to improve BCVA in CRVO patients. Although the efficacy of 1mg and 4 mg IVTA were similar the 1mg dose demonstrated a safety profile superior to that of the 4 mg dose. After IVTA more steroids have been explored for their potential role in similar conditions; flucinolode implant and dexamethasone implant.[39-41]

Dexamethasone is a potent, water-soluble corticosteroid that can be delivered to the vitreous cavity by the dexamethasone intravitreal implant (DEX implant; OZURDEX, Allergan, Inc., Irvine, CA). A DEX implant is composed of a biodegradable copolymer of lactic acid and glycolic acid containing micronized dexamethasone. The drug-copolymer complex gradually releases the total dose of dexamethasone over a series of months after insertion into the eye through a small pars plana puncture using a customized applicator system. In a recent study in eyes with persistent macular edema from several different causes (including RVO), DEX implant 0.7 mg produced improvements in visual acuity, macular thickness, and fluorescein leakage that were sustained for up to 6 months.[39] In a randomized, sham-controlled trial of dexamethasone intravitreal implant in 1,267 patients with macular edema due to retinal vein occlusion. The percentage of eyes with a ≥15-letter improvement in BCVA was significantly higher in both DEX implant groups compared with sham at days 30 to 90 ($P < 0.001$). The percentage of eyes with a ≥15-letter loss in BCVA was significantly lower

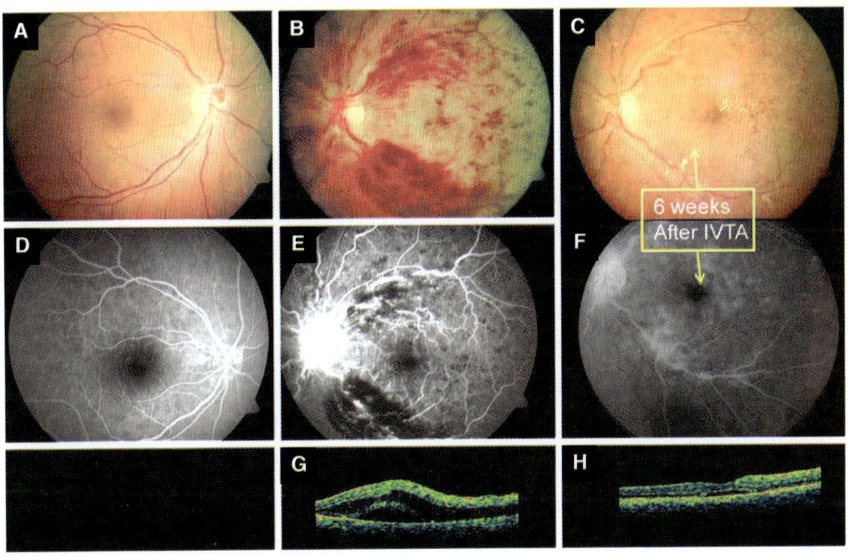

Figs 10.5A to H: Serial Fundus photographs and OCT of a 46 years old female with old CRVO with collaterals (OD) and acute CRVO (OS). Fundus and FFA photographs (A and C) are showing compensated CRVO with collaterals at disk. Fundus and FFA photographs and OCT scans (B, D and E) are showing acute CRVO with macular edema. Fundus, FFA photographs and OCT scans (F to H) at 6 weeks post IVTA injection showing resolution of macular edema, hemorrhages and tortuosity.

in the DEX implant 0.7 mg group compared with sham at all follow-up visits ($P \leq 0.036$).[40] Increased IOP as found in 16% of the cases at day 60 (both doses) and was not different from sham by day 180. Ozurdex received FDA approval for treatment of macular edema secondary to BRVO in 2009.

An implantable fluocinolone acetonide (Retisert, Bausch and Lomb, Rochester, NY) is also being evaluated for the treatment of BRVO and CRVO.[41] These trials help to clarify the role of corticosteroid therapy in the management of BRVO.

Intravitreal Anti-VEGF Drugs

The major stimulus for the formation of macular edema and neovascularization in patients with RVO seems to be hypoxia-induced production of vascular endothelial growth factor (VEGF), an angiogenic factor that promotes angiogenesis and increases permeability.[42] After encountering limitations of IVTA therapy due to high rate of side effects, such as cataract formation or increased intraocular pressure the researchers looked upon VEGF inhibition as an alternative. Since the first report of the efficacy of intravitreal bevacizumab (a recombinant monoclonal antibody binding to all isoforms of VEGF) in a patient with macular edema secondary to CRVO in 2005,[43] several retrospective case series have shown the benefit of this treatment, with an improvement in visual acuity and a decrease of central retinal thickness (CRT) in patients with macular edema associated with both BRVO and CRVO.[44-47]

CURRENT ROLE OF BEVACIZUMAB IN RVO

The initial encouraging results with intravitreal bevacizumab were followed by wide spread use in RVO patients. BRVO patients were found to have more predictable and sustained improvement in visual acuity although it required repeat injections.[47] The report on repeated bevacizumab injections demonstrated early and clinically relevant benefits from bevacizumab injections for complications of CRVO.[46] Visual acuity improved and macular edema decreased after a single injection in the majority of treated patients as early as the 1 week visit. The data also suggested that an injection of intravitreal bevacizumab has a limited beneficial effect of approximately 2 months in most patients and that intermittent reinjection may be needed to sustain the visual benefits. Bevacizumab treatment early after the onset of CRVO was also associated with a statistically significant reduction in venous dilation, tortuosity, optic disc swelling, and macular edema in addition to improvement of VA.[48] However, for CRVO patients the bevacizumab raised some concerns; theoretically, blocking VEGF should avert many of the complications that result from a CRVO. Alternatively, VEGF may be necessary for the formation of collaterals that would allow alternative venous drainage around the central retinal vein thrombosis. If this is the case, blocking VEGF may in fact be detrimental. The long-term role of anti-VEGF agents in the treatment of CME due to CRVO and the role for early intervention in improving outcome and potentially limiting progression to the ischemic variant still remain unanswered. Figure 11.6 shows a case with CRVO and NVG successfully managed with bevacizumab injections and laser photocoagulation.

ROLE OF RANIBIZUMAB

Ranibizumab (Lucentis; Genentech Inc) has been proposed to have potentially increased retinal penetration, because of a smaller molecular size and a higher binding affinity for VEGF than bevacizumab.[49] Spaide et al in a prospective study, evaluated intravitreal injection of ranibizumab as a potential treatment for decreased visual acuity (VA) secondary to central retinal vein occlusion (CRVO).[50] Total 20 eyes of 20 patients with mean age of 72.1 years, a mean VA of 45.8 ETDRS letters, and a mean central macular thickness of 574.6 µm received 3 monthly intravitreal ranibizumab injections. The patients were given additional ranibizumab if they had macular edema as determined by optical coherence tomography or any new intraretinal hemorrhage. At 12 months of follow-up, the mean VA improved to 64.3 letters and the central macular thickness decreased to 186µm (both different than baseline values; $P < 0.001$) using a mean of 8.5 injections. The change in macular thickness was not correlated with the change in VA. At 12 months 56.3% eyes had improvement of three lines or more and 12.5% had an improvement of more than six lines of VA. In one patient with a history of transient ischemic attack, an ischemic stroke developed but no sequel resulted. In another patient, vitreomacular traction developed, but the patient had improved acuity as compared with baseline. There were no infections, retinal tears, or detachments. Interestingly, the prolonged arm-to-early arterial filling time (measured on angiograms) at baseline showed no change at 1 year follow-up. This was despite near normalization of the retinal thickness, retinal appearance, and improvement in VA. This observation led them to hypothesis that the arterial supply into these eyes was compromised. Hypothesis is also supported by an old experiment where reduction of venous outflow with simple ligation of the vein in primates did not produce a picture consistent with severe CRVO; to produce severe CRVO, simultaneous compromise in arterial flow was required.[38]

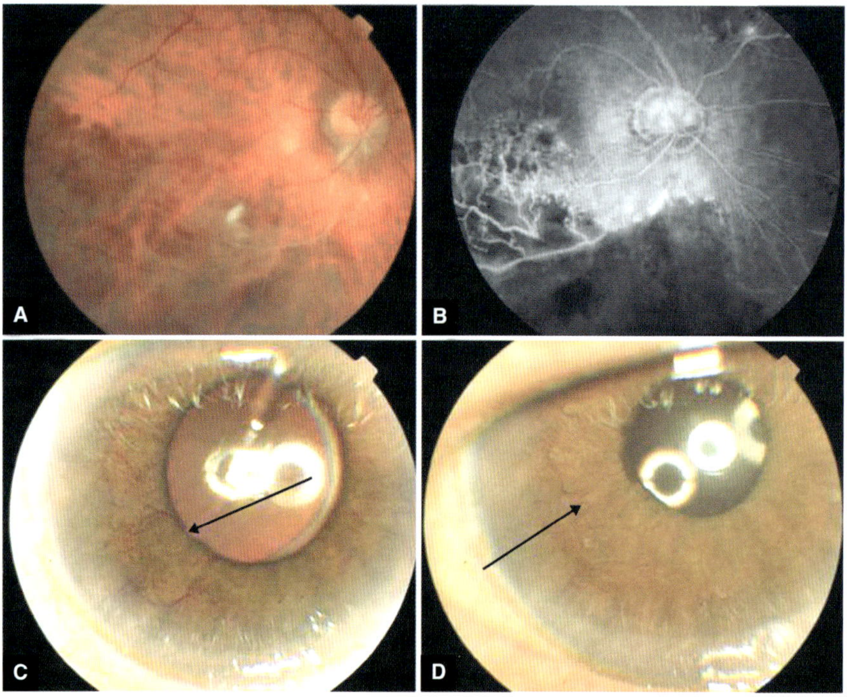

Figs 10.6A to D: Anterior segment and fundus photographs of a 75 years old male with ischemic HRVO leading to neovascular glaucoma. Fundus photographs and FFA (A and B) showing ischemic HRVO. Anterior segment photographs (C and D) showing regression of NVI within 48 hours of bevacizumab injection.

PEGAPTANIB SODIUM

Pegaptanib, a 40 kDa RNA aptamer, binds to VEGF165, the predominant pathological isoform in ischemia mediated ocular neovascularization and in diseases, such as diabetic macular edema.[52-54] Clinical trials have suggested that intravitreous injection of pegaptanib sodium can be effective in the treatment of diabetic macular edema,[55] proliferative diabetic retinopathy,[56] and neovascular age-related macular degeneration.[57,58] A recently published dose-ranging, double-masked, multicenter, phase 2 trial included subjects with CRVO for 6 months' or less duration randomly assigned (1:1:1) to receive pegaptanib sodium or sham injections every 6 weeks for 24 weeks (0.3 mg and 1 mg, n = 33; sham, n = 32). [59]At week 30, 36% subjects treated with 0.3 mg of pegaptanib sodium and 39% treated with 1 mg gained 15 or more letters from baseline as against 28% sham treated subjects. Also subjects treated with pegaptanib sodium were less likely to lose 15 or more letters (9% and 6%; 0.3 mg and 1 mg pegaptanib sodium groups, respectively) compared with sham-treated eyes (31%). Although the difference in the proportion of subjects who gained 15 letters in this trial was not statistically significant, the differences in the proportion of those who lost 15 letters and the mean visual acuity were substantial, providing support for a potential benefit of pegaptanib sodium in visual acuity of patients with macular edema secondary to CRVO. Study also found that fewer eyes in the groups treated with pegaptanib sodium showed retinal or iris neovascularization, a known and frequent complication of CRVO. However, the small sample size and short follow-up (30 weeks) would stop us from making any conclusive inference.

To summarize, almost all reports found beneficial effects of continuous VEGF suppression for macular edema from RVO. The need for repeated injections was also universally felt and most suitable approach seems to be intervening early if central macular thickness exceeds 250 μm and follow the treat and extend approach as used in management of CNVM. The maximum duration for VEG inhibition, ideal injection interval and effect of anti-VEGF drugs on collateral development and conversion from nonischemic to ischemic CRVO are the areas for future studies.

RADIAL OPTIC NEUROTOMY

Radial optic neurotomy is a surgical procedure designed to improve venous outflow in eyes with CRVO. It is proposed to relieve pressure on the occluded vein as it crosses the cribiform plate and scleral outlet.[60] After a standard pars plana vitrectomy, a single radial relaxing incision is made into the scleral ring and adjacent sclera of the optic nerve, typically nasally. The proposed theoretical basis of the procedure remains contentious, with some arguing that a single localized incision is unlikely to cause any meaningful decompression of the lamina cribrosa, which is a relatively rigid interwoven matrix of collagen and elastin.[61-63]Also many cases of CRVO do not have an occlusion at the proposed decompression site. Initial results from a retrospective case series of 10 patients with CRVO and VA 20/400 were promising, with an initial visual improvement in 73%. Another nonrandomized prospective case series of 10 patients and a retrospective case series of 5 patients reported less impressive or no improvement.[64,65] Complications include severe immediate hemorrhage, postoperative neovascularization of the neurotomy site and anterior segment,[64,66] VF defects,[67] and RD [68] originating at the incision site. Some investigators have suggested that RON may facilitate the formation of chorioretinal anastomosis,[69-71] whereas others argue that the results are due to effects from the vitrectomy alone or natural history.[61]

LASER-INDUCED CHORIORETINAL VENOUS ANASTOMOSIS

Up to 14% of eyes with CRVO can spontaneously develop chorioretinal anastomosis over a period of 3 months resulting in resolution of retinal hemorrhages and improvement in perfusion status. Figure 11.7 shows example of such case. In eyes with perfused CRVO, investigators have attempted to bypass the occluded central retinal vein by creating a similar anastomotic outflow channel to the choroidal circulation. It has been suggested that these chorioretinal anastomoses allow transretinal retrograde flow of venous blood from the eye and prevent the development of retinal ischemia.[72,73] Visual acuity may improve as a result of the reduction or resolution of macular edema and/or maintenance of retinal perfusion. The procedure is performed using an argon or neodymium:yttrium-aluminum-garnet (Nd:YAG) laser to rupture Bruch's membrane and the adjacent branch retinal vein, typically nasally and 3 disk diameters away from the optic disk. A few authors have attempted to create chorioretinal anastomoses surgically through a variety of techniques, including transretinal venipuncture, especially in an ischemic CRVO, with variable results.[74,76]

Meanwhile the results of The Central Retinal Vein Bypass Study (CVBS) from Australia were also available in 2010.[76] This was a prospective, randomized, controlled, multicenter clinical trial on 113 consecutive patients with a nonischemic CRVO of >3 months' duration and visual acuity of ≤20/50. A total of 53 control patients and 55 treatment patients completed the study. The 2 groups were comparable for most parameters. A Laser chorioretinal anastmosis (L-CRA) was successfully created in 76.4% of treated patients. Over the 18-month follow-up period, treated eyes had an 8.3 letter mean improvement from baseline compared with control eyes (P = 0.03). Treated eyes that developed a functional L-CRA achieved an 11.7 letter mean improvement from baseline over the control group after 18 months (P = 0.004). Conversion to the ischemic CRVO category occurred in 20.8% of control eyes and in 9.6% of treated eyes overall (P = 0.33). Of the treated group who developed an L-CRA where the retinal ischemia was due to progression of the CRVO, 4.9% progressed to the ischemic category (P = 0.03). Incidence of complications was found to be high with 18.2% of treated patients developing neovascularization at the site of L-CRA and 9.1% of treated eyes requiring vitrectomy surgery because of macular traction or nonresolving vitreous hemorrhage. All complications were successfully managed. Authors have strongly recommended this procedure after suggesting that the risk of these complications should be weighed against the substantial visual morbidity from CRVO, as shown by the CVOS[3] and supported by other studies showing that eyes similar to those enrolled

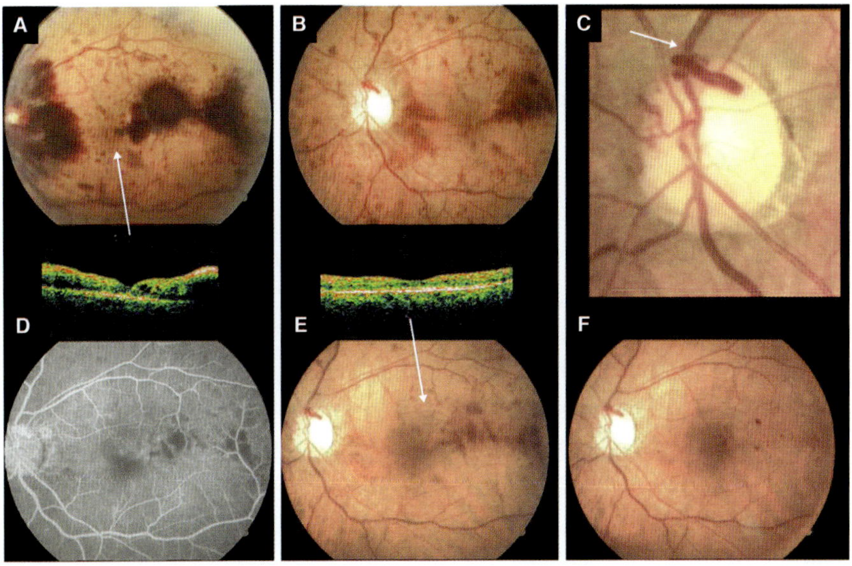

Figs 10.7A to F: Serial Fundus photographs and OCT of 65 years old male with non ischemic CRVO.

FFA and OCT photographs (A to F) showing resolution of retinal hemorrhages and macular edema following spontaneous development of chorioretinal anastomosis (collaterals) at disk. Magnified picture of optic disk (C) showing collaterals (white arrow)

in our study (nonischemic, i.e., <10 DD CNP) have a poor visual prognosis. The study, however, has few limitations like non availability of OCT for assessment of benefit on macular edema and no use of anti-VEGF drugs to address neovascularization associated with L-CRA. Also the purpose-built HGM K3 laser that was used in this study is no longer available. More trials with modern solid-state green wavelength lasers, OCT and Anti-VEGF seem in order.

PARS PLANA VITRECTOMY AND AV SHEATHOTOMY

Arteriovenous sheathotomy has been described as a procedure in which the retinal vein and artery are surgically separated at the arteriovenous crossing by cutting the common adventitial sheath. While many studies report no beneficial effect on visual acuity,[77,78] several case series as well as a nonrandomized controlled study have demonstrated improved CME and/or visual acuity.[79-81] The studies evaluating pars plana vitrectomy (PPV) with removal of the posterior hyaloid, but no sheathotomy, have also found resolution of CME secondary to BRVO.[82,83] Results from a head-to-head comparison study have suggested that PPV with posterior hyaloid removal alone is as effective as combined PPV/sheathotomy in resolving CME and improving visual acuity in BRVO.[84] Complications associated with these procedures include vitreous hemorrhage, intraoperative retinal tears, rhegmatogenous retinal detachment, and cataract development.[85]

HEMODILUTION

The rationale for the use of hemodilution in the treatment of CRVO was based on observations of abnormal red cell deformability, increased plasma viscosity, and hematocrit and fibrinogen levels in some patients with CRVO. It was argued that reducing hematocrit levels lowers plasma viscosity, which may lead to improved retinal microcirculation and perfusion. Several studies (of the RCTs) have reported statistically significant improvements in VA, arteriovenous passage time, and clinical appearance after hemodilution.[86-91] There have been a number of adverse effects including lethargy, fainting spells, and exertional dyspnea may occur but data from these studies indicate that the treatment is generally well tolerated even in elderly patients. Wolf et al,[72] Hansen et al,[88,89] Heinen et al,[88] Poupard et al,[91] and Hehn[92]have all reported improved VAs in patients treated with hemodilution. However, many of these studies have limitations. Most had small numbers, and the protocols, inclusion and exclusion criteria, and end points varied substantially. Small changes in the protocol can have large effects on blood hemodynamics and rheology. All the studies with improved visual outcome required a prolonged period of hospitalization, and the only randomized study that investigated hemodilution in an outpatient setting in CRVO showed no significant benefit.[93]

Isovolemic hemodilution has shown some benefits for eyes with BRVO in randomized studies.[94] This treatment strategy is often not practical, requires great care in patient selection, and is likely not appropriate for those patients with anemia, renal insufficiency, or pulmonary insufficiency.[94]

DIRECT INJECTION OF TISSUE PLASMINOGEN ACTIVATOR INTO THE RETINAL VEIN LUMEN AND OTHER THROMBOLYTICS

No RCT has evaluated the safety and efficacy of this intervention. Adverse effects, such as vitreous hemorrhage in up to a quarter of patients and RD have been reported. Larger studies with concurrent control groups comparing the procedure with vitrectomy alone and standard care are needed before routine use of this procedure can be recommended.

There is limited evidence that any oral or systemic anticoagulation or rheological agent can significantly affect the outcome of CRVO. Although troxerutin and ticlodipine showed a trend for improvement, the evidence supporting these modalities was limited[95,96](level B- III). Ticlodipine has uncommon (0.5%-3%) but very serious hematological toxicity, including neutropenia, thrombocytopenia, and aplastic anemia requiring regular monitoring. Clopidrogel, a newer agent with an almost identical structure and mechanism of action, increasingly is used preferentially due to a reduced incidence of blood disorders and without any regular monitoring. No randomized study has assessed the role of clopidrogel in retinal venous thrombosis, and routine use of these agents is not recommended for CRVO.

References

1. Klein R, Klein BE, Moss SE, Meuer SM. The epidemiology of retinal vein occlusion: the Beaver Dam Eye Study. *Trans Am Ophthalmol Soc.* 2000;98:133-41.
2. Mitchell P, Smith W, Chang A. Prevalence and associations of retinal vein occlusion in Australia: the Blue Mountains Eye Study. *Arch Ophthalmol.* 1996;114:1243-7.
3. Wong TY, Larsen EK, Klein R, et al. Cardiovascular risk factors for retinal vein occlusion and arteriolar emboli: the Atherosclerosis Risk in Communities & Cardiovascular Health studies. *Ophthalmology.* 2005; 112:540-7.
4. Sophie Rogers S, McIntosh R L et al, The Prevalence of Retinal Vein Occlusion: Pooled Data from Population Studies from the United States, Europe, Asia, and Australia. *Ophthalmology.* 2010;117:313-19.
5. Argon laser photocoagulation for macula edema in branch vein occlusion. *Am J Ophthalmol.* 1984;98:271-82.
6. Argon Laser Scatter Photocoagulation for Prevention of Neovascularization and Vitreous Haemorrhage in BRVO. *Arch Ophthalmology.* 1986;104:34-41.
7. The Central Vein Occlusion Study Group: Natural history and clinical management of central retinal vein occlusion. *Arch Ophthalmol.* 1997; 115:486-91.
8. The Central Vein Occlusion Study Group: Evaluation of grid pattern photocoagulation for macular edema in central vein occlusion. The CVOS Group M Report. *Ophthalmol.* 1995;102:1425-1433.
9. The Central Vein Occlusion Study Group: A randomized clinical trial of early panretinal photocoagulation for ischemic central vein occlusion. The CVOS Group N Report. *Ophthalmol.* 1995;102:1434-44.
10. Funk M, Kriechbaum KF, Prager F, et al. Intraocular concentrations of growth factors and cytokines in retinal vein occlusion and the effect of therapy with bevacizumab. Invest Ophthalmol *Vis Sci.* 2009;50(3):1025-32.
11. McIntosh RL, Rogers SL, Lim L, Cheung N, Wang JJ et al, Natural History of Central Retinal Vein Occlusion: An Evidence-Based Systematic Review. *Ophthalmology.* 2010;117:1113-23.
12. Harey SS, Podhajsky PA, Zimmerman MB, Natural History of Visual Outcome in Central Retinal Vein Occlusion. *Ophthalmology.* 2011;118:119-33.
13. O'Mahoney PR, Wong DT, Ray JG. Retinal vein occlusion and traditional risk factors for atherosclerosis. *Arch Ophthalmol.* 2008;126(5):692-9.
14. Poli A, Tremoli E, Colombo A, et al. Ultrasonographic measurement of the common carotid artery wall thickness in hypercholesterolemic patients. A new model for the quantitation and follow-up of preclinical atherosclerosis in living human subjects. *Atherosclerosis.* 1988;70:253-61.
15. Nowak J, Nilsson T, Sylven C, Jogestrand T. Potential of carotid ultrasonography in the diagnosis of coronary artery disease: a comparison with exercise test and variance *ECG. Stroke.* 1998;29:439-46.

16. Brown GC, Shah HG, Magargal LE, Savino PJ. Central retinal vein obstruction and carotid artery disease. *Ophthalmology.* 1984;91:1627-33.
17. Green WR, Chan CC, Hutchins M, Terry JM. Central retinal vein occlusion: a prospective histopathologic study of 29 eyes in 28 cases Trans Am Ophthalmol Soc 1982; LXXIX: 371-422.
18. Matsushima C, Wakabayashi Y, Iwamoto T, Yamauchi Y, Usui M, Iwasaki T, Relationship between Retinal Vein Occlusion and Carotid artery Lesions. *Retina.* 27:1038-43.
19. Glueck CJ, Wang P, Hutchins R, et al. Ocular vascular thrombotic events: central retinal vein and central retinal artery occlusions. *Clin Appl Thromb Hemost.* 2008;14(3):286-94.
20. Rehak M, Rehak J, Mu¨ ller M, et al. The prevalence of activated protein C (APC) resistance and factor V Leiden is significantly higher in patients with retinal vein occlusion without general risk factors. Case-control study and metaanalysis. *Thromb Haemost.* 2008;99(5):925-9.
21. Williamson TH. Central retinal vein occlusion: what's the story? *Br J Ophthalmol.* 1997;81(8):698-704.
22. Yap YC, Barampouti F. Central retinal vein occlusion secondary to protein S deficiency. *Ann Ophthalmol (Skokie).* 2007;39:343-4.
23. Lahey MJ, Tunc M¸ Kearney J, Modlinski B, et al, Laboratory Evaluation of Hypercoagulable States in Patients with Central Retinal Vein Occlusion Who are Less Than 56 Years of Age. *Ophthalmology.* 2002;109:126-31.
24. Janssen MC, den Heijer M, Cruysberg JR, et al. Retinal vein occlusion: a form of venous thrombosis or a complication of atherosclerosis? A meta-analysis of thrombophilic factors. *Thromb Haemost.* 2005;93(6):1021-6.
25. Di Capua M, Coppola A, Albisinni R, et al. Cardiovascular risk factors and outcome in patients with retinal vein occlusion. *J Thromb Thrombolysis.* 2010;30(1): 16-22.
26. Sodi A, Giambene B, Marcucci R, et al. Atherosclerotic and thrombophilic risk factors in patients with recurrent central retinal vein occlusion. Eur *J Ophthalmol.* 2008;18(2):233-8.
27. McCuen BW 2nd, Bessler M, Tano Y, Chandler D, Machemer R. The lack of toxicity of intravitreally administered triamcinolone acetonide. *Am J Ophthalmol.* 1981;91:785-8.
28. Young S, Larkin G, Branley M, Lightman S. Safety and efficacy of intravitreal triamcinolone for cystoid macular edema in uveitis. *Clin Exp Ophthalmol.* 2001;29:2-6.
29. Martidis A, Duker JS, Greenberg PB, Rogers AH, Puliafito CA, Reichel E, Baumal C. Intravitreal triamcinolone for refractory diabetic macular edema. *Ophthalmology.* 2002;109:920-7.
30. Ip M, Kahana A, Altaweel M. Treatment of central retinal vein occlusion with triamcinolone acetonide: an optical coherence tomography study. Semin *Ophthalmol.* 2003 Jun;18(2):67-73.
31. Ip MS, Gottlieb JL, Kahana A, Scott IU, Altaweel MM, Blodi BA, Gangnon RE, Puliafito CA. Intravitreal triamcinolone for the treatment of macular edema associated with central retinal vein occlusion. *Arch Ophthalmol.* 2004 Aug;122(8):1131-6.
32. Bashshur ZF, Ma'luf RN, Allam S, Jurdi FA, Haddad RS, Noureddin BN. Intravitreal triamcinolone for the management of macular edema due to nonischemic central retinal vein occlusion. *Arch Ophthalmol.* 2004 Aug;122(8):1137-40.

33. Krepler K, Ergun E, Sacu S, Richter-Muksch S, Wagner J, Stur M, Wedrich A. Intravitreal triamcinolone acetonide in patients with macular oedema due to central retinal vein occlusion. *Acta Ophthalmol Scand*. 2005 Feb;83(1):71-5.
34. Williamson TH, O'Donnell A. Intravitreal triamcinolone acetonide for cystoid macular edema in nonischemic central retinal vein occlusion. *Am J Ophthalmol*. 2005 May;139(5):860-6.
35. Flynn HW Jr, Scott IU. Intravitreal triamcinolone acetonide for macular edema associated with diabetic retinopathy and venous occlusive disease: it's time for clinical trials. *Arch Ophthalmol* 2005;123:258-9.
36. Ip MS, Oden NL, Scott IU, et al, SCORE Study Investigator Group. SCORE Study report 3: study design and baseline characteristics. *Ophthalmology*. 2009;116:1770-7.
37. SCORE Study Research Group. A randomized trial comparing the efficacy and safety of intravitreal triamcinolone with observation to treat vision loss associated with macular edema secondary to central retinal vein occlusion: the Standard Care vs Corticosteroid for Retinal Vein Occlusion (SCORE) Study Report 5. *Arch Ophthalmol*. 2009;127:1101-14.
38. SCORE Study Research Group. A randomized trial comparing the efficacy and safety of intravitreal triamcinolone with standard care to treat vision loss associated with macular edema secondary to branch retinal vein occlusion: the Standard Care vs Corticosteroid for Retinal Vein Occlusion (SCORE) Study Report 6. *Arch Ophthalmol*. 2009;127:1115-28.
39. Kuppermann BD, Blumenkranz MS, Haller JA, et al, Dexamethasone DDS Phase II Study Group. Randomized controlled study of an intravitreous dexamethasone drug delivery system in patients with persistent macular edema. *Arch Ophthalmol*. 2007;125:309-17.
40. Haller JA, Bandello F, Belfort R Jr, et alfor the OZURDEX GENEVA Study Group. Randomized, sham-controlled trial of dexamethasone intravitreal implant in patients with macular edema due to retinal vein occlusion. *Ophthalmology*. 2010;117(6):1134-46.
41. Ramchandran RS, Fekrat S, Stinnett SS, et al. Fluocinolone acetonide sustained drug delivery device for chronic central retinal vein occlusion: 12-month results. *Am J Ophthalmol*. 2008;146(2):285-91.
42. Aiello LP, Avery RL, Arrigg PG, et al. Vascular endothelial growth factor in ocular fluid of patients with diabetic retinopathy and other retinal disorders. *N Engl J Med*. 1994;331:1480-7.
43. Rosenfeld PJ, Fung AE, Puliafito CA. Optical coherence tomography findings after an intravitreal injection of bevacizumab (avastin) for macular edema from central vein occlusion. *Ophthalmic Surg Lasers Imaging*. 2005;36:336-9.
44. Kreutzer TC, Alge CS, Wolf AH, et al. Intravitreal bevacizumab for the treatment of macular oedema secondary to branch retinal vein occlusion. *Br J Ophthalmol*. 2008;92(3):351-5.
45. Iturralde D, Spaide RF, Meyerle CB, et al. Intravitreal bevacizumab (Avastin) treatment of macular edema in central retinal vein occlusion: a short-term study. *Retina*. 2006;26:279-84.
46. Hsu J, Kaiser RS, Sivalingam A, et al. Intravitreal bevacizumab (avastin) in central vein occlusion. *Retina*. 2007;27:1013-9.
47. Rabena MD, Pieramici DJ, Castellarin AA, et al. Intravitreal bevacizumab (Avastin) in the treatment of macular edema secondary to branch retinal vein occlusion. *Retina*. 2007;27:419-25.
48. Ferrara DC, Koizumi H, Spaide RF. Early bevacizumab treatment of central retinal vein occlusion. *Am J Ophthalmol*. 2007;144:864-71.

49. Ferrara N, Damico L, Shams N, Lowman H, Kim R. Development of ranibizumab, an anti-vascular endothelial growth factor antigen binding fragment, as therapy for neovascular age-related macular degeneration. *Retina*. 2006;26:859-70.
50. Spaide RF, Cang LK, Klancnik JM, Yannuzzi LA, Sorenson J, Slakter JS et al. Prospective Study of Intravitreal Ranibizumab as a Treatment for Decreased Visual Acuity Secondary to Central Retinal Vein Occlusion. Am *J Ophthalmol*. 2009;147:298-306.
51. Hayreh SS, van Heuven WA, Hayreh MS. Experimental retinal vascular occlusion. I. Pathogenesis of central retinal vein occlusion. *Arch Ophthalmol*. 1978; 96:311-23.
52. Ishida S, Usui T, Yamashiro K, et al. VEGF164-mediated inflammation is required for pathological, but not physiological, ischemia-induced retinal neovascularization. *J Exp Med*. 2003;198(3):483-89.
53. Ishida S, Yamashiro K, Usui T, et al. Leukocytes mediate retinal vascular remodelling during development and vaso-obliteration in disease. *Nat Med*. 2003;9(6): 781-88.
54. Ng EW, Adamis AP. Targeting angiogenesis, the underlying disorder in neovascular age-related macular degeneration. *Can J Ophthalmol*. 2005;40(3):352-68.
55. Ng EW, Shima DT, Calias P, Cunningham ET Jr, Guyer DR, Adamis AP. Pegaptanib, a targeted anti-VEGF aptamer for ocular vascular disease. *Nat Rev Drug Discov*. 2006;5(2):123-32.
56. Cunningham ET Jr, Adamis AP, Altaweel M, et al; Macugen Diabetic Retinopathy Study Group. A phase II randomized double-masked trial of pegaptanib, an anti-vascular endothelial growth factor aptamer, for diabetic macular edema. *Ophthalmology*. 2005;112(10):1747-57.
57. Adamis AP, Altaweel M, Bressler NM, et al; Macugen Diabetic Retinopathy Study Group. Changes in retinal neovascularization after pegaptanib (Macugen) therapy in diabetic individuals. *Ophthalmology*. 2006;113(1): 23-28.
58. Gragoudas ES, Adamis AP, Cunningham ET Jr, Feinsod M, Guyer DR; VEGF Inhibition Study in Ocular Neovascularization Clinical Trial Group. Pegaptanib for neovascular age-related macular degeneration. *N Engl J Med*. 2004;351(27):2805-16.
59. Wroblewski JJ, Wells JA, Adamis AP, et al. Pegaptanib Sodium for Macular Edema Secondary to Central Retinal Vein Occlusion. *Arch Ophthalmol*. 2009;127(4): 374-80.
60. Opremcak EM, Bruce RA, Lomeo MD, et al. Radial optic neurotomy for central retinal vein occlusion: a retrospective pilot study of 11 consecutive cases. *Retina*. 2001;21:408-15.
61. Hayreh SS, Opremcak EM, Bruce RA, et al. Radial optic neurotomy for central retinal vein obstruction [letter]. *Retina*. 2002;22:374-7.
62. Hayreh SS. Radial optic neurotomy for central retinal vein occlusion [letter]. *Retina*. 2002;22:827.
63. Hayreh SS. Radial optic neurotomy for nonischemic central retinal vein occlusion [letter]. *Arch Ophthalmol*. 2004;122:1572-3.
64. Weizer JS, Stinnett SS, Fekrat S. Radial optic neurotomy as treatment for central retinal vein occlusion. *Am J Ophthalmol*. 2003;136:814-9.
65. Martínez-Jardón CS, Meza-de Regil A, Dalma-Weiszhausz J, et al. Radial optic neurotomy for ischaemic central vein occlusion. *Br J Ophthalmol*. 2005;89:558-61.

66. Schneider U, Inhoffen W, Grisanti S, et al. Chorioretinal neovascularization after radial optic neurotomy for central retinal vein occlusion. *Ophthalmic Surg Lasers Imaging*. 2005;36:508-11.
67. Schneider U, Inhoffen W, Grisanti S, Bartz-Schmidt KU. Characteristics of visual field defects by scanning laser ophthalmoscope microperimetry after radial optic neurotomy for central retinal vein occlusion. *Retina*. 2005;25:704-12.
68. Samuel MA, Desai UR, Gandolfo CB. Peripapillary retinal detachment after radial optic neurotomy for central retinal vein occlusion. *Retina*. 2003;23:580-3.
69. Nomoto H, Shiraga F, Yamaji H, et al. Evaluation of radial optic neurotomy for central retinal vein occlusion by indocyanine green videoangiography and image analysis. *Am J Ophthalmol*. 2004;138:612-9.
70. García-Arumí J, Boixadera A, Martinez-Castillo V, et al. Chorioretinal anastomosis after radial optic neurotomy for central retinal vein occlusion. *Arch Ophthalmol*. 2003;121:1385-91.
71. Friedman SM. Optociliary venous anastomosis after radial optic neurotomy for central retinal vein occlusion. *Ophthalmic Surg Lasers Imaging*. 2003;34: 315-7.
72. Leonard BC, Coupland SG, Kertes PJ, Bate R. Long-term follow-up of a modified technique for laser-induced chorioretinal venous anastomosis in nonischemic central retinal vein occlusion. *Ophthalmology*. 2003;110:948-54, discussion 955.
73. Fekrat S, Goldberg MF, Finkelstein D. Laser-induced chorioretinal venous anastomosis for nonischemic central or branch retinal vein occlusion. *Arch Ophthalmol*. 1998;116:43-52.
74. Peyman GA, Kishore K, Conway MD. Surgical chorioretinal venous anastomosis for ischemic central retinal vein occlusion. *Ophthalmic Surg Lasers*. 1999;30:605-14.
75. Mirshahi A, Roohipoor R, Lashay A, et al. Surgical induction of chorioretinal venous anastomosis in ischaemic central retinal vein occlusion: a non-randomised controlled clinical trial. *Br J Ophthalmol*. 2005;89:64-9.
76. McAllister IL, Gillies ME, Smithies LA, et al. The Central Retinal Vein Bypass Study: a trial of laser—induced chorioretinal venous anastomosis for central retinal vein occlusion. *Ophthalmology*. 2010;117(5):954-65.
77. Cahill MT, Kaiser PK, Sears JE, et al. The effect of arteriovenous sheathotomy on cystoid macular oedema secondary to branch retinal vein occlusion. *Br J Ophthalmol*. 2003;87(11):1329-32.
78. Le Rouic JF, Bejjani RA, Rumen F, et al. Adventitial sheathotomy for decompression of recent onset branch retinal vein occlusion. *Graefes Arch Clin Exp Ophthalmol*. 2001;239(10):747-51.
79. Mason J 3rd, Feist R, White M Jr, et al. Sheathotomy to decompress branch retinal vein occlusion: a matched control study. *Ophthalmology*. 2004;111(3): 540-5.
80. Mester U, Dillinger P. Vitrectomy with arteriovenous decompression and internal limiting membrane dissection in branch retinal vein occlusion. *Retina*. 2002;22(6):740-6.
81. Opremcak EM, Bruce RA. Surgical decompression of branch retinal vein occlusion via arteriovenous crossing sheathotomy: a prospective review of 15 cases. *Retina*. 1999;19(1):1-5.
82. Saika S, Tanaka T, Miyamoto T, et al. Surgical posterior vitreous detachment combined with gas/air tamponade for treating macular edema associated

with branch retinal vein occlusion: retinal tomography and visual outcome. *Graefes Arch Clin Exp Ophthalmol.* 2001;239(10):729-32.

83. Tachi N, Hashimoto Y, Ogino N. Vitrectomy for macular edema combined with retinal vein occlusion. *Doc Ophthalmol.* 1999;97(3-4):465-9.
84. Figueroa MS, Torres R, Alvarez MT. Comparative study of vitrectomy with and without vein decompression for branch retinal vein occlusion: a pilot study. *Eur J Ophthalmol.* 2004;14(1):40-7.
85. Chung EJ, Lee H, Koh HJ. Arteriovenous crossing sheathotomy versus intravitreal triamcinolone acetonide injection for treatment of macular edema associated with branch retinal vein occlusion. *Graefes Arch Clin Exp Ophthalmol.* 2008;246(7): 967-74.
86. Wolf S, Arend O, Bertram B, et al. Hemodilution therapy in central retinal vein occlusion: one-year results of a prospective randomized study. *Graefes Arch Clin Exp Ophthalmol.* 1994;232:33-9.
87. Brunner R, Heinen A, Konen W, et al. Therapy of retinal vascular disorders by modification of blood viscosity—a randomized double-blind study [in German]. *Fortschr Ophthalmol.* 1984;81:440-3.
88. Heinen A, Brunner R, Hossmann V, et al. Changes in hemorheologic and physiologic coagulation parameters in different methods of therapy of retinal vascular disorders—a randomized double-blind study [in German]. *Fortschr Ophthalmol.* 1984;81:444-8.
89. Hansen LL, Wiek J, Wiederholt M. A randomised prospective study of treatment of non-ischaemic central retinal vein occlusion by isovolaemic haemodilution. *Br J Ophthalmol.* 1989;73:895-9.
90. Hansen LL, Danisevskis P, Arntz HR, et al. A randomised prospective study on treatment of central retinal vein occlusion by isovolaemic haemodilution and photocoagulation. *Br J Ophthalmol.* 1985;69:108-16.
91. Poupard P, Eledjam JJ, Dupeyron G, et al. Role of acute normovolemic hemodilution in treating retinal venous occlusions [in French]. *Ann Fr Anesth Reanim.* 1986;5:229-33.
92. Hehn F. Isovolaemic haemodilution and naftidrofuryl versus naftidrofuryl in treatment of retinal vein occlusion [in French]. *Ophthalmologie.* 1995;9:309-12.
93. Luckie AP, Wroblewski JJ, Hamilton P, et al. A randomised prospective study of outpatient haemodilution for central retinal vein obstruction. *Aust N Z J Ophthalmol.* 1996;24:223-32.
94. Chen HC, Wiek J, Gupta A, et al. Effect of isovolaemic haemodilution on visual outcome in branch retinal vein occlusion. *Br J Ophthalmol.* 1998; 82(2):162-7.
95. Glacet-Bernard A, Coscas G, Chabanel A, et al. A randomized, double-masked study on the treatment of retinal vein occlusion with troxerutin. *Am J Ophthalmol.* 1994;118:421-9.
96. Houtsmuller AJ, Vermeulen JA, Klompe M, et al. The influence of ticlopidine on the natural course of retinal vein occlusion. *Agents Actions Suppl.* 1984;15:219-29.

11

chapter

Nidhi Relhan
Subhadra Jalali

Macular Dystrophies

ABSTRACT

Hereditary macular dystrophies are a common cause of bilateral progressive low vision, usually seen in young children and adolescents and rarely in older individuals. Progression is variable but often the central vision is substantially affected. Fundus photography, visual electrophysiology, ocular coherence tomography, fundus autofluorescence, and sometimes fundus angiography are helpful in identifying the precise phenotype and provide appropriate prognostic information. Appropriate counseling, careful refraction, and low vision aids assessment are keys to the successful management of patients with macular dystrophies.

Introduction

There are several forms of hereditary disorders that affect the macular area in children, teenagers, and young adults. These macular dystrophies often present with failing vision that progress variably and result often in severe loss of central vision and rarely the peripheral vision. Patients can progress to legal blindness. Peripheral residual vision is very often preserved even in late stages of the macular dystrophies. Common conditions include X-linked retinoschisis, Best's vitelliform dystrophy, Stargardt's with or without fundus favimaculatus, pattern dystrophy, macular cone dystrophy, dominant cystoid macular edema (CME). Some of the generalized retinal dystrophies can have associated changes in the macular area and are not discussed here. These include Lebers' congenital amaurosis (LCA) that can have macular colobomas or macular atrophy, and retinitis pigmentosa (RP) that can have a variety of macular changes, including CME, macular holes, epiretinal membrane and atrophy and rarely a central pigmentary retinopathy or central RP.

Definition of Hereditary Macular Dystrophies

A group of hereditary disorders that are defined as bilaterally symmetrical usually present during childhood or early adulthood involving the macular area and sparing the peripheral retina and characterized by a typical fundus picture especially in moderately advanced stages of the condition that almost always has normal retinal vessels often with associated electrophysiological test abnormalities[1-4] Figures 11.1 to 11.4 show normal visual electrophysiology waveforms of retinal pathways for understanding the subsequent abnormal electrophysiogy.[4] The diseases involve early and premature cell changes and cell death for which no clearly demonstrable cause except genetic abnormalities has been determined.

Classification

Macular dystrophies can be classified on the basis of:

1. Anatomical layers of the retina (Table 11.1) or
2. Inheritance pattern (Table 11.2)

Some of the important macular dystrophies are described below.

Autosomal Dominant Macular Dystrophies

BEST'S VITELLIFORM DYSTROPHY

Best's vitelliform macular dystrophy[1-4,5-7] (Figs 11.5 and 11.6) a commonly seen autosomal dominant dystrophy of the retinal pigment epithelium characterized by a distinctive, if not pathognomonic, "egg yolk cyst" in the foveal area, and is associated with a normal flash electroretinogram (ERG) but an abnormal light peak/dark trough ratio on the electrooculogram (EOG).

Genetic mutation: Bests' disease results from a mutation in the *Vitelliform macular dystrophy 2 (VMD2) gene*. In families in which the EOG is a distinguishing marker, all members of the family bearing the gene can be identified by EOG testing and at least one member would show the 'egg-yolk cyst' phenotype.

Ophthalmoscopic Staging and Visual Function[5]

There is wide phenotypic variability in expression of the fundus lesions, both in the fovea and in the extrafoveal retina. The five stages of the disease and the sequalae are:

1. Carrier state
2. Vitelliform

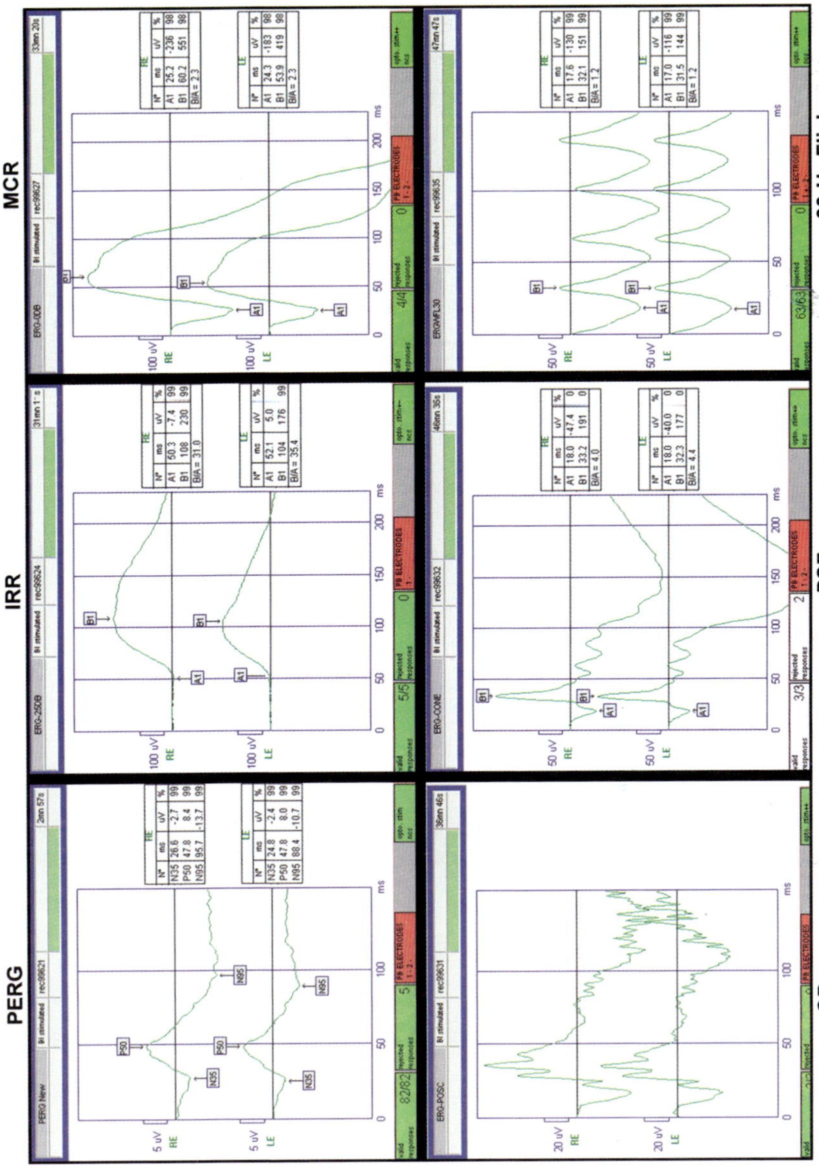

Fig. 11.1: Normal flash ERG in an emmetropic subject with visual acuity 20/20. PERG: Pattern ERG for macular function, IRR: Isolated rod inner retinal response; MCR: Maximal combined rod-cone response, OPs: Oscillatory potentials from inner retina, PSF: Photopic single flash cone response

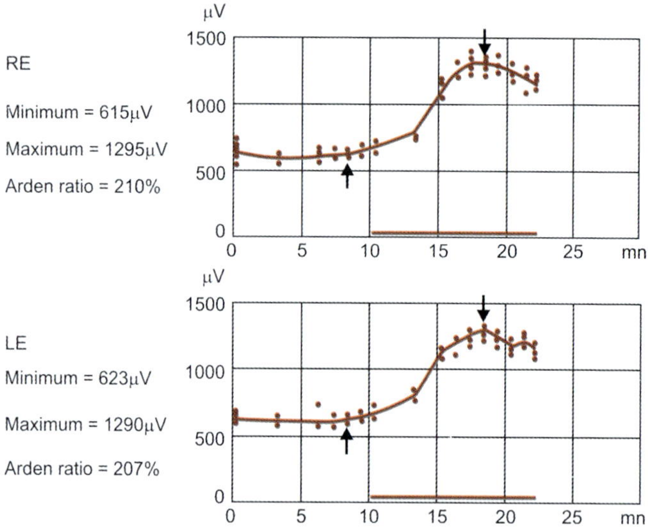

Fig. 11.2: An EOG graph with the light rise and normal Arden ratio of >200% in each eye

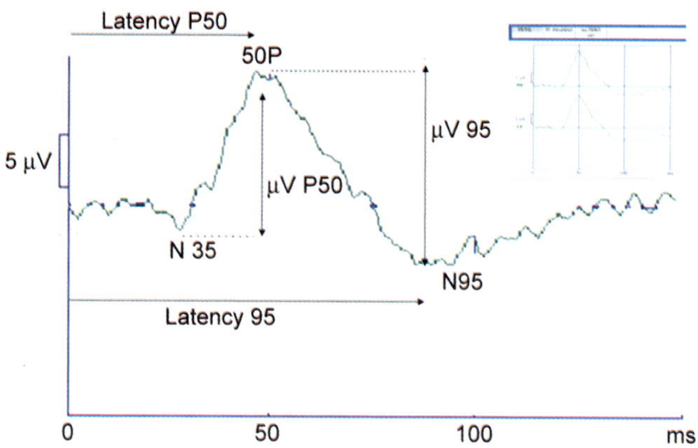

Fig. 11.3: PERG measurements Inset shows actual PERG recording.

3. Scrambled egg
4. Pseudohypopyon
5. Atrophic
6. Cicatricial or choroidal neovascular

In most infants and children, the fundus is normal at birth, although some individuals could demonstrate an appearance of foveal hypoplasia appearing as an abnormal neuroretinal light reflex (stage 0). This is possibly similar to the "carrier state" in older adults who can genetically transmit

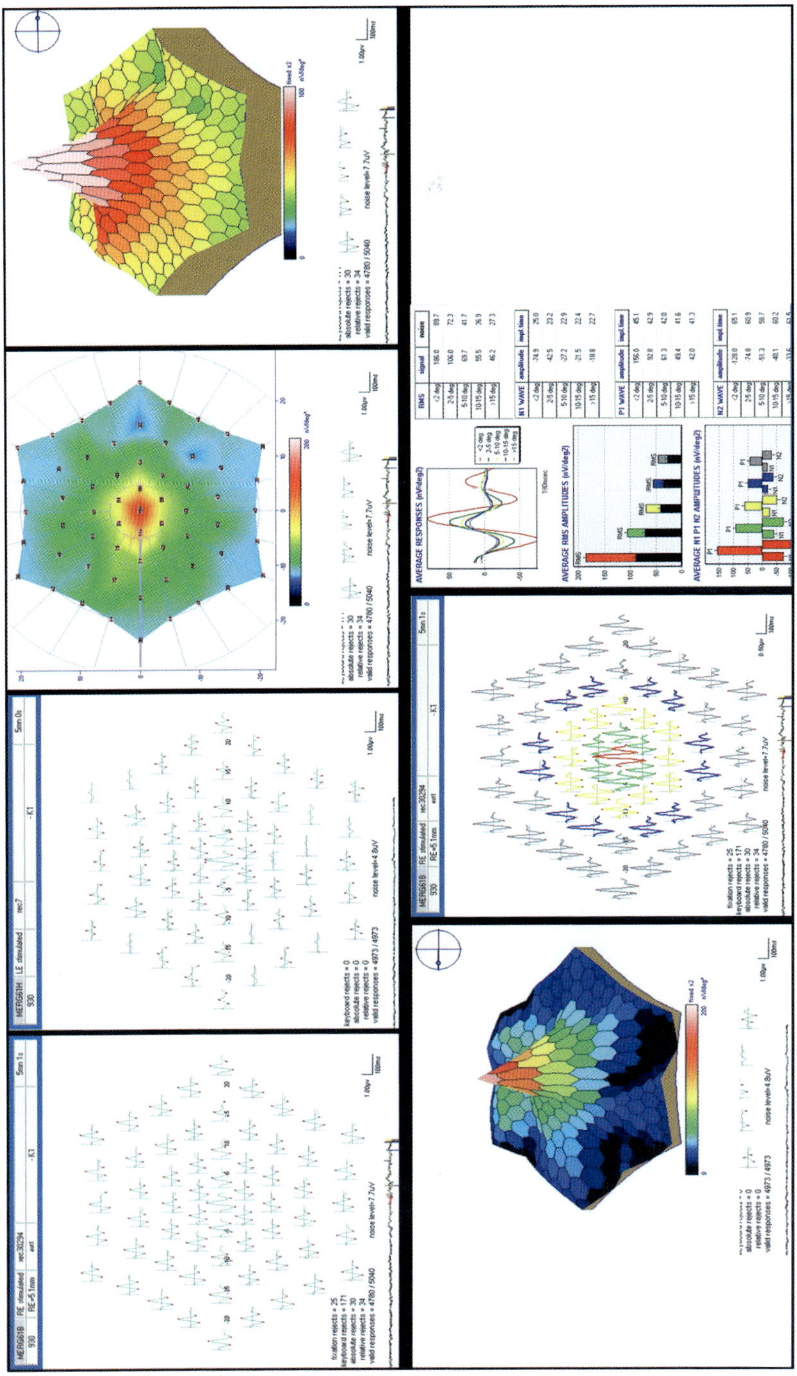

Fig. 11.4: Various displays available for mfERG in a normal eye. Clockwise from top left trace arrays of two eyes, colored density plot, 3D scalar plot, scalar plot compared to normative data base, ring averages, average values of N1, P1 and P2

TABLE 11.1: Classification of hereditary macular dystrophies based on retinal layers affected

1. Nerve fiber layer
   - X-linked juvenile retinoschisis
2. Photoreceptors and retinal pigment epithelium (RPE)
   - Stargardt's disease (atrophic macular dystrophy with fundus flavimaculatus)
   - Pericentral retinitis pigmentosa
   - Progressive atrophic macular dystrophy
   - Cone (-rod) dystrophy
3. Retinal pigment epithelium
   - Bests' vitelliform dystrophy
   - Fundus flavimaculatus
   - Butterfly-shaped pigment dystrophy, or pattern dystrophy
   - Reticular dystrophy
   - Dominant cystoid macular dystrophy (DCMD)
   - Familial grouped pigmentations
   - Benign concentric annular macular dystrophy
   - Dominant drusen
4. Bruch's membrane
   - Pseudoinflammatory dystrophy
   - Angioid streaks
   - Age-related macular dystrophy
   - Myopic macular degeneration
5. Choroid
   - Central areolar choroidal dystrophy

TABLE 11.2: Classification of heredomacular dystrophies based on Inheritance patterns

1. Autosomal dominant
   - Best's disease
   - Pattern dystrophy
   - Adult onset vitelliform macular dystrophy
   - Central areolar dystrophy
   - Dominantly inherited drusens
   - North Carolina macular dystrophy
   - Progressive foveal dystrophy
   - Cystoid macular edema
2. Autosomal recessive
   - Stargardt's disease (fundus flavimaculatus)
   - Sjogrens reticular dystrophy
   - Bietti's crystalline dystrophy
3. X linked
   - X-linked familial foveal retinoschisis
   - Familial foveal hypoplasia
4. Hereditary cone and rod dysfunction syndromes
   - Dominantly inherited cone dysfunction syndrome
   - Autosomal recessive cone dysfunction syndrome
   - X-linked cone dysfunction syndrome

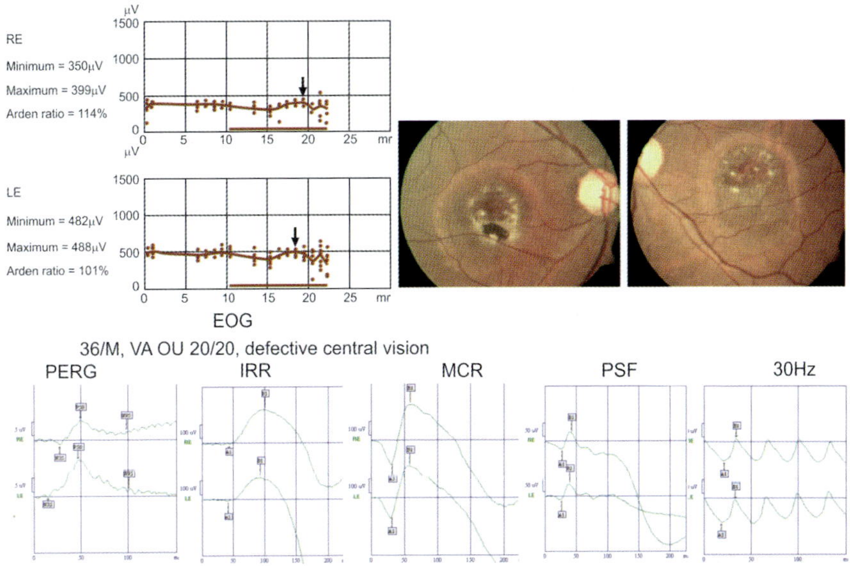

Fig. 11.5: Absent light-rise on EOG and normal ERG in Best's Disease.

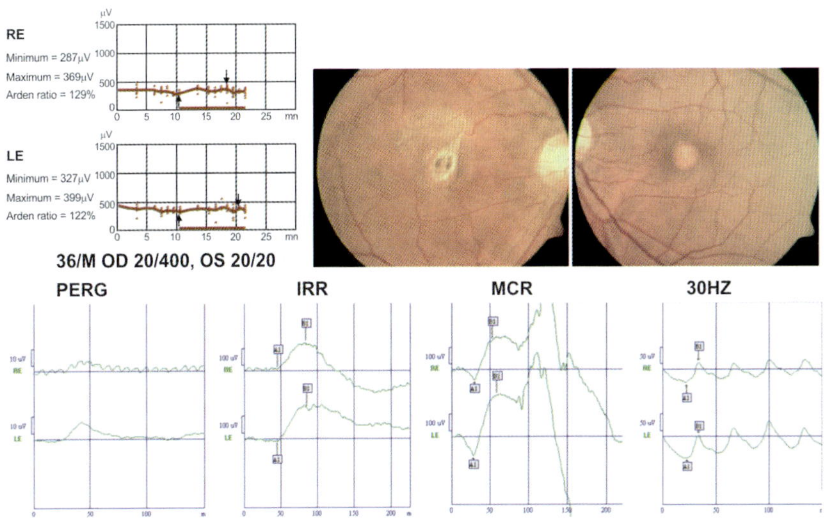

Fig. 11.6: Atrophic stage in right eye and egg-yolk stage in left eye in Best's disease

the disease to their offspring, have an abnormal EOG, but who themselves have no visible ophthalmoscopic lesions.

The earliest visible lesion, the "previtelliform stage" (stage 1) shows a fine yellow speckled pigment disturbance under the central fovea. This can appear as early as one week of age. A subtle window defect on fundus fluorescein angiography (FFA) may be present at this point. Thereafter, usually between 4 and 10 years of age, but occasionally, later, a yellow orange "cyst" like an 'intact egg yolk' evolves (stage 2). This is centered in and under the foveal neuroepithelium and ultimately progresses to about one disk-diameter in size. Although usually bilateral and symmetrical, asymmetries of both extent and size can be seen. FFA may show blocked choroidal fluorescence. Usually, there are no visual complaints at this stage.

The vitelliform "cyst" may remain intact into middle age with little disturbance in visual function, and most patients may retain visual acuity of better than 20/40. The intact vitelliform cyst may sometimes "break up" and flatten, having the appearance of a "scrambled egg" (stage 3) often with the slight reduction of visual acuity. Alternatively, it may evolve into a secondary macular retinal detachment with layering of the yellow material as a pesudohypopyon (stage 4). This yellow lipofuscin-like material gravitates inferiorly in the subretinal space and shifts with changing head positioning and is compatible with good (including 20/20) visual acuity. Peripheral visual fields and dark adaptation remain normal.

A disparity between fundus appearance and visual function should raise the suspicion of Best's diseases.

Following the pseudohypopyon stage, a variety of alternatives may occur. Resorption of the yellow material may leave an indistinct area of retinal pigment epithelial atrophy, orange to red in color due to increased visibility of the choroidal vasculature resembling central areolar choroidal sclerosis and can occur in the middle-aged and older individuals. On FFA, large choroidal vessels may become visible in the atrophic stage. Sometimes, choroidal neovascular membrane (CNVM) with subretinal pigment epithelium or subretinal hemorrhagic detachment of macula may occur even as early as at 6–10 years old. FFA and OCT help to delineate and monitor treatment of CNVM. A fibrous white central diskiform scar may develop that sometimes can retain remarkably good visual function, sometimes in the 20/40 to 20/60 range. Some eyes may have severe reduction of central vision.

Extrafoveal vitelliform lesions, unilaterally or bilaterally, may develop in some patients. Variations include drusen-size lesions, sometimes in clusters and belts, to large vitelliform cysts eccentric to the fovea, single or multiple. Uncommonly, pseudohypopyon and eccentric diskiform scars develop in these extrafoveal lesions.

Because of the wide variability of phenotypic expression, family screening by retinal examination and EOG may help to establish the diagnosis.

Pathology: Retinal pigment epithelium defect leads to accumulation of lipofuscin granules in the RPE cells and macrophages in the subretinal space and PAS positive, finely granular material in the photoreceptors

EOG and flash ERG: For Best's disease both flash ERG[6] and EOG always need to be performed. The disparity between the presence of a normal Flash ERG and an abnormal, distinctly pathological, light peak/dark trough ratio on EOG is an important diagnostic criterion for Best's disease. Only butterfly epithelial dystrophy of the fovea has similar coincidentally normal responses on flash ERG with abnormal EOG. In virtually all other diseases, the EOG is abnormal only when the ERG is abnormal. Thus, there is no merit in performing an EOG if the ERG is abnormal, since no useful information can be derived from such an abnormal EOG. The EOG abnormality may precede ophthalmoscopic findings and can help identify genetic "carriers" with normal retinal examination who can transmit disease to the next generation but do not express the macular change.

PATTERN DYSTROPHY

Pattern dystrophy[1,2,7-11] is an autosomal dominant macular dystrophy usually starts in midlife. A variety of patterns of deposits of yellow, orange, grey pigment in macular area have been described. Rarely, these could be associated with systemic conditions like myotonic dystrophy and pseudoxanthoma elasticum.

Following four groups of pattern dystrophy have been described; all characterized by normal flash ERG and EOG.

1. Group 1: Adult onset foveomacular vitelliform dystrophy
2. Group 2: Butterfly-shaped pigment dystrophy
3. Group 3: Reticular dystrophy of the pigment epithelium
4. Group 4: Coarse pigment mottling in the macula.

Foveomacular Vitelliform Dystrophy—Adult Type

Foveomacular vitelliform dystrophy—adult type is an autosomal dominant disease with mild symptoms of decreased visual acuity and metamorphopsia beginning in the fourth and fifth decades in one or both eyes, although rarely as early as age 20 years. It progresses slowly. Clinically, one can see pseudovitelliform lesions approximately, one-quarter to one-third disk. diameter in size. It is horizontally oval, slightly elevated, yellowish subretinal lesion with a surrounding ring of white or gray depigmentation and a central brown to gray dot of hyperpigmentation. There may be a few small yellow flecks paracentrally.

The histopathology in pattern dystrophies shows that the central pigmented spot consists of a clump of large pigment-laden cells and extracellular melanin, while the surrounding white/gray ring consists of granular, eosinophilic, PAS-positive material lying between the atrophic RPE and Bruch's membrane.

Color vision, ERG and EOG are normal for the patient's age and are not diagnostic. Fluorescein angiography shows a blocked center corresponding to the gray brown central pigment dot and a ring of surrounding fluorescence without secondary retinal detachment. Other reported findings are eccentric, nonfoveal lesions which on FFA block fluorescein centrally and may have a small surrounding halo window defect. Progression to severe vision loss is rarely reported.

Butterfly-shaped Pigment Pattern Dystrophy

Gray or yellow pigment is seen arranged in a well organized triradiate pattern confined to the center of the macula in the shape of a butterfly. FFA reveals hyperfluorescent margin of the non fluorescent pigment figure. The disease is moderately progressive with most patients having moderate loss of vision.

Reticular Dystrophy of the Pigment Epithelium

The pigmentation starts in the foveal area and slowly extends into the periphery of the macula in a knotted fishnet fashion. It can be seen in 10–20 % patients of pseudoxanthoma elasticum.

Coarse Pigment Mottling in the Macula

The macular area shows prominent, coarse, mottling of the pigment epithelium in the central macular area. The condition leads to moderate loss of central vision.

CENTRAL AREOLAR CHOROIDAL AND PIGMENT EPITHELIAL ATROPHY

Central areolar dystrophy[1-4] is commonly seen after 45–50 years of age. The visual acuity, fields, ERG and EOG are normal initially. Later, they develop mild-to-moderate visual loss. Retinal examination shows fine, mottled depigmentation in the macular region. This slowly evolves into symmetric, sharply outlined, bull's eye oval or round areas of geographic atrophy of the RPE in the absence of flecks/drusen. FFA shows varying degree of loss of choriocapillaris within the area of RPE atrophy. Multifocal ERG would show corresponding reduction of amplitudes (Fig. 11.7).

FAMILIAL DOMINANT DRUSEN

Familial dominant drusen[1,2,12] is an autosomal dominant disease. It is characterized by widespread drusen extending beyond the macula, especially nasal to the optic disk. It is commonly seen during routine dilated retinal screening in the fourth to fifth decades. It is generally a benign condition but some patients can develop macular atrophy or CNVM leading to a central scotoma on visual field evaluation. FFA shows atrophy of RPE and the drusen appear more extensive than seen clinically. Dark adaptation and ERG remain normal while EOG may be subnormal in some cases.

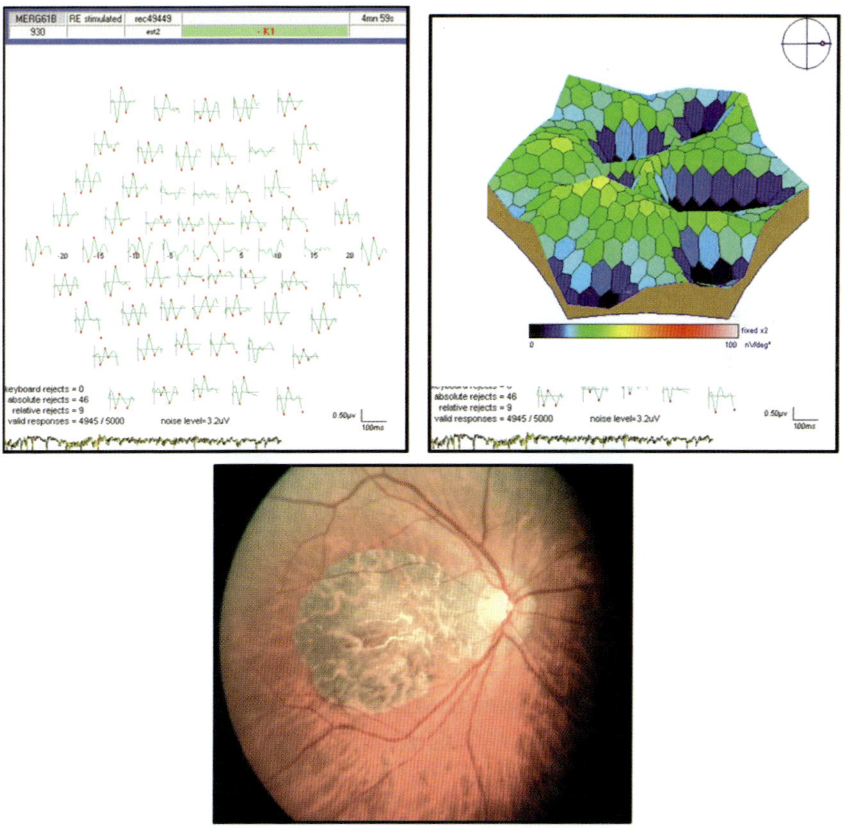

Fig. 11.7: Central areolar atrophy

Histopathology shows round accumulation of hyaline in the pigment epithelium that is continuous with the inner layer of Bruch membrane. Later on, the choroid and the neural retina show atrophy. The disease gene has been mapped to chromosome 2.

NORTH CAROLINA MACULAR DYSTROPHY

North Carolina macular dystrophy[1,2] is a rare autosomal dominant macular degeneration. It is characterized by macular coloboma with well demarcated atrophy of RPE and choriocapillaris, and pigment deposition in macular area. Visual acuity remains relatively better and can range from 6/6 to 6/60 (mean 6/18). The gene has been mapped to chromosome 6q.

PROGRESSIVE FOVEAL DYSTROPHY[1,2]

Progressive foveal dystrophy[1,2] has a dominant mode of inheritance. It shows atrophy of the pigment epithelium in the macula and flecks similar to those seen in fundus flavimaculatus. The visual loss varies from mild to severe and the disease progresses with age. There is normal cone/ and rod ERG and EOG. Color defects also present later in life.

AUTOSOMAL DOMINANT INHERITED CME

Autosomal dominant inherited CME[1,2,7] is seen in hyperopic patients at a young age. Progressive decrease in VA (<6/36) is found in 50% cases by fourth decade. It progresses to atrophy and pigmentary changes in macula which can be confirmed on FFA. Normal ERG and abnormal EOG suggest poor prognosis.

Autosomal Recessive Macular Dystrophies

STARGARDT'S DISEASE AND FUNDUS FLAVIMACULATUS

This group of diseases[1-4,13,14] is characterized by bilateral presence of peculiar yellowish flecks within the RPE. Most commonly school going children complain of recent reduction of central vision. They are unable to copy from the school board while earlier they were able to do so. Correction of refractive error does not provide 20/20 vision. At the very early stage, the flecks may be difficult to visualize ophthalmoscopically and patients may be subjected to various tests for macular and optic nerve diseases and indeed may be labeled as malingerers. Males and females are equally affected.

Classically, when flecks were distributed throughout the fundus and the onset was in adulthood, it was called as *fundus flavimaculatus*. If the

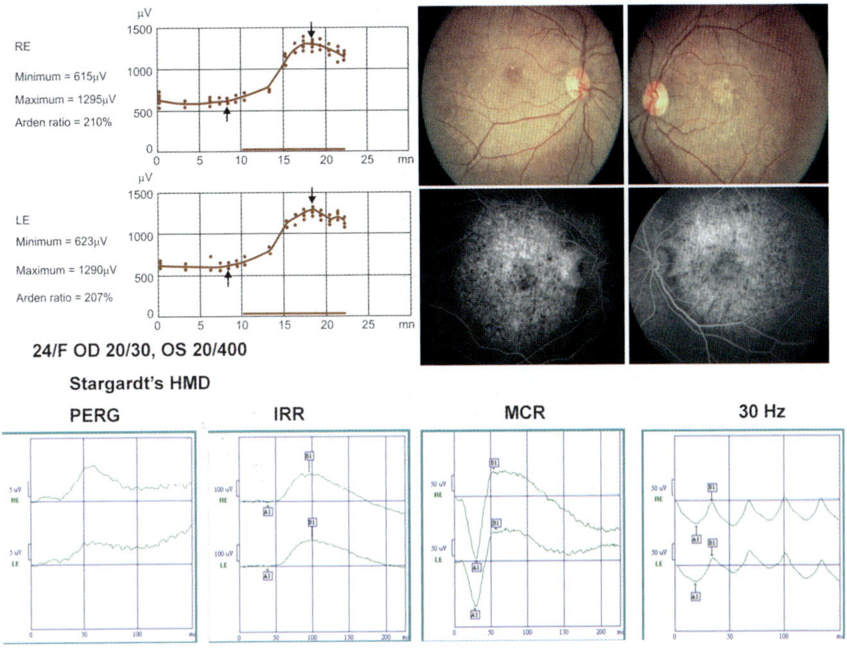

Fig. 11.8: Vermillon fundus and silent choroid on FFA with normal flash ERG, and EOG in Stargardt's dystrophy. Pattern ERG is abnormal in both eyes more in left eye that has developed atrophic changes around the fovea

flecks were confined to the posterior pole and were present relatively early in life, it was called as *Stargardt's disease*. Pathology shows excessive accumulation of lipofuschin within the RPE that prevents visualization of choroidal details. The condition has in recent years been divided into following four groups:

Group 1: Vermillon fundus and hidden choroidal fluorescence
Group 2: Atrophic maculopathy with or without flecks
Group 3: Atrophic maculopathy with late signs and symptoms of retinitis pigmentosa
Group 4: Flecks not associated with macular atrophy

***Vermillon Fundus and Hidden Choroidal Fluorescence* (Fig. 11.8)**

The heavily pigmented RPE obscures choroidal details. The FFA shows prominent retinal vessels especially the retinal capillary network against a dark background of minimal choroidal fluorescence called as the *'silent choroid.'* The optic disk and retinal vessels are normal.

***Atrophic Maculopathy with or without Flecks* (Fig. 11.9)**

The degree and pattern of atrophy of the central macular RPE vary. It may show a beaten metal (bronze) appearance or marked geographic atrophy

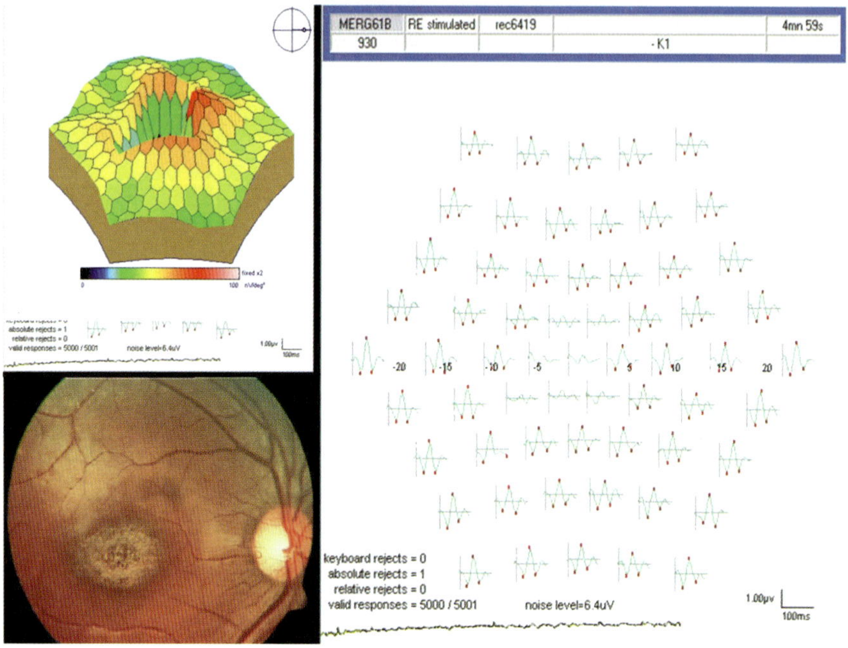

Fig. 11.9: Beaten-metal appearance of macular lesion with normal vessels and surrounding retina. Corresponding multifocal ERG in Stargardt's dystrophy.

often as a diffuse oval lesion and very rarely as a bull's eye pattern. The optic disk and retinal vessels are normal.

Atrophic Maculopathy with Late Signs and Symptoms of Retinitis Pigmentosa (RP)

The fundus appearance is similar to atrophic maculopathy with or without flecks. In addition there are signs and symptoms of RP. This includes nyctalopia, loss of pigment from RPE, narrowing of retinal vessels, pigment migration and abnormal scotopic and photopic ERG.

Flecks Not Associated With Macular Atrophy

Paracentral and central flecks are associated with minimal biomicroscopic and angiographic evidence of atrophy of the RPE. The visual acuity may be normal if the center of the fovea is not involved by a fleck. FFA shows blocked florescence due to flecks and minimal hyperflorescence due to the RPE atrophy. FFA shows more flecks than visible clinically.

The progression of symptoms in this group of disorders is variable. Visual acuity slowly decreases till it reaches around 20/40 after which there is a relative rapid progression till it reaches 20/200. By 50 years of age, almost 50% patients have 20/200 visual acuity. Eventually, visual acuity usually stabilizes between 20/200 and 20/400 in all cases.

Autofluorescence is a very useful non-invasive tool to diagnose early disease, and monitor its severity and progression. Multifocal ERG is also very useful for functional assessment of these eyes.

Genetics and clinical trials: Flecks not associated with macular atrophy is an autosomal recessive condition. It is due to mutations in the ABCA 4 gene, which normally causes production of a protein involved in the visual cycle. The dysfunctional protein produced due to ABCA 4 mutation leads to lipofuscin accumulation in the RPE cells. Gene therapies with a normal ABCA 4 gene are just starting that are believed to help in restoration of production of the normal proteins. Administration of the drugs that slow down the lipofuscin build up in retina is likely to delay the visual loss in the various stages of development of the disease.

BIETTI'S CRYSTALLINE DYSTROPHY

Bietti's crystalline dystrophy[1,2,15,16] is characterized by crystalline deposits in all the layers of retina. It has autosomal recessive inheritance. There is varying degrees of choriocapillary and RPE loss especially in the macula. Some eyes would show associated superficial limbal corneal crystals. The crystals are cholesterol and complex lipid deposits. It is a slowly progressive disorder. We recently reported tortuous vessels and subfoveal neurosensory detachment (Fig.11.10) in this condition.[16]

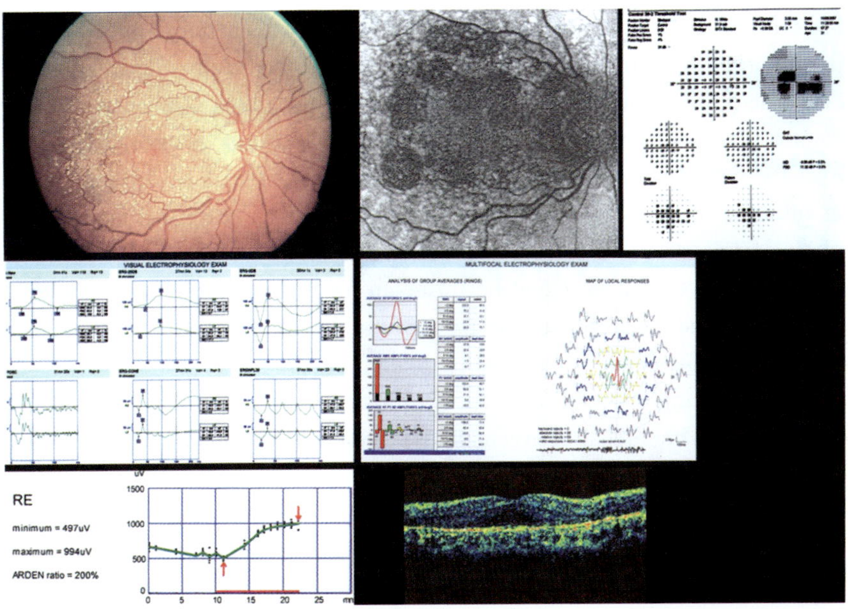

Fig. 11.10: Fundus photo, autofluorescence visual field, visual electrophysiology and OCT in Bietti's Crystalline retinal dystrophy (First published by Padhi TR, Kesarwani, Jalali S, in Doc Ophthalmologica 2011, Jun 122(3): 199-206)

SJÖGREN'S RETICULAR DYSTROPHY OF THE RPE

Sjögren's reticular dystrophy of the RPE[1,2] is a rare autosomal recessive condition characterized by accumulation of pigment in a fishnet like network at the level of the RPE. It often starts centrally and slowly extends to the peripherally in later stages. The visual acuity is affected minimally. The EOG and flash ERG are normal. FFA shows blocked choroidal fluorescence due to the pigment.

X-linked Recessive Diseases

JUVENILE X-LINKED RETINOSCHISIS

Juvenile X-linked retinoschisis[1-4,17] is characterized by typical stellate, radial schisis of the foveal tissue, often associated with surrounding radial retinal striae. One-half of all patients may also have peripheral retinoschisis cavities, usually not extending to the ora serrata. These peripheral retinoschisis are seen at presentation or develop later in life.

Clinical Features

Juvenile X-linked retinoschisis has been reported across races and ethnic groups including Asian Indians. It may be one of the most common causes of subnormal vision due to macular disease in male children and adolescents. In a clinic a bimodal age of presentation is seen in 6–10 year old school boys or in 30–50 year old adults. In schoolboys, the common mode of presentation is an inability to read the classroom board or in current times, being detected during school vision screening programs. The visual acuity cannot often be corrected beyond 20/40 to 20/60 and deteriorates slowly over the next three decades to about 20/200. Sometimes a severe congenital or infantile retinoschisis, which may evolve rapidly into retinal detachment in the first year of life, can be seen. This may sometimes present as a leukokoria or esotropia, and be mistaken for retinoblastoma or congenital retinal dysplasia. Careful ultrasonography and detailed examination of both eyes under anesthesia can usually make the diagnosis apparent.

Fundus changes are seen in the fovea and in the periphery (Figs 11.11 and 11.12). The foveal lesion called *foveal schisis* initially appears as a cluster of small radially arranged pattern of "cysts" (Figs 11.12 and 11.13). Occasionally, a few radial folds of the inner limiting membrane are also seen. FFA typically shows no leakage from the macular area (Fig. 11.12). OCT shows typical cystic changes and splitting of nerve fiber layer (Fig. 11.12) and ganglion cell layers, involving the fovea with thinning of the superficial layers. Autofluorescence imaging also highlights the foveal cystic lesions in a non-invasive manner (Fig.11.12).

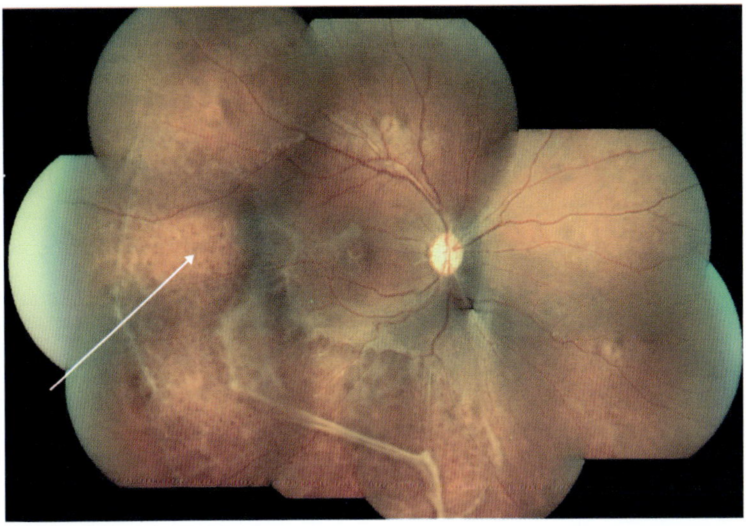

Fig. 11.11: X-linked retinoschisis with foveal and peripheral schisis. Note the dark brown, pinhead size, rounded appearance of the split retinal layers in area of the schisis, due to rupture of the Muller cells across the schisis cavity (arrow). Retinoschisis does not extend to ora

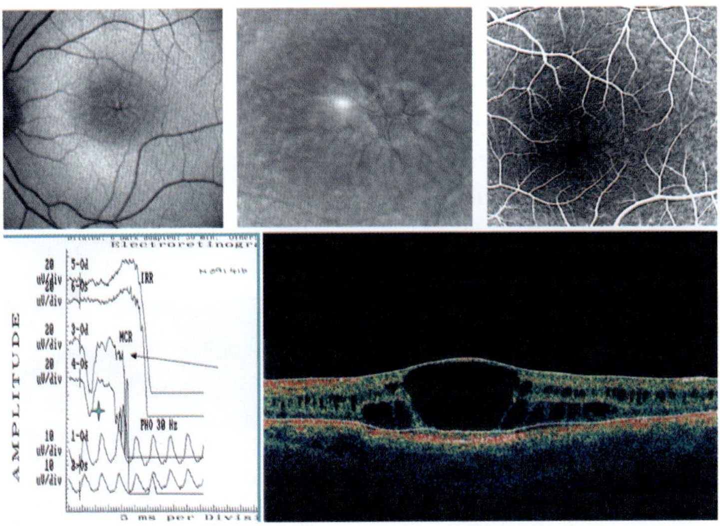

Fig. 11.12: Area of altered Autoflourescence in low and high magnification depicting cystoid and stellate pattern of foveal schisis changes. FFA shows minimal pooling of dye in the schitic stellate lesions without any obvious leakage that helps to differentiate from inflammatory CME where profuse leakage is seen. OCT of foveal schisis showing a split in the inner retina and thinning of the overlying retinal layers. Flash ERG shows a negative ERG with much reduced scotopic b-wave of inner retina (arrow) and nearly normal photoreceptor a-wave (star)

With increasing age, the characteristic radial folds in the fovea disappear as the microcysts enlarge or coalesce, forming an irregular shredded appearance, occasionally resembling a foveal hole. In late stages, foveal atrophy and thinning is seen with nonspecific pigmentary change and retinal vascular pattern changes around the fovea. Diagnosis may be difficult in such eyes. A high degree of suspicion, presence of peripheral lesions, family screening, pedigree charting and ERG provide useful clues to the disease condition.

True peripheral retinoschisis is commonly present in the inferior temporal quadrant (Fig. 11.11) and never extends to the ora serrata, unlike retinal detachments. Silver-gray, glistening spots are also seen scattered throughout the retina and may represent the first pathological changes in the retinal periphery due to splitting of the Muller cells across the retinal split (Fig. 11.13). Other fundus changes include arborescent gray-white and dendritiform figures, particularly within areas of peripheral schisis, perivascular phlebitis, vitreous veils with or without enclosed retinal vessels, "pseudopapilledema" or "pseudoneuritis," apparently caused by glial tissues spreading onto the borders of the disc. Later, clumped pigmentation suggestive of an old chorioretinitis or a spontaneously attached retinal detachment is observed.

Other long-term complications include vitreous hemorrhage, avulsed retinal vessels, vitreous veils, peripheral cysts with intracystic or vitreous hemorrhages, and both inner and outer retinal holes with resultant rhegmatogenous retinal detachment (Fig. 11.13). These would need surgical intervention in many cases. Female carriers have normal retina, normal electrophysiology and normal psychophysiology and are hence difficult to detect.

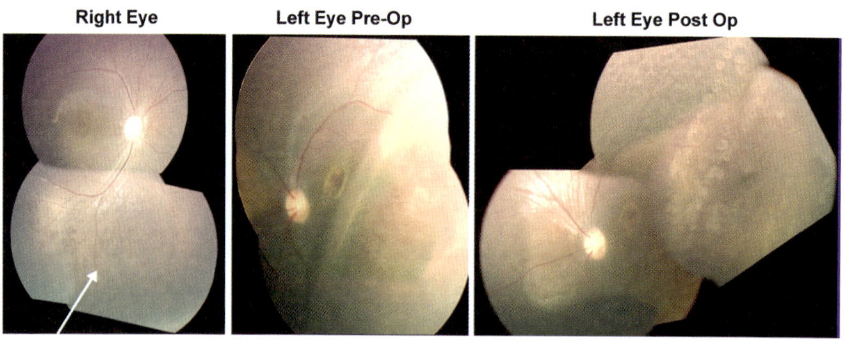

Fig. 11.13: Infantile retinoschisis: Arrow shows early peripheral schisis in right eye. Foveal schisis is seen in both eyes. The patient has recent onset left esotropia due to retinal detachment. Esotropia disappeared after surgical reattachment.

Visual Fields

Nonspecific and nondiagnostic field changes include relative central scotoma and some mild concentric constriction, Peripheral visual field reduction is seen often in the superonasal quadrant from the inferotemporal schisis. Rhegmatogenous retinal detachment would cause an absolute field defect while retinoschisis causes a relative field defect.

ERG and EOG

In flash ERG, the a-wave is generally intact but the b-wave is characteristically subnormal. The scotopic recordings are more disturbed than the photopic. ERG shows a 'negative ERG' with reduced amplitudes and prolonged implicit time of the scotopic b-wave, normal a-wave and reduced oscillatory potentials (Fig. 11.12). Other causes of inner retinal dysfunction can also appear as 'negative ERG" and need to be excluded such as congenital stationary night blindness (CSNB). With progression of the retinal pathology, all Ganzfeld voltages deteriorate and rarely, the ERG becomes non-recordable at which stage the normal EOG of retinoschisis eyes also becomes abnormal. EOG is hence not a useful diagnostic procedure.

NON-SEX-LINKED FOVEAL SCHISIS

Non-sex-linked foveal schisis[18] that affects females and males from pedigrees with autosomal dominant inheritance are also reported. In such eyes the foveal changes resemble the CME of RP rather than of retinoschisis, though peripheral retina also shows schisis in some eyes.

A. HEREDITARY CONE AND ROD DYSFUNCTION SYNDROMES

Non congenital dominantly inherited, autosomal recessively inherited and X-linked recessive cone dysfunction syndromes have been described.[1-4,7,19]

The dominantly inherited disease is most widely studied. The syndrome is characterized by a gradual progressive, reduction of visual acuity starting often in the second decade. There is no nystagmus and patients are not symptomatic in earlier years. There are associated abnormal color vision (often hue) problems and photo aversion or hemeralopia. In the initial stages, retina looks normal and visual acuity is often 20/30 or so. This is followed by early temporal disk pallor and patient may undergo VEP and neuroimaging to rule out optic nerve diseases. Macular ERG (multifocal/focal or pattern ERG) techniques can diagnose the condition to be retinal in origin at an early stage. Later stages of the disease show classical pigment stippling in the perifoveal area that evolves into a round or ovoid bulls'eye like lesion. FFA can show diffuse stippled hyperfluorescence in patients with pigment stippling. In the bulls' eye lesion, a zone of hyperfluorescence is seen that surrounds a hypofluorescent center. Some of the dystrophies may be confined to the macular area, macular cone dystrophies (Fig.11.14) or be associated with a more generalized cone dysfunction (Fig.11.15) as diagnosed by flash and macular ERG techniques. Rod responses are usually normal or subnormal with stable waveforms. Peripheral visual fields remain normal while central fields may show scotoma corresponding to the clinical lesions. Prognosis is generally better than in RP and cone-rod dystrophy. Often the patient gets benefit by tinted glasses worn according to the lighting conditions. Some patients report relief of glare with antioxidants such as betacarotene and lutein. Late-onset X-linked patients have a tapetal-like bright sheen in the inferior retina

MANAGEMENT OF HEREDOMACULAR DYSTROPHY

Initially and each subsequent visit, all patients with heredomacular dystrophy (HMD) must have detailed comprehensive eye examination, including refraction, slit-lamp biomicroscopy, ocular motility and alignment, pupillary reactions, intraocular pressure measurement, and dilated lens and fundus evaluation. Fundus evaluation should include optic nerve, macula, peripheral retina, vitreous, and retinal vasculature. It should not be forgotten that patients with HMD can develop any other ocular pathology, including glaucoma, CNS tumors, neovascular pathologies, etc. that need to be diagnosed and

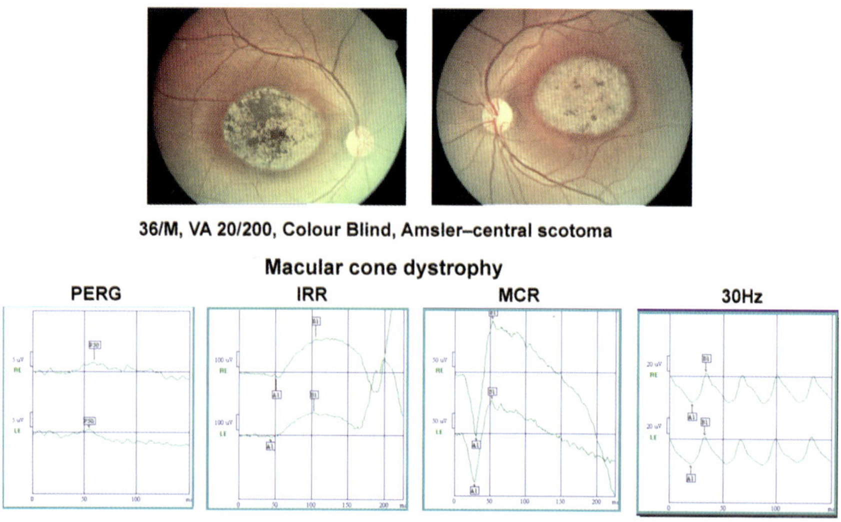

Fig. 11.14: Well circumscribed ovoid macular lesions with markedly reduced PERG and normal peripheral cone ERG responses showing localized macular cone dystrophy

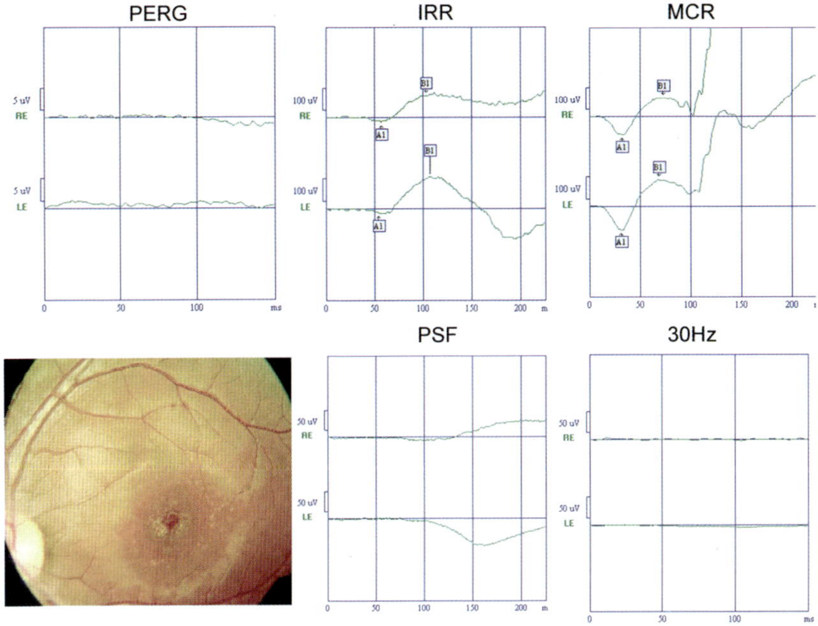

Fig. 11.15: Macular changes with absent PERG, absent photopic cone ERG and normal rod waveforms in a 47 year–female with VA of 20/400, central scotoma and defective color vision due to generalized cone dystrophy

treated. A question often asked is what should be the frequency of eye evaluations after the diagnosis is confirmed. In children and teenagers, we usually follow every year to evaluate their visual status and address their functional, educational, social and vocational needs in tandem with the low vision specialists. In adulthood, we see every 2–3 years if condition is stable and no complications are envisaged. In conditions that are known to develop complications like RD or CNVM, evaluations could be more frequent and discussion about sign/symptoms is reinforced.

While making a diagnosis especially in the early stages of HMD, it may be required to exclude optic nerve diseases, generalized retinal degenerations like retinitis pigmentosa,[1-4,20] solar retinopathy, drug toxicity and other acquired disorders including nutritional problems, trauma and drug abuse. Proper pedigree charting, family history of consanguinity and vision problems and evaluation of family members are desirable.

Detailed visual functional history should include information about nyctalopia, color vision especially matching colors, peripheral vision, light sensitivity, impaired contrast sensitivity, current and past eye poking behavior.

The history of onset and progression of visual disturbance should be noted. A general review of systems including skeletal, auditory, balance, skin, neurology, and gastroenterology are mandatory.

Investigations should start with noninvasive ones like color vision, visual fields, fundus autofluorescence, OCT and visual electrophysiology. Invasive investigations like FFA are used sometimes for diagnosis, such as in Stargardt's disease or to evaluate presence of CNVM that can be seen in Best's disease, dominant drusens and pattern dystrophy.

Detailed evaluation by a low vision specialist is critical in these patients as there are limited treatment options. Using modern technological low vision aids, most patients are able to lead near-normal educational and vocational lives. Vocational counseling and rehabilitation services are now available in many larger cities but are still to percolate down to eye hospitals in smaller towns and cities. An optometrist or vision technician can learn some basic skills of managing low vision through short term courses. Support groups are facilitated by physicians to help in advocacy and the educational, social and psychological needs of the patient.

The physician should discuss regarding proper diet rich in vitamins and minerals. Avoidance of retinal and optic nerve toxic substances, including tobacco and certain drugs may help to avoid additional causes of visual loss. There is some evidence that sunlight may cause further harm to eyes with retinal degenerations and so use of U-V blocking sunglasses or sun-protection measures like use of umbrellas/hats/caps/ dupatta, etc. are generally recommended for outdoors. Dark glasses reduce the contrast and are generally not preferred by most patients with retinal diseases, except those with a predominant cone dysfunction.

Counseling and explanation are a very important aspect in management of these potentially incurable diseases. Unfortunately, most physicians either do not have the time or patience to talk in detail to the patient or, are more often embarrassed to talk about a condition where they can offer no 'treatment'! Patients and care givers are often upset and shocked that except for telling that the disease is genetic, incurable and progressive, no further explanation or support was provided by the physician who diagnosed the condition. Realistic and correct information of nature of condition, underlying etiology, rate of progression, longterm prognosis and recent advances towards cure must be conveyed to the patient and family members. Genetic counseling regarding mode of inheritance and risk to other family members is required but unfortunately only few trained genetic counselors are available in larger cities in India currently.

References

1. Newsome DA. Retinal degenerations and dystrophies. Raven press, New York, 1998.
2. Heckenlively JR, Arden GB (editors). Principles and Practice of Clinical electrophysiology of vision. Second edition, MIT Press 2006.
3. Krill AE, Deutman AF. Hereditary retinal and choroidal dystrophies. Hagerstown Md. Harper and Row 1977.
4. Jalali S, Holder GE, Ram LSM, Vedantham V. Visual electrophysiology in the clinic: A basic guide to recording and interpretation. AIOS CME series number 17, January 2009 (available at www.aios.org).
5. Mohler CW and Fine SL. Long-term evaluation of patients with Best's vitelliform dystrophy. *Ophthalmology.* 1981;88:688-92.
6. Deutman AF. Electro-oculography in families with vitelliform dystrophy of the fovea. *Arch Ophthalmol.* 1969;81:305-16.
7. Shetty NS, Sharma T, Shanmugam MP, Bhende MP, Gopal L, Samant P, Gopal L. The Sankara Nethralaya atlas of fundus fluorescein angiography. Jaypee Brothers Medical publishers; New Delhi, 2004.
8. Bloom IH, Swanson DE, Bird AC. Adult vitelliform macular degeneration. *Br J Ophthalmol.* 1981;65:800-01.
9. Hsieh CR, Fine BS, Lyons JS. Patterned dystrophies of the retinal pigment epithelium. *Arch Ophthalmol.* 1977;95:429-35.
10. Marmor MF, Byers B. Pattern dystrophy of the pigment epithelium. *Am J Ophthalmol.* 1977;84:32-44.
11. Ayazi S, Fagan R. Pattern dystrophy of the pigment epithelium. *Retina.* 1981;1:287-9.
12. Deutman AF, Jansen LM. Dominantly inherited drusen of Bruch's membrane. *Br J Ophthalmol.* 1970;54:373-82.
13. Fishman GA, Farber M, Patel BS, Derlacki DJ. Visual acuity loss in patients with Stargardts' Macular Dystrophy. *Ophthalmology*. 1987;94:809-14.
14. Glazer LC, Dryja TP. Understanding the etiology of Stardgardt's disease. *Ophthalmol Clin N Am.* 2002;15:93-100.
15. Welch RB. Bietti's tapetoretinal degeneration with marginal corneal dystrophy and crystalline retinopathy. *Trans Am Ophth Soc.* 1977;75:164-79.
16. Padhi TR, Kesarwani S, Jalali S. Bietti's Crystalline retinal dystrophy with subfoveal neurosensory detachment and congenital tortuosity of retinal vessels. *Doc Ophthalmologica.* 2011;122(3):199-206.
17. Kellner U, Brummer S, Forester MH, Wessing A. X-linked congenital retinoschisis. *Graefes' Arch Clin Exp Ophthalmol.* 1990;228:432-7.
18. Noble KG, Carr RE, Siegel IM. Familial foveal retinoschisis associated with a rod-cone dystrophy. *Am J Ophthalmol.* 1978;85:551-7.
19. Heckenlively JR. RP cone-rod degeneration. *Trans Am Ophthalmol Soc.* 1987; 85: 438-70.
20. Jalali S. Retinitios Pigmentosa. In LC Dutta, editor. Modern Ophthalmology, 3rd edition. New Delhi; Jaypee Publication; 2005.

12
chapter

Meena Chakrabarty
Arup Chakrabarty
Sonia S John

Macular Hole

ABSTRACT

This chapter outlines the pathogenesis, clinical features, and current concepts in the management of macular holes. The results of macular hole surgery and gas tamponade as well as the role of internal limiting membrane (ILM) peeling and the relative merits and demerits of the various ILM staining techniques are highlighted.

Introduction

A macular hole is a defect of the foveal retina involving its full thickness from the internal limiting membrane (ILM) to the outer segment of the photoreceptor layer. The condition was first described by Knapp[1] in 1869 in a patient who sustained blunt trauma to the eye. Subsequent case reports and series pointed to antecedent episodes of ocular trauma such that the two were customarily linked to each other. In the present century, ophthalmologists increasingly have recognized that the condition occurs more commonly in atraumatic settings and have differentiated these macular holes from trauma-induced holes by describing them as idiopathic full-thickness macular holes. In fact, case series as far back as the 1970s reported that more than 80% of macular holes are idiopathic and that only less than 10% are associated with history of trauma to the eye.

The overall prevalence macular hole is approximately 3.3 cases in 1000, in persons older than 55 years. Peak incidence of idiopathic macular hole is found in the seventh decade of life, and women typically are affected more than men. Reasons for sex difference are not known. Cardiovascular disease, hypertension, and a history of hysterectomy have been reported as risk factors. However, none of these has been proven to have any significant effect on macular hole formation. The prevalence rate of macular hole in India is reported to be 0.17%, with a mean age 67 years.[2] The Beijing Eye Study[3] found the rate of macular holes to be 1.6 out of 1000 elderly Chinese, with a strong female predilection.

The natural history of a macular hole varies based on its current clinical stage. It has been reported that around 50% of stage 0 and stage 1 macular hole (Fig. 12.1A) may resolve both in the anatomic changes and the symptoms. Stage 2 holes progress in most cases to stage 3 or stage 4 (Fig. 12.B), resulting in worsening vision (Table 12.1). Occasionally, a full-thickness macular hole may spontaneously close with resultant good vision.[4]

An estimate for the incidence of development of an idiopathic full-thickness macular hole in the fellow eye is approximately, 12%.[5]

The figures in the Table 12.1 suggest that the natural history of macular hole is that of deterioration over a few years with subsequent stabilization of both visual acuity and size of the hole.

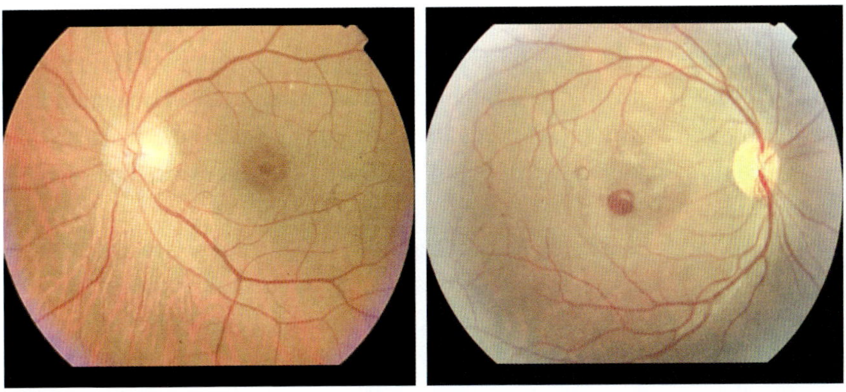

Figs 12.1A and B: Fundus photographs of stage 1 (A) and stage 4 (B) macular holes. Note the presence of localized subretinal fluid around (B)

TABLE 12.1: Natural course of idiopathic macular holes
• Nearly 50% of holes undergo spontaneous vitreofoveal separation, relief of retinal traction and show no further progression • About 8–10% holes show spontaneous resolution and one-third of these cases have visual improvement • About 40% progress to early small macular hole within several months Most stage 2 holes progress to larger stage 3 holes

Pathogenesis of Macular Hole

The exact pathogenesis of macular holes remains unknown. The first reported macular holes in the late 19th century were believed to result from trauma that caused cystoid changes in the macula. Concurrent with the discovery around 1970 that the majority of macular holes were not associated with trauma, the predominant thought was that macular hole etiology was related to the presence of cystoid macular edema (CME), including any condition, which may lead to CME.

The vitreomacular traction theory of pathogenesis of macular hole gained in popularity with the recognition that peripheral retinal breaks occur secondary to vitreoretinal traction and that strong adhesion exists between the vitreous and fovea. The recognition of a temporal association between posterior vitreous detachment (PVD) and full-thickness macular hole assisted Gass [7] in the development of the grading scheme. Optical coherence tomography has enhanced our understanding of the orientation of this traction, which is now thought to be predominantly anteroposterior (A-P) in direction.

There is also mounting evidence that A-P traction may not be the only factor in macular hole formation. Researchers have documented macular hole formation after complete PVD/vitrectomy as well as spontaneous closure of macular hole in eyes without PVD (documented by OCT). Such observations led to the development of other theories of macular hole pathogenesis, such as the hydrodynamic model, in which the macular hole is formed or maintained by fluid flow caused by the macular retinal pigment epithelium pump.

The hydration theory of pathogenesis of macular holes was put forward in 2003 by Tornambe et al.[8] In this theory, posterior hyaloidal traction on fovea resulting in a tear in inner fovea was the first step in the genesis of macular holes. Seepage of fluid vitreous into the spongy layers of the macula through this defect resulted in the creation of a cavity in inner retina, enlargement of hole and spread of fluid to outer retina. Resistance is offered by RPE and Bruchs membrane to the seepage of fluid vitreous. Therefore, the swollen retina remains elevated and retracted.

In reality, the etiology of macular hole is probably multifactorial, and determining the primary event may be less important than the recognition that vitreomacular traction, foveolar dehiscence, and other factors are likely to play a role.

Macular hole has long been recognized as a female-predominant disease, yet despite extensive research, the reason for such a gender predilection is unclear, and there is no strong evidence to support an association between estrogen replacement[9] and macular hole.

Staging of Macular Holes

Gass classified macular hole in following stages:

- **Stage 1a:** Tangential vitreous traction results in the elevation of the fovea marked by presence of foveal detachment and increased clinical prominence of xanthophyll pigment. This stage is occasionally referred to as the *yellow dot stage* and can also be seen in cases of central serous chorioretinopathy, cystoid macular edema, and solar retinopathy.
  Fundus photograph of a stage 1a macular hole presents characteristic yellow spot at the center of the fovea.
- **Stage 1b:** As the foveal retina elevates to the level of the perifovea, the yellow dot of xanthophyll pigment changes to a donut-shaped yellow ring. Persistent traction on the fovea leads to dehiscence of deeper retinal layers at the umbo.
- **Stage 2:** This is the first stage when a full-thickness break in the retina exists. It is defined as a full-thickness macular hole less than 400 μm in size. The full-thickness defect may appear eccentric, and there may be a pseudo-operculum at this stage if there has been spontaneous vitreofoveolar separation. These opercula have been examined and found to be vitreous condensation and glial proliferation without harboring any retinal tissue.
- **Stage 3:** A full-thickness macular hole in the retina exists. It is greater than 400 μm in size and is still with partial vitreomacular adhesion/traction.
- **Stage 4:** A full-thickness macular hole exists in the presence of a complete separation of the vitreous from the macula and the optic disk. There is recent evidence, however, that, even in the presence of an apparent posterior vitreous detachment, a thin shell of residual cortical vitreous may still remain and contribute to the macular hole.

The advent of ocular coherence tomography (OCT) has provided *in vivo* structural support to the hypotheses focused on vitreous traction underlying idiopathic macular holes. Both biomicroscopic examination and OCT can evaluate the various stages of the macular holes (Fig. 12.2). The OCT has allowed careful evaluation of the vitreoretinal interface demonstrating persistent adhesion on the fovea resulting in oblique traction on the fovea even with a partial posterior vitreous detachment. The persistent traction on the fovea prior to anatomic changes to the fovea has been referred to as stage 0.[10] The clinical appearance may resolve without progression in 40–50% of patients.

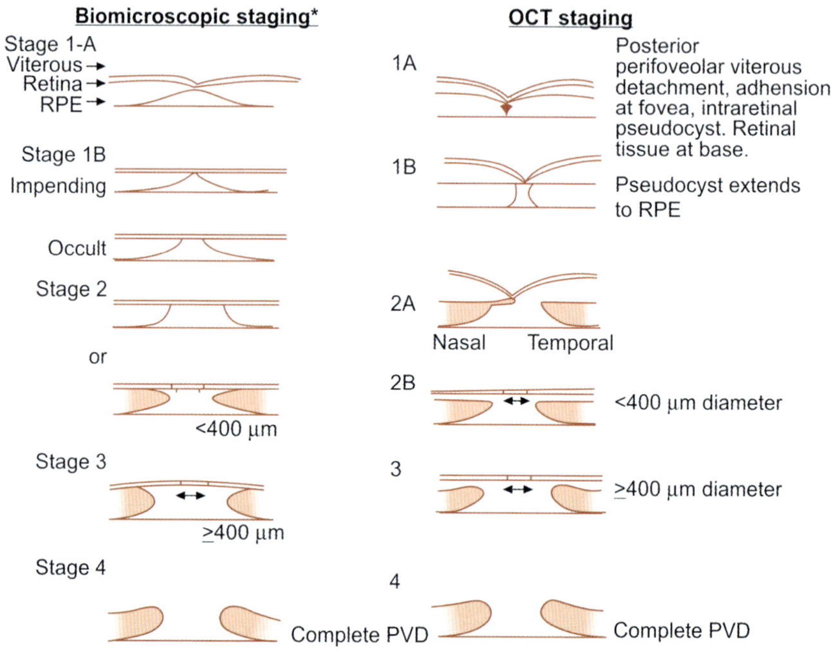

Fig. 12.2: Comparison between the biomicroscopic and OCT staging of macular holes (Adapted from Ryan SJ, ed. *Retina*. 1994:1169-85)

STAGE 1A: Perifoveal PVD with central adherence. Intraretinal pseudocysts with retinal tissue at base

STAGE 1B: Impending hole with pseudocyst extending to RPE.

STAGE 2A: Full-thickness with partial opening of roof. And focal vitreous adhesion to flap of <400 microns size

STAGE 2B: Full-thickness operculated MH <400 microns with traction on fovea released

STAGE 3: Full-thickness operculated > 400 micron with Vitreous traction released

STAGE 4: Full-thickness MH with Complete PVD

Screening of eye[11, 12] at regular intervals can document progression macular hole in the eye (Figs 3A to D). In eyes without preexisting PVD the cumulative risk of developing macular hole is 4.6% in 3 years, 6.5% in 5 years, and 7.1 % in 6 years. In eyes with PVD the risk is negligible.

Visual dysfunction in patients with macular hole [13] is directly related to the absence of retinal tissue in the fovea. However, visual dysfunction may seem out of proportion to the size of the macular hole and potentially may also be related to the presence of a cuff of subretinal fluid with associated photoreceptor atrophy.

Patients with idiopathic macular holes present with a variety of symptoms. Initial symptoms include blurred central vision or metamorphopsia. Patients may characterize these symptoms as being mild and only apparent when

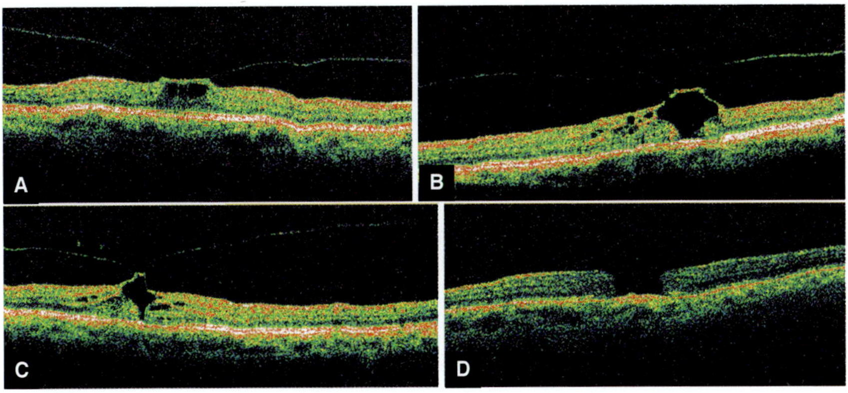

Figs 12.3A to D: Showing the serial OCT follow up of a 60-year-old female patient during 9-month holes progression to full-thickness MH occurred

reading or driving. Because the initial changes may be mild and gradual, it may be some time before the patient discovers that something is wrong with their vision. Macular holes may only be discovered when patients cover one eye and notice blurred vision and metamorphopsia in the opposite eye. Rarely, some patients may describe the exact moment at which the hole developed, but more commonly, they describe the onset as slow and gradual if at all noticeable. Later, a larger macular hole may produce a central defect, or scotoma, in the central vision of the patient[14.] Some patients may be asymptomatic, and the hole is diagnosed only on routine ophthalmologic examination.The visual acuity of the patient varies according to the size, location, and the stage of the macular hole. Patients with small, eccentric holes may retain excellent visual acuity in the range of 6/9 to 6/12. In addition, a macular hole that is not full thickness can have very good visual acuity in the range of 6/18 to 5/60. However, once a macular hole is well developed or full thickness, the usual range of visual acuity is from 6/24 to 2/60, averaging at 6/60[15] (Table 12.2).

A full-thickness macular hole visualized with direct ophthalmoscope [16] is characterized by a well-defined round or oval lesion in the macula with yellow-white deposits at the base. These yellow dots probably represent lipofuscin-laden macrophages or nodular proliferations of the underlying pigment epithelium with associated eosinophilic material. With biomicroscopic (slit-lamp) examination, [17] a round excavation with well-defined borders interrupting the beam of the slit-lamp can be observed.

In most patients, an overlying semitranslucent tissue, representing the pseudo-operculum, can be seen suspended over the hole. There is often a surrounding cuff of subretinal fluid. Cystic changes of the retina also

TABLE 12.2: Clinical features of various stages of Macular Holes

Clinical features	Stage 1A and 1B	Stage 2	Stage 3	Stage 4
Inital symptoms	Metamorphopsia mild loss	>6/12	6/12-6/60	>1/60
Microscopy/ OCT	VMT/ Preifoveolar detachment	VMTTR on flap pseudo-operculum	Pseudo-operculum	PVD
Fundus	Foveolar depression yellow spot/ ring (100-300)	Central/ eccentric small, 400 μm full thickness	>400 μm neurosensory RD	400–1500 μm neurosensory RD
FFA	Hyper-fluorescence	Hyper-fluorescence	Hyper-fluorescence	Hyper-fluorescence

may be evident at the margins of the hole. The retinal pigment epithelium is usually intact and normal in acute stages but may undergo chronic changes, such as atrophy and hyperplasia, with time. Fine crinkling of the inner retinal surface caused by an epiretinal membrane may be present and sometimes may even distort the appearance of the hole.

The most useful diagnostic tests for ophthalmologists to distinguish full-thickness macular holes from other lesions are the Watzke-Allen and the laser aiming beam tests. The Watzke-Allen test[18] is performed at the slit-lamp using a macular lens and placing a narrow vertical slit-beam through the fovea. A positive test is elicited when patients detect a break in the bar of light that they perceive. This reaction is due to the fact that there is a lack of retinal element in the area of the hole, thus producing a central defect or scotoma. Narrowing or distortion of the bar of light is not diagnostic of full-thickness macular holes and should be interpreted with caution. The laser aiming beam test also is performed similarly, but this time a small 50 μm spot size laser aiming beam is placed within the lesion. A positive test is obtained when the patient fails to detect the aiming beam when it is placed within the lesion but is able to detect it once it is placed onto normal retina. In addition, some slit-lamps are equipped with a setting to project a small test object, often a star, onto the fovea. Again, the patient is asked whether they perceive the test object.

Etiology of Macular Hole

TRAUMA

Approximately 6% of patients experiencing a contusion injury of the eye, develop a macular hole following the trauma. Trauma[19-22] is also commonly associated with commotio retinae involving the macula, subretinal hemorrhage, and intraretinal hemorrhage.

PROGRESSIVE HIGH MYOPIA (FOVEAL SCHISIS)

Patients with high myopia[23-26] may develop foveal schisis, which can progress to a full-thickness macular hole. Of those patients in whom foveal schisis identified, 31% developed macular holes. Risk factors include axial eye length, macular chorioretinal atrophy, and vitreoretinal interface factors.

PRECEDING RHEGMATOGENOUS RETINAL DETACHMENT REPAIR

Less than 1% of patients with a successfully repaired rhegmatogenous retinal detachment[27] will present with macular holes several years later.

DIFFERENTIAL DIAGNOSIS

The macular hole must be differentiated from the following conditions:

1. Pseudo hole due to epimacular membrane[28]
2. Cystoid macular edema[29]
3. Lamellar macular hole[30,31]

Primary consideration should be given to conditions that may mimic the appearance of a macular hole. While most of these conditions are readily apparent clinically, subtle presentations may present as a macular hole. These conditions include any disease that can cause the development of cystoid macular edema (eg. choroidal neovascularization, retinal vein occlusions, retinitis pigmentosa). An appropriate work-up and examination should identify these conditions. Ocular coherence tomography (OCT) allows high-resolution cross-sectional imaging of the retina. OCT allows the physician to detect the presence of a macular hole as well as changes in the surrounding retina. OCT can distinguish lamellar holes and cystic lesions of the macula from macular holes. Also, the status of the vitreomacular interface can be evaluated. This allows the clinician to evaluate the earliest of the stages of a macular hole as well as evaluate for other vision-limiting conditions associated with macular holes, such as a surrounding cuff of subretinal fluid and epiretinal membranes. Fluorescein angiography (FA) may be a useful test in differentiating macular holes from masquerading lesions, such as cytoid macular edema (CME) and choroidal neovascularization (CNVM). Full-thickness stage 3 holes typically produce a window defect early in the angiogram. The arteriovenous phase of the angiogram best demonstrates a granular hyperfluorescent window associated with the overlying pigment layer changes. No leakage or accumulation of dye is observed as opposed to other lesions. In CME, a gradual accumulation of dye occurs in the cystoid spaces, eventually demonstrating a petaloid appearance late in the angiogram. B-scan ultrasonography may be helpful in elucidating the relationship of the macula to the vitreous; therefore, it may be helpful in staging the disease but is not sensitive to distinguish a true macular hole from masquerading lesions.

Investigations

- ***Amsler grid abnormalities,***[32] although sensitive for macular lesions, are not specific for macular holes. Plotting of small central scotomas caused by full-thickness macular holes using the Amsler grid is difficult because of the poor fixation in the affected eye. However, bowing of the lines and micropsia frequently are appreciated. This could be attributable to the surrounding area of retinal edema and intraretinal cysts, which can be seen in macular holes as well as other lesions like CNV.
- ***Microperimetry***[33] and ***multifocal electroretinography***[34] have also been used to evaluate patients with idiopathic macular holes. These studies show loss of retinal function corresponding to the macular hole with subsequent recovery of function following surgical repair of the hole.

MEDICAL CARE

No current medical treatment exists for macular holes. Historically, therapy for macular holes has evolved from pharmacologic interventions, such as anxiolytics and vasodilators, to an assortment of surgical techniques, such as cerclage, scleral buckles, direct photocoagulation of the hole edges, and intraocular gas tamponade without the aid of vitrectomy. In 1982, Gonvers and Machemer[35] were the first to recommend vitrectomy, intravitreal gas, and prone positioning for retinal detachments secondary to macular holes.

Kelly and Wendel[36] reported that vision might be stabilized or even improved if it were possible to surgically relieve tangential traction on the macula, reduce the cystic changes, and reattach the cuff of detached retina surrounding the macular hole. They proposed that by performing this surgery, they could flatten the retina and possibly reduce the adjacent cystic retinal changes and neurosensory macular detachment.

In 1991, Kelly and Wendel[37] demonstrated that vitrectomy, removal of cortical vitreous and epiretinal membranes, and strict face-down gas tamponade could successfully treat full-thickness macular holes. The overall results of their initial report were a 58% anatomic success rate and visual improvement of 2 or more lines in 42% of eyes. A succeeding report showed a 73% anatomic success rate and 55% of patients improving 2 or more lines of visual acuity. Present anatomic success rates range from 82 to 100% depending on the series.[38-42] Possible mechanisms to explain why vitrectomy and fluid-gas exchange can close a macular hole include relief of traction (tangential and A-P) and stimulation of fibroglial proliferation to plug the hole. Histopathology evidence has revealed hyperplastic RPE and fibroglial cells associated with spontaneously closed macular holes. A variety of adjuvant therapies have been used at the time of surgery in an effort to enhance glial proliferation. Prospective, randomized studies of transforming growth factor beta (TGF-β) [43] and autologous platelets[44] have, however, shown little benefit in terms of anatomic closure or final visual acuity. Case reports exist that describe the use of autologous plasmin for idiopathic and traumatic macular holes. Ongoing clinical trials are evaluating the role of plasmin[45] as a means of "chemovitrectomy." In these studies, case illustrations have demonstrated resolution of idiopathic macular holes following intravitreal injection of plasmin and no surgical intervention.

There are several controversies regarding the surgical management of macular holes

1. How soon to advice surgical intervention?

OCT will help to detect stage 1 and stage 2 macular holes. It is best to observe eyes with VA 6/6 and monitor progression (<6/12).

Some stage 2A holes can be closed with out surgical intervention by inducing vitreofoveolar separation by air injection and maneuvering the air bubble under the flap to detach the posterior hyaloid phase adherent to the flap. This was demonstrated by Chang and associates[46] with OCT demonstration of vitreofoveolar separation. Surgical results are best for macular holes <1 year duration. But some chronic holes do well as demonstrated by Steele et al[47] who achieved a closure rate of 83% in holes of >4.2 years duration; and 39% of these eyes achieved a final vision of >20/70)

Thus, it is reasonable to offer surgery for macular holes of 1–5 years duration especially if the fellow eye has a visually debilitating and progressive macular or optic nerve pathology. The potential for better vision, as well as the 12% chance that the fellow eye will develop another macular hole, has prompted ophthalmologists to seek for a viable treatment of this condition.

Indications for consideration in the surgical management of macular holes are based on the presence of a full-thickness defect. Once this defect has developed, the potential for spontaneous resolution is low. Thus, surgical management is recommended with documentation of a stage 2 or higher, full-thickness macular hole. Stage 1 holes and lamellar holes are managed conservatively with observation at this time.

Lamellar holes cause symptoms but minimal loss of central visual acuity. Management has historically been conservative. Garretson et al[48] reported a series of successfully repaired lamellar macular holes, wherein 93% eyes demonstrated improved visual acuity. The mean improvement was 3.2 Snellen lines.

Some aspects of the surgery may vary, but the basic technique is the same. The anterior and middle vitreous is removed via a standard 3-port pars plana vitrectomy. Patients with macular hole frequently undergo vitrectomy using smaller gauge vitrectomy systems (i.e., 25 gauge, or the 23 gauge). The critical step appears to be the removal of the perimacular traction. Factors contributing to this traction, such as the posterior hyaloid, the ILM, and coexisting epimacular membranes, need to be addressed. The traction exerted by the posterior hyaloid on the macula should be relieved by either removing just the perimacular vitreous or combining it with the induction of a complete posterior vitreous detachment. Various surgical techniques have been described to accomplish this task, including the use of a soft-tipped silicon cannula or the vitrectomy cutter using suction alone. A "fish-strike sign"[49] or bending of the silicon cannula has been described as a sign that the posterior hyaloid has been engaged. Then, it may be released from the underlying retina and removed with the vitrectomy cutter.

2. To peel or Not to peel internal limiting membrane?

The removal of ILM is considered to be a contributing factor in the success of macular hole surgeries. ILM peeling may be accomplished via a "rhexis" not unlike that of a capsulorrhexis in lens surgeries.[50] Very fine forceps may be used to peel the ILM from the underlying retina. Care should be taken not to include the deeper layers in the forceps' grasp, which may further damage the surrounding retinal tissues. Many surgeons use vital dyes to stain the ILM making it easier to visualize and manipulate.

Peeling of epiretinal membrane (ERM) or ILMD, through release of cytokines, is thought to induce a similar fibroglial proliferation in order to facilitate macular hole closure.[51] ILM peeling may also remove any contractile ERM formed above it, thereby, relieving tangential traction. In addition, membrane removal can enhance mobility of the hole edges, thereby, facilitating re-approximation. Data on whether the benefit of ILM peeling is translated into improved anatomical and functional results are not available. Several retrospective studies suggest that ILM peeling is beneficial [52-56] in attaining improved visual acuity and anatomic closure in macular holes of less than six months duration. A multicenter controlled randomized trial[57] showed a significant increase in closure rates with ERM peeling, but no effect on visual acuity. Accordingly, there has been some concern regarding damage to the retina secondary to membrane peeling. Another study[58]showed that internal limiting membrane peeling at the time of macular hole surgery significantly improves the closure rate of macular holes larger than 400 μm in diameter but has no effect on the closure rate of smaller macular holes. Based on an association between ERM formation and late hole reopening, some have postulated that ILM peeling may prevent macular hole recurrence. Indocyanine green dye[59] has been successfully used to facilitate visualization during ILM peeling; however, several studies have demonstrated significant retinal toxicity and decreased visual acuity results associated with this technique. A recent review[60] showed that the use of ICG during macular hole surgery is not associated with worse visual outcome, suggesting that retinal toxicity may not be clinically significant.

One study using scanning laser ophthalmoscopy[61] revealed paracentral scotomas in more than half of patients after ILM peeling. However, a prospective study[62] with five-year follow-up revealed that macular hole surgery with ILM peeling is a safe and effective procedure with 95% of patients achieving anatomic closure and 92% achieving improvement in visual acuity. In that study, the majority of patients (97%) were pseudophakic at five years, but there were no cases of late hole reopening or ERM formation after successful hole closure. The absence of a large randomized clinical trial likely accounts for the lack of consensus regarding the efficacy of and indications for ILM peeling.

Use of vital dyes for internal limiting membrane peeling

Indocyanine green (ICG) dye was the first vital dye used for macular surgery. There is considerable literature questioning the toxicity of ICG dye to the retina and retinal pigment epithelium (RPE). Despite the laboratory and literature cautioning the use of ICG dye, an equal amount of literature documented good surgical and visual results. ICG dye is still used by surgeons with care taken to limit the exposure of the retina and, potentially more importantly, the RPE to the dye (Table 12.3)

Trypan blue has also been used to stain the ILM without the literature suggesting toxicity. On the other hand, trypan blue does not appear to stain the ILM as effectively as ICG dye. Triamcinolone acetonide has also been used to facilitate peeling of the ILM.

TABLE 12.3: Comparative analysis of the efficacy and toxicity of ICG used for ILM staining in MHS and ERM peels

S. No	Authors	Year	Procedure	ICG Effect	Complication
1.	Sheidow et al[63]	2003	MHS	Worse visual acuity when ICG used as adjuvant	
2.	Gass et al[64]	2003	MHS	Worse visual acuity when ICG used as adjuvant	
3.	Ando et al[65]	2004	MHS	Worse visual acuity when ICG used as adjuvant	Optic atrophy
4.	HillenKamp J et al[66]	2006	ERM	No difference with and without ICG	Optic atrophy
5.	Lochead et al[67]	2004	MHS	No adverse effects	
6.	Slaughter and Lec[68]	2004	MHS	No adverse effects	
7.	Rodrigues and Meyer[69]	2007	MHS	No difference in anatomic outcome	Worse functional outcome

Brilliant blue G is less toxic to the retinal pigment epithelium and stains both ERM and ILM well.

Majority of studies used ICG in higher concentration and this factor could be responsible for the toxicity. We suggest following safety measures when using ICG for ILM peeling:

1. Perform a fast surgical procedure in order to minimize the duration of contact with RPE cells and to minimize the ICG exposure to light from endo illuminator.
2. Use ICG concentrations lower than 0.5 mg/ml to minimize the risk of RPE damage and possible retinal toxicity.
3. Avoid ICG injection direct through the macular hole by any method to control ILM staining (slow injection, use of the 20 gauge, prototype painting brush called vitreoretinal internal limiting membrane color enhancer (VINCE)[70] or by use of perfluorocarbons over the macular hole, etc).
4. Epiretinal membranes, if present, also should be removed.

Techniques in completing this procedure vary from surgeon to surgeon.

3. Are adjuvants necessary to optimize surgical outcome?

Bovine TGF-β,[71] Recombinant TGFβ[72] platelets,[73] autologous serum,[74] and plasmin[75] are adjuvants commonly used in macular hole surgery. Which one is effective? Does it have effect on late reopening? Does ILM peeling create adjuvants? are all partially answered questions with various studies demonstrating a positive outcome or no added effect following use of adjuvant. Use of adjuvant[76] may be necessary in recurrent holes, myopic holes, ruptured cyst, traumatic holes, chronic holes, and pediatric holes, The use of pharmacologic adjuncts, such as a transforming growth factor-beta (TGF-beta) and autologous serum, to facilitate hole closure has not been proven to have any added benefit as compared to controls and hence their use has not gained much popularity.

4. Which gas to be used intraocular for temponade?

After careful indirect ophthalmoscopic examination of the peripheral retina for tears, a total air-fluid exchange is performed to desiccate the vitreous cavity. A nonexpansile concentration of a long-acting gas is exchanged for air. Studies have shown that a longer period of internal tamponade equated to a higher success rate.[78]

Sterile air and varying concentrations of either perfluoropropane or sulfur hexafluoride have been used based on surgeon preference for internal tamponade. The primary difference achieved using different gases is the duration of action of the gas bubble and, consequently, the amount of internal tamponade achieved within the first several days after surgery.

The rate of hole closure of idiopathic macular holes is based on many important factors mentioned below:

1. Size of the hole.
2. Duration of symptoms.
3. Whether ILM peeling has been performed or not.
4. Type of Tamponade (air/C3F8, SF6, or silicone oil).
5. Length of face-down position.

The mechanism by which the gas bubble closes the hole is not really known. It was initially thought that the buoyancy of the gas was what reattached the retina. Berger et al [79] successfully proved that the buoyancy exerted by the intraocular gas bubble is small. It was later postulated that it was the interfacial tension rather than the buoyancy that reattached the retina. Therefore, if surface tension is all that is important, the gas must be in contact with the hole all the time.

Longer-acting gas like C3F8 allows for 2–3 weeks of contact between hole and gas if supine position is avoided. Hence, there is more leeway in positioning. Shorter acting gas therefore requires more rigorous positioning to achieve hole/gas contact as bubble dissipates. Positioning may actually be more critical as the bubble dissipates. Majority of surgeons use C3F8 (64% C3F8 versus 33% SF6). Intraocular tamponade with C3F8 gas produces 6 weeks of visual debility which is as cumbersome to the patient as the prone positioning. Ulnar neuropathy has also been reported in patients on prolonged face down positioning.

The duration for which face-down prone positioning is advocated is also variable. Majority of surgeons[80] advocate at least 2 weeks of face down positioning (63%) while 25% advice only 1 week of prone positioning (Tables 12.4A and B).

Historically, strict face-down positioning had been recommended for patients for up to 4 weeks, with consequent difficulties of compliance and patient's quality of life during that period. Traditionally, it has been believed that the shorter the period of face-down positioning, the lower the rate of successful hole closure. In 1997, Tournambe et al described a pilot study of patients without face-down positioning. They reported a success rate with one surgery of 79% and suggested that pseudophakia was necessary for consideration of liberalization of positioning requirements. The advent of ILM peeling has encouraged a second look at minimal to no face-down positioning. Rubinstein et al[90] described a case series of 24 eyes of patients who underwent ILM peeling and then did not position postoperatively. In this case series, 22 eyes were successfully closed and had visual improvement. Both eyes that failed were stage 4 large holes. Others have reported comparable, if not better, results in patients with only 1 day of positioning.

TABLE 12.4A: Showing duration of face-down prone position reported by various authors

Author	Patients	Size/Duration	ILM	Gas	Position	Closure
Park 1999	58	All	+	Air	4 days	91%
Isomae 2002	21	Recent	–	C3F8	1 day	91%
Sato 2003	23	Small	+	Air	1 day	91%
Krohn 2005	24	All	–	C3F8	3 days	87.5%
Wickens 2006	21	All	+	Mostly C3F8	3 days	95%

TABLE 12.4B: Meta analysis of available literature on results of macular hole surgery sans positioning

Author	Patients	Size/Duration	ILM	Gas	Position	Closure
Tornambe 1997	33	21% chronic	_	C3F8		79%
Simcock 2001	20	STAGE 2 &3	_	C2F6		90%
Tranos 2007	16	ALL	+	C3F8		88%
Merkur 2007	72	RECENT	+	C3F8		92%

Dhawahir-Scala et al[91] suggests that a critical factor is the size of the gas bubble on postoperative day 1 being greater than 70%.Tranos et al[83] showed, however, that there may be more rapid progression of cataract formation with less face-down positioning. Tranos et al were among several authors who recommended combined phacovitrectomy for phakic patients to allow less stringent positioning requirements.

Macular hole surgery is generally associated with good anatomical success. Various periods of face down positioning have been suggested to allow for anatomical closure. The addition of ILM peeling has been reported to increase the rate of anatomical hole closure.

Histologic analysis of ILM specimens removed during macular hole surgery indicated that with higher stages of macular holes there was an increased amount of myofibroblasts. ILM peeling may reduce the tangential tractional forces by assuring that any remaining cortical vitreous or surface myofibroblasts are removed. As the edges of the hole become more mobile, the hole closes in a shorter period, allowing for a reduced period of face down positioning. In addition to reducing tangential traction, other investigators have suggested that ILM removal may increase cytokine release and thus enhance glial proliferation that leads to hole closure. Previous reports have evaluated the necessity of extended periods of face down positioning. Krohn[88] found similar hole closure rates for 3-day and 1-week face down positioning with vitrectomy, gas tamponade, and no ILM peeling. Macular holes closed when surgery was performed with vitrectomy, ILM peeling, intravitreous air, and face down positioning for 4 days.[89] Tornambe et al[81] described macular hole surgery without any face down positioning. In a series of 33 macular holes, 79% closed when surgery was performed with 15% C3F8, no ILM peeling, and no face down requirements. In a single case observation, Sato et al reported with optical coherence tomographic images that a fullthickness macular hole closed completely within 3 days after ILM peeling and gas tamponade. These studies support a shortened period of face down positioning. A difficulty with macular hole surgery is often motivating the patient to accept face down positioning. Extended periods of face down positioning often produce neck or back pain. There have been reports of complications, including ulnar nerve neuropathy and pressure sores. In addition to these medical complications, there are the financial costs of lost time from work, caregiver requirements, and expensive medical equipment. These associated costs of macular hole surgery may be reduced if a shorter period of for postoperative positioning of patient, such as the reina recovery system face down positioning were required.

A shortened prone positioning period offers patients decreased risk of medical complication, increases patient convenience, and lowers the indirect costs of macular hole surgery.

In the surgical management, we often use air or gas bubble, long acting gas, ILM peeling and vitrectomy depending on the stage and duration of mucular hole. Old patients seldom follow instructions regarding facedown positioning. Our results in terms of anatomical closure of the hole and visual improvement are encouraging (Figs 12.4A to D)

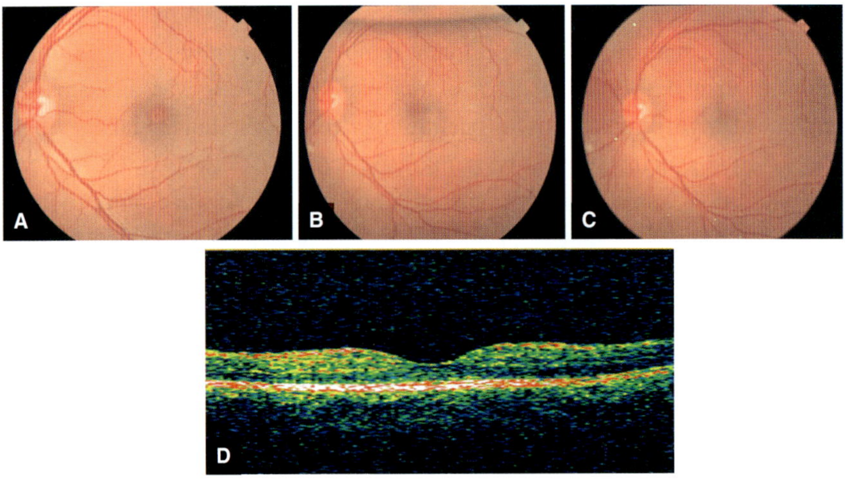

Figs 12.4A to D: A. Preoperative stage 3 Macular hole and postoperative B. appearance on day 20 and at C. 1 month and D. OCT after surgery

Long-acting gas with face down positioning for up to three weeks was used earlier in the development of surgery for macular hole. There is evidence, however, that macular holes can be effectively closed without strict positioning regimens. One study of stage 3 and 4 macular holes revealed a 90% closure rate with significant improvement in visual acuity one year after vitrectomy combined with ILM peeling, instillation of C3F8 gas, and 15 day postoperative period avoiding the supine position. OCT has demonstrated anatomic resolution beginning as soon as one day after surgery. Infusion of silicone oil or a gas bubble theoretically provides a scaffolding or template for fibroglial proliferation. Face-down positioning is commonly used to facilitate macular hole tamponade and closure postoperatively.

Silicone oil has also been used as an internal tamponade for patients with difficulty positioning or altitude restrictions. However, the use of silicone oil necessitates a second subsequent surgery to remove the oil. Furthermore, the visual results are not comparable to the use of gas tamponade, possibly as a result of silicone oil toxicity at the level of the photoreceptors and RPE.

Tafoya et al[92] showed, at 1 year, a final postoperative visual acuity difference of 20/96 (LogMAR 0.208) for silicone oil eyes versus 20/44 (LogMAR 0.453) for gas treated eyes. Lai et al[93] also showed the visual acuity advantage of gas tamponade with a smaller difference (20/70 vs. 20/50). However, Lai et al also showed the rate of single operation closure being only 65% for silicone oil and 91% for gas tamponade Thus, unless limited by patient circumstances, gas tamponade for macular hole repair is preferable to silicone oil tamponade. It has been suggested that silicone oil may improve the tamponade effect and decrease the need for face-down positioning; however, there is evidence that success rates with gas are superior. One study[94] demonstrated greater one-surgery anatomic success and superior visual acuity with gas tamponade compared to silicone oil.

20-gauge versus 23-gauge versus 25-gauge vitrectomy systems

While no one system poses a significant long-term advantage, smaller gauge vitrectomy systems, with frequently self-sealing wounds, avoid induced astigmatism from suturing sclerotomies, resulting in a more rapid recovery of vision. An initial increase in endophthalmitis[95] appears to have been addressed by changing the means of wound construction but may still be considered a disadvantage to small gauge vitrectomy systems. Smaller gauge vitrectomy systems, especially 25-gauge systems, lack shaft stiffness because of the smaller barrel and also complicate the actual vitrectomy surgery for surgeons trained using 20-gauge systems.

Important predictor of postoperative vision

1. Preoperative visual acuity and duration of macular hole.
2. Preoperative minimum hole diameter and base diameter (Fig. 12.5) are prognostic factors.

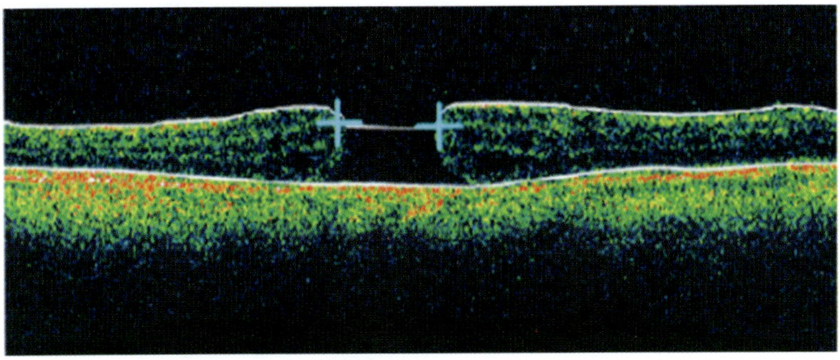

Fig. 12.5: Measurement of macular hole

3. The larger the size of the macular hole and the longer its duration, the final anatomic as well as functional outcome is adversely affected

SURGICAL COMPLICATIONS

With improving surgical techniques, we have seen a decline in complication rates of the macular hole surgery. A review of three multicenter[97-99] randomized, controlled trials found the following complications to be most prevalent: cataract (>75%), late macular hole reopening (2 to 10%), retinal detachment (3%), and endophthalmitis (<1%). Because the rate of cataract formation is so high, some surgeons remove the lens prior to or simultaneous with the macular hole surgery. A study [100] of 631 eyes revealed a high rate of peripheral retinal tears, but a significantly lower rate of retinal detachment (2%), less than reported in previous studies. Visual field defects are another reported complication of macular hole surgery. These deficits have been hypothesized to occur secondary to mechanical injury and/or dehydration of the nerve fiber layer during intraoperative air-fluid exchange.

REOPERATION

Reoperations are considered for failed primary surgery and reopened macular hole.[101,102] Failed primary surgery is seen in 1–15% of cases.[103] The incidence of primary failures decrease with increasing experience, use of adjuvants and ILM peel. Reopened macular holes have an incidence of 4–9%[104] operated cases. Increase in axial length, pseudophakia and presence of ERM[105] are the risk factors for late reopening of operated macular holes may respond to same surgery with visual improvement.

The various combinations of procedures which can be carried out to improve the anatomical success rate in reoperations are given in Table 12.5.

TABLE 12.5: Procedure for reoperations
• Repeat standard PPV
• PPV + ILM PEEL
• PPV + ILM PEEL + DYE
• Operate FAE with laser to RPE
• Use longer-acting gas as tamponade
• Stress on face-down positioning
• Silicone oil tamponade

The pattern of hole closure and foveal contour has a definite relation to the visual prognosis. The patterns of hole closure that are commonly seen are;[106]

1. U-pattern: Normal foveal contour
2. V-pattern: Steep foveal contour
3. W-pattern: Foveal defect of neurosensory retina

The visual prognosis is best with a U pattern of closure.It progressively worsens with V- and W-patterns of closure (U<V<W).

Summary

A summary of current management strategies of macular holes is presented in Table 12.6.

TABLE 12.6: Current treatment strategies
• Almost all macular holes can achieve success
• ILM peel improves hole closure rate (85-90%-95%)
• ILM peel slows visual recovery
• Use of dye staining facilitates complete peel
• Prone positioning: duration decreased with ILM P
• 1 Week gas adequate in most eyes
• Long-term (5+ years) results excellent: 60% >6/12

Since macular holes were first recognized in the 19th century, there have been many developments in our understanding and treatment of the condition. This evolution has been facilitated by advancing theories of pathogenesis, improved imaging modalities, including OCT, as well as refinement of surgical technique. Accordingly, outcomes for patients with macular hole have improved dramatically since surgical results were initially reported in 1991. However, many questions remain unanswered and are currently being investigated regarding the pathogenesis and optimal surgical techniques for macular hole.

REFERENCES

1. Aaberg T.M. Macular Holes a review. *Survey Ophthalmol.* 1970;15:139-62.
2. Sen P, Bhargava A, Vijaya L, et al. Prevalence of idiopathic macular hole in adult rural and urban south Indian population. *Clin Experiment Ophthalmol.* 2008;36:257-60.
3. Wang S, Xu L, Jonas JB. Prevalence of full-thickness macular holes in urban and rural adult Chinese: the Beijing Eye Study. *Am J Ophthalmol.* 2006;141(3): 589-91.
4. Freund KB, Ciardella AP, Shah V, Yannuzzi LA, Fisher YA. Optical coherence tomography documentation of spontaneous macular hole closure without posterior vitreous detachment. *Retina.* 2002;22:506-9.
5. Spaide R . Measurement of the posterior precortical vitreous pocket in fellow eyes with posterior vitreous detachment and macular holes. Retina 2003;23:481-5.

6. Casuso LA, Scott IU, Flynn HW, et al. Long-term follow-up of unoperated macular holes. *Ophthalmology.* 2001;108:1150-55.
7. Johnson RN, Gass JD. Idiopathic macular holes. Observations, stages of formation, and implications for surgical intervention. *Ophthalmology.* 1988; 95(7):917-24.
8. Tornambe PE. Macular hole genesis (the hydration theory). *Retina*. 2003;23: 421-4.
9. The Eye Disease Case-Control Group. Risk factors for idiopathic macular holes. *Am J Ophthalmol.* 1994;118:754-61.
10. Azzolini C, Patelli F, Brancato R. Correlation between optical coherence tomography data and biomicroscopic interpretation of idiopathic macular hole. *Am J Ophthalmol.* 2001;132:348-55.
11. Ezra E, Wells JA, Gray RH, et al. Incidence of idiopathic full-thickness macular holes in fellow eyes (a 5-year prospective natural history study). *Ophthalmology.* 1998;105:353-9
12. Lewis ML, Cohen SM, Smiddy WE, Gass JDM .Bilaterality of idiopathic macular holes. *Grafes Arch Clin Exp Ophthalmol.* 1996;234:241-5.
13. Madreperla SA, Geiger GL, Funata M, de la Cruz Z, Green WR. Clinicopathologic correlation of a macular hole treated by cortical vitreous peeling and gas tamponade. *Ophthalmology.* 1994 Apr;101(4):682-6.
14. Judson PH, Yannuzzi LA. Macular hole. In: Ryan SJ, ed. *Retina* Vol 2. 1994:1169-85.
15. Chew EY, Sperduto RD, Hiller R, et al. Clinical course of macular holes (the eye disease case-control study). *Arch Ophthalmol.* 1999;117:242-6.
16. Krzystolik M, Ciulla TA, Frederick AR. Evolution of a full-thickness macular hole. *Am J Ophthalmol.* 1998;125:245-7.
17. Ho AC. *Macular hole. Retina Vitreous Macula.* Vol 2. 1999:217-29.
18. Ho AC, Guyer DR, Fine SL. Macular hole. *Surv Ophthalmol.* 1998;42(5):393-416.
19. Cox MS, Schepens CL, Freeman HM. Retinal detachment due to ocular trauma.
20. Rubin J S,Glaser B M, Thomson J T, et al. Vitrectomy, fluid-gas exchange and transforming growth factor â for the treatment of traumatic macular holes.Ophthalmology. 1995;102:1840-5.
21. Margheria R R,Schepens CL: Macular breaks: diagnosis,etiology and observation. *Am J Ophthalmol.* 74:219;1972.
22. Wilkinson CP,Rice T A,Michels retinal detachment, St Louis, Mosby 1997.
23. Gaucher D, Haouchine B, Tadayoni R, et al. Long-term follow-up of high myopic foveoschisis: natural course and surgical outcome. *Am J Ophthalmol.* 2007;143(3):455-62
24. Blakenship G W,Ibanez-Langlois S,Treatment of myopic macular hole and detachment: intravitreal gas exchange. *Ophyhalmology*. 1987;94:333-6;.
25. Croll U and Croll M ,Hole in the macula. *Am J Ophthalmol.* 1950;33: 249-52.
26. Campo RV, Lewis RS: Lightning induced macular holes. *Am J Ophthalmology.* 1984;97:792-4.
27. Benzerroug M, Genevois O, Siahmed K, et al. Results of surgery on macular holes that develop after rhegmatogenous retinal detachment. *Br J Ophthalmol.* 2008;92(2):217-9.
28. Gass JDM, Joondeph BC. Observations concerning patients with suspected impending macular holes. *Am J Ophthalmol.* 1990;109:638-46.
29. Rao PK, Shah G, Blinder KJ. Bilateral macular hole formation in a patient with retinitis pigmentosa. *Ophthalmic Surg Lasers.* 2002;33:152-4.

30. Garretson BR, Pollack JS, Ruby AJ, et al. Vitrectomy for a symptomatic lamellar macular hole. *Ophthalmology*. 2008;115(5):884-6.
31. Smiddy WE, Michels RG, Glaser BM, de Bustros S. Vitrectomy for impending idiopathic macular holes. *Am J Ophthalmol*. 105:371-6.
32. Guyer DR, Fine SL, Ho AC. Macular holes—major review. *Surv Ophthalmol.* 1998;42;393-416.
33. Sjaarda R N. Macular hole Int *Ophthalmol Clinic*. 1995;35:105-22.
34. Smiddy WE, Gass JDM. Masquerades of macular holes. *Ophthalmic Surg.* 1995;26:16-24.
35. Gonvers and Machemer R.Anew approach to treating retinal detachment with macular holes. *Am J Ophthalmol*. 1982;94:468-472.
36. Kelly NE, Wendel RT. Vitreous surgery for idiopathic macular holes. *Arch Ophthalmol.* 1991;109:654-9.
37. Kelly NE, Wendel RT. Vitreous surgery for idiopathic macular holes. Results of a pilot study. *Arch Ophthalmol*. 1991;109(5):654-9.
38. De Bustro S. Vitrectomy for prevention of macular holes: results of a randomized multicentre clinical trial.Vitrectomy for prevention of macular holes study group. *Ophthalmology*. 1994;101:1055-9.
39. James M,Feeman S.S.Macular holes. *Graefes Arch Clin Exp Ophthalmol.* 1980; 215:59-63.
40. Morgan CM,Schatz H. Idiopathic macular holes. *Am J Ophthalmol.* 1985;99: 437-44.
41. Gass JDM. Stereoscopic Atlas of Macular Diseases: Dignosis and Treatment. ed 4, St Louis, Mosby, 1996.
42. Freeman WR. Vitrectomy surgery for full-thickness macular holes. *Am J Ophthalmol.* 1992;2:233-5.
43. Thompson JT, Glasser BM, Sjaarda RN, Murphy RP. Progression of nuclear sclerosis and long-term visual results of vitrectomy with transforming growth factor beta-2 for macular holes. *Am J Ophthalmol.* 1995;119:48-54.
44. Faude F, Edel E, Dannhauer M, Petzel C, Meier P, Wiedemann P. Autologous thrombocyte administration in treatment of idiopathic macular foramen. *Ophthalmologe.* 1997;94:877-81.
45. Sakuma T, Tanaka M, Inoue M, et al. Efficacy of autologous plasmin for idiopathic macular hole surgery. *Eur J Ophthalmol.* 2005;15(6):787-94.
46. Ruiz-Moreno JM, Staicu C, Pinero DP, et al. Optical coherence tomography predictive factors for macular hole surgery outcome. *Br J Ophthalmol*. 2008;92(5): 640-4.
47. Steele et al. Prognosis of macular hole surgery. *Ophthalmology*. 2001;108: 1471-78.
48. Garretson BR, Pollack JS, Ruby AJ, et al. Vitrectomy for a symptomatic lamellar macular hole. *Ophthalmology.* 2008;115(5):884-6.e1.
49. Wendel RT, Patel NC, Kelly NE.Vitreous surgery for macular holes. *Ophthalmology*. 1993;100:1671-76.
50. Meena Chakrabarti, Arup Chakrabarti et al. Macular Hole surgery in the Young. *KJO* 2007;17:23-26.
51. Smiddy WE, Feuer W, Cordahi G. Internal limiting membrane peeling in macular hole surgery. *Ophthalmology*. 2001;108:1471-8.
52. Kumagai K, Furukawa M, Ogino N, et al. Vitreous surgery with and without internal limiting membrane peeling for macular hole repair. *Retina*. 2004;24: 721-7.

53. Smiddy WE, Feuer W, Cordahi G. Internal limiting membrane peeling in macular hole surgery. *Ophthalmology*. 2001;108:1471-8.
54. Brooks HL Jr. Macular hole surgery with and without internal limiting membrane peeling. *Ophthalmology*. 2000;107:1939-49.
55. Rodriguez EB, Meyer CH et al. Intravitreal staining of ILM using ICG in the treatment of macular holes. *Ophthalmologica*. 2005;219:251-62.
56. Nakamura.T, Murata T et al. Ultra structure of the vitreoretinal interface following the removal of ILM using ICG. *Curr Eye Research*. 2004;27: 395-9.
57. Hillenkamp J, Saikia P, Herrmann WA et al. Surgical removal of idiopathic ERM with or without the assistance of ICG: a randomised controlled clinical trial. *Graefes Arch Clin Exp Ophthalmol*. 2006;21.
58. Rodriguez EB, Meyer CH et al.Intravitreal staining of ILM using ICG in the treatment of macular holes. *Ophthalmologica*. 2005;219:251-62.
59. Maia.M, Haller JA, Pieramici DJ et al. Retinal pigment epithelial abnormalities after internal limiting membrane peeling guided by ICG staining. *Retina*. 2004;24:157-60.
60. Guo S, Tutela AC, Wagner R, Caputo AR. A comparison of the effectiveness of four biostains in enhancing visualization of the vitreous. *J Pediatr Ophthalmol Strabismus*. 2006;43:281-4.
61. Haritoglou C, Gass CA, Schaumberger M, et al. Macular changes after peeling of the internal limiting membrane in macular hole surgery. *Am J Ophthalmol.* 2001;132:363-8.
62. Kim JW, Freeman WR, Azen SP, El-Haig W, Klein DJ, Bailey IL. Prospective randomized trial of vitrectomy or observation for stage 2 macular holes. *Am J Ophthalmol.* 1996;121:605-14.
63. Sheidow TG, Blinder KJ, Holekamp N, et al.Outcome results of macular hole surgery: an evaluation of internal limiting membrane peeling with and without indocyanine green. *Ophthalmology.* 2003;110:1697-1701.
64. Gass CA, Haritoglou C, Schaumberger M, et al. Functional outcome of macular surgery with and without indocyanine green assisted peeling of the ILM Graefes *Arch clin Exp Ophthalmol*. 2003;241:716-20.
65. Ando.F, Sasano. K, Ohba N, et al. Anatomic and visual outcomes after ICG assisted peeling of the retinal ILM in Indiopathic macular hole surgery. *Am J Ophthalmol.* 2004;137:744-6.
66. Hillenkamp J, Saikia P, Herrmann WA et al. Surgical removal of idiopathic ERM with or without the assistance of ICG: a randomised controlled clinical trail. *Ophthalmology*. 2005;146:432-35.
67. Lochhead J, Jones E, Chui D et al. Outcome of ICG assisted ILM peel in macular hole surgery. *Eye*. 2004; 18: 804-8.
68. Slaughter K, Lee IL. Macular hole surgery with and without ICG assistance. *Eye.* 2004;8;376-8.
69. Rodrigues EB, Meyer CH. Meta analysis of chromovitrectomy with ICG in macular hole surgery. *Ophthalmologica.* 2007;114:587-90.
70. Meyer CH, Rodrigues EB vet al. A novel applicator for the selective painting of pre-retinal structures during vitreo retinal surgery. *Graefes Arch Clin Exp Ophthalmol.* 2005;243:487-9.
71. Thompson JT, Smiddy WE, Williams GA, Sjaarda RN, Flynn HW Jr, Margherio RR, et al. Comparison of recombinant transforming growth factor-beta-2 and placebo as an adjunctive agent for macular hole surgery. *Ophthalmology.* 1998;105: 700-06.

72. Minihan M, Goggin M, Cleary PE. Surgical management of macular holes: results using gas tamponade alone, or in combination with autologous platelet concentrate, or transforming growth factor beta 2. *Br J Ophthalmol.* 1997;81:1073-9.
73. Dosquet C et al. Effect of autologous platelet concentrate in surgery for idiopathic macular hole: results of a multicenter, double-masked, randomized trial. Platelets in Macular Hole Surgery Group. *Ophthalmology.* 1999;106:932-8.
74. Blumenkraz MS, et al Use of autologous plasmathrombin mixture as adjuvant therapy for macular holes. *Ophthalmology.* 1994;101(suppl)69
75. Liggett PE, et al. Human autologous serum in the treatment of idiopathic macular holes. *Ophthalmology*. 1993;102:1071-6.
76. Lansing MB, Glaser BM. The effect of transforming growth factor beta 2 without epiretinal membrane peeling in full-thickness macular holes. *Ophthalmology*. 1993;100:868-72.
77. Kotobelnik, et al. Autologous platelet concentrate as an adjunct in macular hole healing: a pilot study. *Ophthalmology.* 1996;103:590-4.
78. Thompson JT, Smiddy WE, Glaser BM. Intraocular tamponade duration and success of macular hole surgery. *Retina*. 1996;16:373-82.
79. Berger JW, et al. Buoancy of gas bubble in macular hole surgery. *Ophthalmology*. 1997;113:390-4.
80. Benson WE, Cruickshank KC, Fong DS. Surgical management of macular holes; a report by the American academy of Ophthalmology. *Ophthalmology.* 2001;108:1328-35.
81. Tornambe PE, Poliner LS, Grote K. Macular hole surgery without face-down positioning. A pilot study. *Retina*. 1997;17:179-85.
82. Krohn et al. Macular Hole Surgery with shortened face down positioning. *Am J Ophthalmol.* 2005;146:285-7.
83. Tranos PG, Peter NM, Nath R, et al. Macular hole surgery without prone positioning. *Eye*. 2007;21(6):802-6.
84. Merkur AB, Tuli R. Macular hole repair with limited nonsupine positioning. *Retina*. 2007;27(3):365-9.
85. Park DW, Sipperley JO, Sneed SR, et al. Macular hole surgery with internal-limiting membrane peeling and Intravitreous air. *Ophthalmology.* 1999;106:1392-8.
86. Isomae et al Macular hole repair with ILM peeling and limited positioning. *Am J Ophthalmol.* 2002;136:185-7.
87. Sato H, Kawasaki R, Yamashita H. Observation of idiopathic full-thickness macular hole closure in early postoperative period as evaluated by optical coherence tomography. *Am J Ophthalmol.* 2003;136:185-7.
88. Wickens, et al. Macular hole surgery with internal-limiting membrane peeling and Intravitreous C3F8 and shortened 3 day positioning 2005
89. Simcock, et al, Macular hole surgery without internal-limiting membrane peeling and Intravitreous C2F6 and shortened positioning for Stage 2 & 3 holes: 2001.
90. Rubinstein A, Ang A, Patel CK. Vitrectomy without postoperative posturing for idiopathic macular holes. *Clin Experiment Ophthalmol*. 2007;35(5):458-61.
91. Dhawahir-Scala FE, Maino A, Saha K, Mokashi AA, McLauchlan R, Charles S. To posture or not to posture after macular hole surgery. *Retina*. 2008;28(1): 60-65.
92. Tafoya ME, Lambert HM, Vu L, Ding M. Visual outcome of silicone oil versus gas tamponade for macular hole surgery. Semin 2003;18(3):127-31.

93. Lai JC, Stinnett SS, McCuen BW. Comparison of silicone oil versus gas tamponade in the treatment of idiopathic full-thickness macular hole. *Ophthalmology*. 2003;110:1170-4.
94. Goldbaum MH, McCuen BW, Hanneken AM, Burgess SK, Chen HH. Silicone oil tamponade to seal macular holes without position restrictions. *Ophthalmology.* 1998;105(11):2140-2148.
95. Park SS, Marcus DM, Duker JS, et al. Posterior segment complications after vitrectomy for macular hole. *Ophthalmology.* 1995;102(5):775-81.
96. Kusuhara S, Teraoka Escano MF, Fujii S, et al. Prediction of postoperative visual outcome based on hole configuration by optical coherence tomography in eyes with idiopathic macular holes. *Am J Ophthalmol.* 2004;138(5):709-16 97.
97. Chen CJ. Glaucoma after macular hole surgery. *Ophthalmology*. 1998;105: 94-100.
98. Poliner LS, Tornambe PE. Retinal pigment epitheliopathy after macular hole surgery. Ophthalmology. 1992;99:1671-7.
99. Sjaarda RN, Glaser BM, Thompson JT, Murphy RP, Hanham A. Distribution of iatrogenic retinal breaks in macular hole surgery. *Ophthalmology.* 1995; 102:1387-92.
100. Hutchins RK. Complications of macular hole surgery. *Ophthalmology.* 1998;105:762.326.
101. Pasques S, Passin P Visual field loss after vitrectomy for full thickness macular holes. *Am J Ophthalmol.* 1997;124:88-94.
102. Pendergast SD, McCuen BW. Visual field loss after Vitrectomy for full thickness macular holes. *Ophthalmology.* 1996;103:1069-71.
103. Johnson RN, McDonald HR, Schatz H, Ai E. Outpatient postoperative fluid-gas exchange after early failed vitrectomy surgery for macular hole. *Ophthalmology*. 1997;104:2009-13.
104. Ohana E, Blumenkranz MS. Treatment of reopened macular hole after vitrectomy by laser and outpatient fluid-gas exchange. *Ophthalmology*. 1998;105:1398-1403.
105. Park SS, Marcus DM, Duker JS, Posterior segment complications after vitrectomy for macular holes. *Ophthalmology*. 1995;102:775-81.
106. Baba T, Yamamoto S, Arai M, et al. Correlation of visual recovery and presence of photoreceptor inner/outer segment junction in optical coherence images after successful macular hole repair. *Retina.* 2008;28(3):453-8.

13

chapter

Ajit Majjhi

Proliferative Vitreoretinopathy

ABSTRACT

Proliferative vitreoretinopathy (PVR) is characterized by the growth and contraction of cellular membranes in the vitreous and inner or outer surfaces of the retina following development of rhegmatogenous retinal detachment (RRD) or ocular trauma. RRDs are particularly at risk of developing PVR if associated with giant retinal tear, large or multiple retinal breaks, signs of uveitis, aphakia, vitreous hemorrhage and choroidal detachment. PVR is found in 5–10% of RRDs. Of these patients 20–40% has recurring episodes of PVR. PVR occurs in up to 20% of cases following various vitreoretinal surgeries. The goals of reattachment surgery for PVR remain same as those for conventional retinal surgery. However, these goals are more difficult to achieve in PVR and the difficulty increases with the severity of PVR. The silicone study confirmed the superiority of silicone oil over SF6, but not over C3F8 in terms of reattachment rates or achieving a visual acuity of >5/200 in RDs complicated by severe grades of PVR. The anatomic success ranges from 60 to 80% depending on the severity of PVR.

Introduction

Proliferative vitreoretinopathy (PVR) is a complex cellular process that has many similarities to a wound healing response involving inflammation, cell migration, proliferation resulting in extracellular matrix production, fibroblastic transformation and contraction of fibrocytes.[1] Clinically, proliferative vitreoretinopathy is characterized by the growth and contraction of cellular membranes within the hyaloid, the vitreous and on both retinal surfaces.[2] These membranes result in traction, which may cause a traction retinal detachment that reopens otherwise successfully treated retinal breaks or may create new retinal breaks.[3] Membrane contraction may also cause macular pucker. Proliferative vitreoretinopathy comprises variety of different intraocular cellular proliferations, including epiretinal membranes, subretinal strands, and retinal detachments in combination with star folds, vitreous traction and anterior loop traction (anterior PVR).[4-6]

Pathogenesis

The pathogenesis of proliferative vitreoretinopathy is similar to wound healing consisting of inflammation, proliferation and modulation of scar (Fig.13.1). Proliferative vitreoretinopathy occurs when cellular migration in the presence of inflammation resulting in membrane formation in the vitreous and inner or outer surfaces of the retina following development of rhegmatogenous retinal detachment (RD) or ocular trauma.[2] PVR is characterized by the migration and proliferation of retinal pigment epithelial (RPE) cells along with synthesis of extracellular matrix (ECM) proteins, such as collagen or fibronectin which organizes into an epiretinal or subretinal membrane.[7] Various reactions may be discerned in the development of PVR, including chemotaxis and cellular migration, cellular proliferation, membrane formation and contraction. These membranes are composed of RPE cells, glial cells (primarily Muller cells and astrocytes), fibroblasts and inflammatory cells.[8,9]

The cellular components involved in PVR include RPE cells, hyalocytes and glial cells.[8] Proinflammatory cytokines involved in PVR include interleukin-8, Monocyte chemotactic protein-1, interleukin-1, interleukin-6, tumor necrosis factor a (TNF α) and interferon-γ.[10,11] Growth factors involved in PVR include platelet derived growth factor (PDGF), transforming growth factor-β (TGF-β) epidermal growth factor (EGF) and fibroblast growth factor (FGF).[12,13]

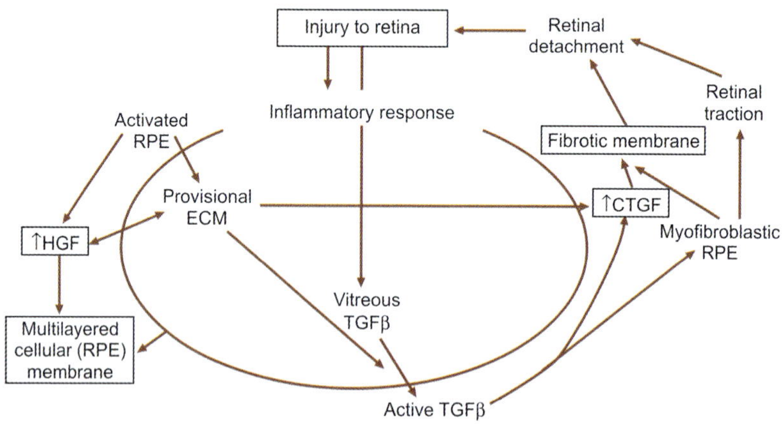

Fig. 13.1: Flowchart showing pathogenesis of PVR.

The extracellular matrices involved in PVR are thrombospasmodin, laminin and vetreonectin.[7,8,14] The inflammatory cells involved in PVR include macrophages, lymphocytes and fibroblasts.[15] Proliferation and migration of the cells (mainly RPE cells and/or glial cells) form sheets of differentiated cells within a provisional extracellular matrix that contains fibronetin, laminin and vitreonectin.[8] These cellular membranes become progressively paucicellular and fibrotic.[9] After the retinal break formation the inflammatory cells are drawn to the lesion and secrete TNF α.[16] TNF α acts as mediator of RPE activation, PDGF acts as an important mitogen, chemoatractant and mediator of cellular contraction.[3, 12] TGF β is an important contributor for tissue fibrosis (Fig. 13.1).[17]

Terminology and Classification

PVR has been termed in the past as *massive vitreous retraction* by Havener, *massive preretinal retraction* by Tolentino et al and *Massive preretinal proliferation* by Machemer and Laqua.[18] The term *proliferative vitreoretinopathy* was coined in 1983 by the Retina Society Terminology Committee,[19] The Retina Society Terminology Committee proposed a new classification of PVR (Table 13.1). The new classification modified the one proposed by Machemer in 1978.[18] Unlike the 1978 classification the 1983 classification avoided any reference to the extension and/or intensity of PVR. Substituting the word *massive* for the term proliferative, referred to its pathogenesis. The term vitreoretinopathy was selected to identify the location of the disease. The Retina Society classification is widely accepted today. This classification has been revised by the silicone study group to

TABLE 13.1: Retina society classification of retina detachment with the proliferative vitreoretinopathy

Grade	Name	Clinical Signs
A	Minimum	Vitreous haze, vitreous clumps (Fig. 13.2A)
B	Moderate	Wrinkling of the inner retinal surface, rolled edge of retinal break, retinal stiffness, vessel tortuosity (Fig. 13.2B)
C	Marked	Full thickness fixed retinal folds in:
C-1		One quadrant (Fig. 13.2C)
C-2		Two quadrants (Fig. 13.2D)
C-3		Three quadrants (Fig. 13.2E)
D	Massive	Fixed retinal folds in four quadrants
D-1		Wide funnel shape (Fig. 13.2F)
D-2		Narrow funnel shape* (Fig. 13.2G)
D-3		Closed funnel (optic nerve head not visible) (Fig. 13.2H)

* Narrow funnel shape exists when the anterior end of the funnel can be seen by indirect ophthalmoscopy within the 45° field of a +20 D condensing lens (Nikon or equivalent).

include anterior PVR as well as quantitative assessment of amount of PVR to provide a description of PVR relevant to modern vitreoretinal surgery, which involves both anterior and posterior forms of proliferative vitreoretinopathy.[20]

The recognition of the anterior form of PVR is one of the most important contributions of the Silicone Study group classification.[21] Retina Society classification has been updated (Tables 13.2 and 13.3) after the Silicone Study group classification and results of a major randomized trial (Silicone Study results) to evaluate the efficacy of silicone oil compared to prolonged intraocular gas tamponade.[20,22]

The Silicone Study group has evaluated the reproducibility and prognostic utility of the Retina Society and the Silicone Study classification systems

TABLE 13.2: Modified Retina Society classification of retina detachment with the proliferative vitreoretinopathy

Grade	Features
A B	Vitreous haze; vitreous pigment clumps; pigment clusters on inferior retina Wrinkling of inner retinal surface; retinal stiffness; vessel tortuosity; rolled and irregular edge of retinal break; decreased mobility of vitreous
C P 1-12	Posterior to equator; focal diffuse or circumferential full-thickness folds*; subretinal strands*
C A 1-12	Anterior to equator; focal diffuse or circumferential full-thickness folds*; subretinal strands*; anterior displacement*; condensed vitreous with strands

*Expressed in the number of clock hours involved

TABLE 13.3: Grade C PVR of Modified Retina Society classification described by contraction type

Type	Location (in relation to equator)	Features
1. Focal	Posterior	Star fold posterior to vitreous base
2. Diffuse	Posterior	Confluent star folds posterior to vitreous base. Optic disk may not be visible
3. Subretinal	Posterior/ Anterior	Proliferations under the retina; Annular strand near disk; linear strands; motheaten-appearing sheets
4. Circumferential	Anterior	Contraction along posterior edge of vitreous base with central displacement of the retina: peripheral retina stretched; posterior retina in radial folds
5. Anterior displacement	Anterior	Vitreous base pulled anteriorly by proliferative tissue; peripheral retinal trough; ciliary processes may be stretched, may be covered by membrane; iris may be retracted

of PVR.[23] Reproducibility of Silicone Study classification system was 64% for the type of contraction, 77% for the number of clock hours, 67% for the posterior PVR, 88% for the anterior and posterior PVR and 94% for the anterior, posterior and sub retinal PVR. The reproducibility of Retina Society classification system was 99%. Thus Retina Society classification was highly reproducible. However the Silicone Study classification predicted postoperative visual acuity (P = 0.004) and incidence of hypotony (P = 0.01) better than the Retinal Society classification.[23] Both Silicone Study classification and Retina Society classification do not provide information about biologic activity or risk factors in progression of PVR; number and location of retinal breaks. The individual evaluator can make an additional note of these findings to give completeness to the current classification of PVR.

Risk Factors

Retinal detachments are particularly at risk of developing PVR if they have any of the following characteristics: giant retinal tear, large or multiple retinal breaks, signs of uveitis, aphakia, vitreous hemorrhage and preoperative choroidal detachment.[24, 25] Postoperative PVR is most strongly associated with the preoperative presence of PVR grades A and B, uveitis, vitreous hemorrhage (intra- or postoperative), excessive cryotherapy, diathermy or photocoagulation, repeated surgical procedures, loss of vitreous during drainage of subretinal fluid, missed or untreated retinal breaks, use of air or SF_6 and postoperative choroidal detachment.[1, 24-27] PVR is the main reason for failures of vitreoretinal surgery.[18] PVR occurs up to 20% of cases following various vitreoretinal surgical procedures.[28] PVR is found in 5–10% of rhegmatogenous retinal detachments.[24] Of these patients 20-40% have recurring episodes of PVR.[5] Several studies have shown that successful sealing of all retinal breaks does not necessarily provide complete protection against post-operative PVR.[24,25]

Clinical Features

Clinical signs of proliferative vitreoretinopathy depend on the stage and vary from mild haze and pigment clumps in the vitreous in grade A PVR to epiretinal, vitreous or subretinal bands and intrinsic retinal contraction in grade C (modified Retina Society classification). The different signs were detailed along with the grading of PVR in Tables 13.2 and 13.3. Grade A PVR is clinically characterized by the presence of vitreous haze and pigment clumps in the presence of rhegmatogenous RD (Fig. 13.2A). The

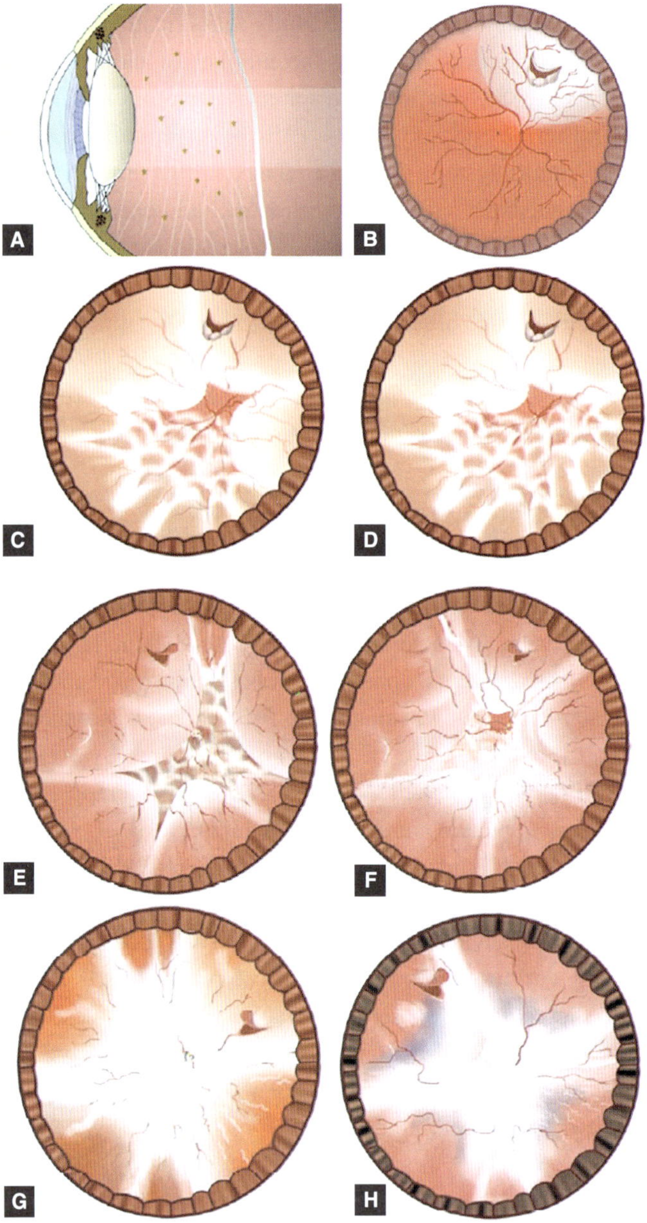

Figs 13.2A to H: Diagramatic representation of grades of proliferative vitreoretinopathy (PVR) with rhegmatogenous retinal detachment. **A:** Grade A with pigment clumps in the anterior vitreous. **B:** Grade B with rolled edges of a retinal break. **C to E:** Grade C with full thickness retinal fixed folds in one quadrant (PVR C1, C), two quadrants (PVR C2, D) and three quadrants (PVR C3, E). **F to H:** Grade D with full thickness retinal fold in all 4 quadrants with wide-funnel (PVR D1, F), narrow-funnel (PVR D2, G) and closed-funnel (PVR D3, H).

retinal surface is undulated in the detached areas of retina, but devoid of any surface wrinkles and the retinal breaks have sharp margins. In grade B PVR, wrinkles are observed in the surface of the detached retina with partial restricted mobility and fine pigmented membranes over the surface of the detached retina. The margins of retinal breaks characterised by rolled edges with fine pigmented membrane extending from the edge of the retinal break (Figs 13.2B and 13.3A) over to the retinal surface in PVR grade B or more. In grade C PVR, the fine transparent pigmented membrane of grade B turns more opaque and contracted, forming either star fold if the membrane is small or a diffuse retinal fold in case of a large membrane (Figs 13.2 C to H and 13.3B). Depending upon the location of these membranes in relation to the equator, they form a part of anterior or posterior PVR. Subretinal membranes usually appear in the form of cords, extending across the quadrants. If the cord like subretinal membrane is located in the posterior pole surrounding the disc, it forms a napkin ring configuration. Rarely the subretinal membranes form sieve like sheets under the retina, especially when they are located anterior to the equator. PVR membranes in the region of vitreous base form different configurations depending on the location and extent of the epiretinal membranes. They may assume a circumferential contraction sheet or as sheets of fibrous membranes pulling the vitreous base or ciliary body anteriorly. One should observe the regions anterior and posterior to equator

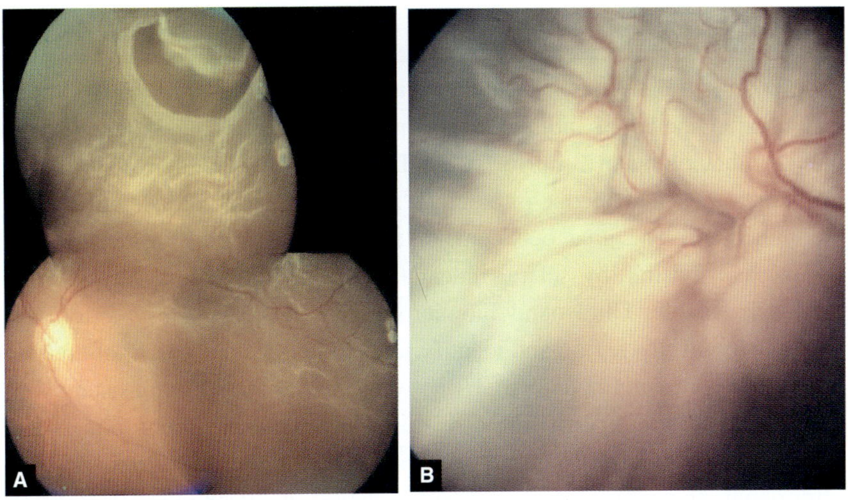

Figs 13.3A and B: A: Color fundus photograph showing rhegmatogenous retinal detachment with retinal break in superotemporal quadrant with rolled edges indicative of grade B proliferative vitreoretinopathy. **B:** Color fundus photograph showing retinal detachment with full thickness retinal folds and closed funnel RD indicative of PVR D3.

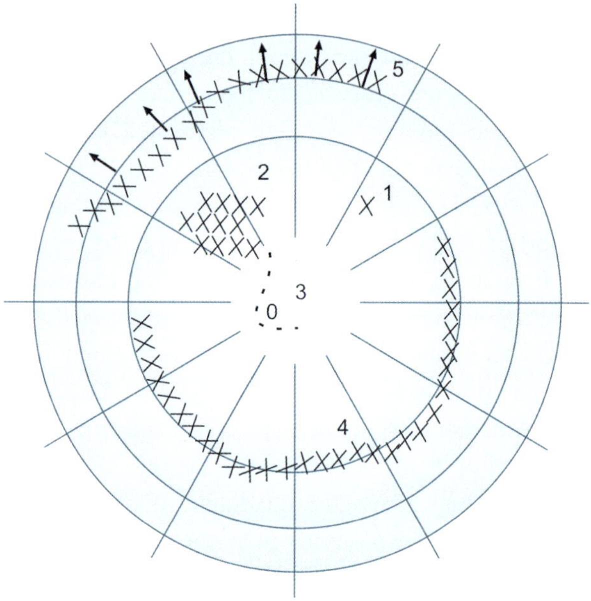

Fig. 13.4: Retina diagram to represent various types of full thickness retinal folds. Type 1: focal = X, Type 2: diffuse = XXX, Type 3: subretinal = —, Type 4: circumferential = xxx and Type 5: anterior displacement = x-x-x-

as well as each clock hour to know the complete extent of PVR (Fig.13.4).[21,22]

Investigations

Proliferative vitreoretinopathy is best diagnosed and graded by good clinical examination including indirect ophthalmoloscopy, slit-lamp biomicroscopy along with Goldmann 3-mirror or 78 D or 90 D contact/non contact lens examination. When media is cloudy "A" or "B"-scan ultrasonography is recommended. The area between ora serrata and the retro-iridian region is not easily visible by scleral indentation or ultrasonography; even when fundus is visible. Ultrasound biomicroscopy (UBM) is a useful tool for examination of this region and identifying the presence and extent of anterior proliferative vitreoretinopathy.[29] UBM was found to be 92% consistent with surgical observation.[29] In silicone oil filled eye ultrasonography images get attenuated due to reflections and attenuation of sound waves. Prone position ultrasonography is shown to yield better images in silicone oil filled eyes.[30] Silicone oil filling does not influence UBM imaging of the eyeball wall.[29] Optical Coherence Tomography (OCT) is useful during postoperative period, to assess the macular attachment status and to correlate anatomic results with functional outcomes.[31-33]

Management

PROPHYLAXIS

Trans-scleral cryopexy has been shown to release viable RPE cells and also causes inflammation and fibrin formation. All three components have been implicated in pathogenesis of PVR. To lessen the risk of PVR one need to consider methods other than cryotherapy, to create chorioretinal adhesion in patients with a high risk of PVR.[34] In this regard laser photocoagulation is better than cryopexy, and one should consider laser photocoagulation instead of cryopexy, whenever possible.

Any procedure that produces thermal adhesion of retina induces cell necrosis, inflammation and fibrocellular proliferation. Efforts have been made to find nonthermal ways of retinal break closure with synthetic tissue adhesives, such as cyanoacrylates, polysiloxanes and acetate polymers or biological tissue adhesives like fibrin, recombinant cytokine TGF-β.[35,36] However, their use has been very limited in clinical setting. Recurrent retinal detachment with open retinal breaks is one of the major risk factor for development of proliferative vitreoretinopathy.[24] Successful reattachment of retina with single surgical intervention avoids development of PVR. One should aim at achieving complete attachment of retina in the first attempt.

SURGICAL MANAGEMENT

The goals of retinal reattachment surgery for PVR remain same as those for conventional retinal re-attachment surgery, i.e. to close all retinal breaks and relieve vitreoretinal traction. However, these goals are more difficult to achieve in PVR and the difficulty increases as the severity of PVR increases. The surgical steps in PVR surgery may include scleral buckle/external encircling procedure,[37] standard pars plana vitrectomy with seperation of posterior hyaloid till the vitreous base with or without use of chromo-vitrectomy techniques,[8, 28,38,39] peeling of epiretinal membranes,[5] release of anterior traction membranes,[40] retinotomy/retinectomy;[41-48] release of subretinal membranes,[43] intraoperative use of perfluorocarbon liquids,[49-53] internal tamponading agents (SF6/ C_3 F_8/ silicone oil/heavy silicone oil),[20, 21, 23, 42,54-61] endophotocoagulation[62] and use of adjuvant antiproliferative agents.[63-66] A detailed description of each of these procedures is beyond the scope of this chapter. The readers are advised to read the relevant references given at the end of this chapter, so as to obtain an in depth understanding of surgical management.

A surgical approach to a patient with retinal detachment with proliferative vitreoretinopathy depends largely on grade of PVR, type, number, and location of retinal breaks and media clarity. With the advent of advances in vitreous surgery, it is preferred over scleral buckle for even initial grades of PVR especially in pseudophakic and aphakic eyes.[67] Scleral buckling technique alone may achieve a sustained retinal re-attachment with good closure of retinal breaks and relief of traction in early (grades A and B) PVR. There are no clear indications for treating PVR with standard scleral buckling procedure, but PVR grades up to C_1 (Retina Society classification) can be tried if the detachment is associated with small peripheral retinal break unassociated with dynamic traction or an area of proliferative vitreoretinopathy.

Prasplana vitrectomy is indicated in patients with RD with early grades of PVR if there is traction from the epi- or subretinal membranes in patients in whom the retinal breaks cannot be appropriately sealed by scleral buckling. Vitrectomy is preferred over scleral buckling in pseudophakic and aphakic eyes or if the retinal breaks are located posterior to the equator.[68] Suture less vitrectomy without belt buckle may be considered for patients with rhegmatogenous retinal detachment with grade A or B proliferative vitreoretinopathy.[69-71] However, proliferative vitreoretinopathy grade C or worse would warranty belt buckle along with pars plana vitrectomy.[72]

In patients with retinal detachment with PVR grades more than C_1 (Retina Society classification) and/or those associated with anterior PVR, vitrectomy with membrane peeling and a gas or silicone oil tamponade is essential. The silicone study confirmed the superiority of silicone oil over SF6, but not over perfluoropropane gas in terms of retinal reattachment rates or achieving a visual acuity of 5/200 or greater in patients of retinal detachment complicated by severe grades of PVR.[73-77]

Prevalence of anterior PVR is significantly greater in eyes with prior vitrectomy than in eyes without a prior vitrectomy (88% vs 73%).[21, 78,79] Eyes with anterior PVR and clinically significant posterior PVR changes (>PVR D_1) had a better visual prognosis if silicone oil rather than C_3F_8 gas was used.[21] Patients with severe grades of PVR often require bimanual surgery, removal of the lens and rertinotomy or retinectomy.[40,43,80]

Vitrectomy has improved the surgical results.[81-84]The anatomic success ranges from 60 to 80% depending on the severity of PVR. Eyes with posterior PVR had better outcome at 6-month postoperative follow-up than eyes with anterior PVR.[21, 37] Of the anatomically successful patients 40–80% might recover at least ambulatory vision. Vision may be poor because of macular changes (cystoid macular edema, macular pucker, subretinal membranes) in a high percentage of patients.[42, 56,85,86] The likelihood of achieving a visual acuity of 5/200 or better was greater in eyes when the retinal reattachment was achieved with a single procedure (60%) than in those who required multiple operations (32%).[42]

In our hands surgical intervention either sclera buckling or parsplana vitrectomy along with other procedures has resulted in 86% (80/93) of eyes with single intervention and 95.6% (89/93) of eyes with second intervention. However, good visual outcomes have been observed only in 61.2% (57/93) of eyes (unpublished data).

ADJUVANT THERAPY

Intraoperative use of perfluorocarbon liquids has been widely in practice after their introduction in 1980s.[50-52] The perfluorocarbon liquid is unfolds the retinal flap in giant retinal tears, displaces the subretinal fluid or blood anteriorly and by applying counter traction stabilizes the retina during membrane peeling in eyes with proliferative vitreoretinopathy.[49,87,88] Heavy silicone oil (silicone oil-RMN_3 mixture), with density heavier-than-water (1.03 g/cm^3 and viscosity of 3,800 cps) is useful in complicated retinal detachments with inferior retinal tears.[89-95] Triamcinolone acetonide is shown to be useful as an adjuvant tool in delineation of posterior hyaloid and ERMs, allowing a more complete and safer removal of PVR membranes.[96,97] However, corticosteroids are not associated with improved results in terms of prevention or recurrence of proliferative vitreoretinopathy.[28]

Several antiproliferative agents have been considered in treatment of PVR. 5-fluorouracil in isolation or in combination with low-molecular-weight heparin was tried with limited success.[64,65,98,99] Daunorubicin infusion was found non-toxic, but the results were not encouraging.[63,100] Gene therapy based strategies have also been tried in animal models and were found useful in prevention of proliferative vitreoretinopathy.[7,101,102] However, good clinical trials are lacking to suggest their clinical application.

References

1. Asaria RHF, Kon CH, Bunce C, et al. How to predict proliferative vitreoretinopathy. *Ophthalmology.* 2001;108:1184-6.
2. Ryan SJ. The pathophysiology of proliferative vitreoretinopathy in it's management. *Am J Ophthalmol.* 1985;100:188-93.
3. Pastor JC. Proliferative vitreoretinopathy. An overview. *Surv Ophthalmol.* 1998; 43:3-18.
4. Lopez PF, Grossniklaus HE, Aaberg TM, et al. Pathogenetic mechanisms in anterior proliferative vitreoretinopathy. *Am J Ophthalmol.* 1992;114:257-79.
5. Aaberg TM. Management of anterior and posterior proliferative vitreoretinopathy. XIV Edward Jackson memorial lecture. *Am J Ophthalmol.* 1988;106:519-32.
6. Lewis H, Aaberg TM. Anterior proliferative vitreoretinopathy. *Am J Ophthalmol.* 1988;105:277-84.

7. Ikuno Y, Kazlauskas A. An in vivo gene therapy approach for experimental proliferative vitreoretinopathy using the truncated platelet-derived growth factor alpha receptor. *Invest Ophthalmol Vis Sci.* 2002;43:2406-11.
8. Charteris DG. Proliferative vitreoretinopathy: Pathobiology, Surgical management and adjunctive treatment. *Br J Ophthalmol.* 1995;79:953-60.
9. Hiscott PS, Grierson J, Mc Leod D. Natural history of fibrocellular epiretinal membrane: a anantitative, antoradiographic and immunohistochemical study. *Br J Ophthalmol.* 1985;11:810-23.
10. Limb GA, Little BC, Meager A, et al. Cytokines in proliferative vitreoretinopathy. *Eye.* 1991;5:686-93.
11. La Heij EC, Van de Wearenburg MPH, Blaauwgeers HGT, et al. Basic fibroblast growth factor, Glutamine synthetase and interleukin -6 in vitreous fluid from eyes with retinal detachment complicated by proliferative vitreoretinopathy. *Am J Ophthalmol.* 2002;134:367-75.
12. Wiedemann P. Growth factors in retinal diseases: Proliferative vitreoretinopathy, proliferative diabetic retinopathy and retinal degeneration. *Surv Ophthalmol.* 1992;36:373-84.
13. Ogata N, Nishikawa M, Nishimura T, et al. Inverse levels of pigment epithelium derived factor and vascular endothelial growth factor in the vitreous of eyes with rhegmatogenous retinal detachment and proliferative vitreoretinopathy. *Am J Ophthalmol.* 2002;133:851-2.
14. Hinton DR, He S, Jin ML, et al. Novel growth factors involved in the pathogenesis of proliferative vitreoretinopathy. *Eye.* 2002;16:422-8.
15. Charteris DG, Hiscott P, Robey HL, et al. Inflammatory cells in proliferative vitreoretinopathy subretinal membranes. *Ophthalmology.* 1992;99:1364-7.
16. Jin ML, He S, Worpel V, et al. Promotion of adhesion and migration of RPE cells to provisional extracellular matrices by TNF-µ. *Invest Ophthalmol Vis Sci.* 2000;41:4324-32.
17. Connor TB Jr., Roberts AB, Sporn MB, et al. Correlation of fibrosis and transforming growth factor beta type 2 levels in the eye. *J Clin Invest.* 1989;83: 1661-6.
18. Machemer R. Pathogenesis and classification of massive periretinal proliferation. *Br J Ophthalmol.* 1978;62:737-47.
19. The retina society terminology committee. The classification of retinal detachment with proliferative vitreoretinopathy. *Ophthalmology.* 1983;90:121-5.
20. The silicone oil study group. Classification of proliferative vitreoretinopathy used in the silicone study. *Ophthalmology.* 1989;96:765-71.
21. The silicone oil study group. Anterior proliferative vitreoretinopathy in the silicone study. Silicone study report number 10. *Ophthalmology.* 1996;103:1092-99.
22. Machemer R, Aaberg TM, Freeman HM, et al. An updated classification of retinal detachment with proliferative vitreoretinopathy. *Am J Ophthalmol.* 1991;112: 159-65.
23. The silicone study group. The prognostic utility of the silicone study classification system. Silicone study report 9. *Arch Ophthalmol.* 1996;114:286-92.
24. Girard P, Mimoun G, Karpouzas I, Montefiore G. Clinical risk factors for proliferative vitreoretinopathy after retinal detachment surgery. *Retina.* 1994;14:417-24.
25. Cowley M, Conway BP, Campochiaro PA, et al. Clinical risk factors for proliferative vitreoretinopathy. *Arch Ophthalmol.* 1989;107:1147-51.
26. Tseng W, Cortez RT, Ramirez G, Stinnett S, Jaffe GJ. Prevalence and risk factors for proliferative vitreoretinopathy in eyes with rhegmatogenous retinal detachment but no previous vitreoretinal surgery. *Am J Ophthalmol.* 2004; 137(6):1105-15.

27. Mitry D, Singh J, Yorston D, et al. The predisposing pathology and clinical characteristics in the Scottish retinal detachment study. *Ophthalmology.* 2011;118(7):1429-34.
28. Ryan SJ. Traction retinal detachment. X LIX Edward Jackson memorial lecture. *Am J Ophthalmol.* 1993;115:1-20.
29. Liu W, Wu Q, Haung S, Tang S. Ultrasound biomicroscopic features of anterior proliferative vitreoretinopathy. *Retina*. 1999;19:204-12.
30. Kumar A, Sharma N, Singh R. Prone position ultrasonography in silicone filled eyes. *Acta Ophthalmol Scand*. 1998;76:496-8.
31. Odrobina DC, Michalewska Z, Michalewski J, Nawrocki J. High-speed, high-resolution spectral optical coherence tomography in patients after vitrectomy with internal limiting membrane peeling for proliferative vitreoretinopathy retinal detachment. *Retina*. 2010;30(6):881-6.
32. Kiss CG, Richter-Müksch S, Sacu S, Benesch T, Velikay-Parel M. Anatomy and function of the macula after surgery for retinal detachment complicated by proliferative vitreoretinopathy. *Am J Ophthalmol.* 2007;144(6):872-7.
33. Benson SE, Grigoropoulos V, Schlottmann PG, Bunce C, Charteris DG. Analysis of the macula with optical coherence tomography after successful surgery for proliferative vitreoretinopathy. *Arch Ophthalmol.* 2005;123(12):1651-6.
34. Glasser BM, Vidaurri-Leal J, Michels R, Campochiaro PA. Cryotherapy during surgery for giant retinal tears and intra-vitreal dispersion of retinal pigment epithelial cells. *Ophthalmology*. 1993;100:466-70.
35. Gilbert CE. Adhesives in retinal detachment surgery. *Br J Ophthalmol*. 1991;75:309-10.
36. Coleman DJ, Lucas BC, Fleischmann JA, et al. A biologic tissue adhesive for vitreo-retinal surgery. *Retina*. 1988;8:250-6.
37. Hanneken AM, Michels RG. Vitrectomy and scleral buckling methods for proliferative vitreoretinopathy. *Ophthalmology*. 1988;95:865-9.
38. Farah ME, Maia M, Rodrigues EB. Dyes in ocular surgery: principles for use in chromovitrectomy. *Am J Ophthalmol*. 2009;148(3):332-40.
39. Teba FA, Mohr A, Eckardt C, et al. Trypan blue staining in vitreoretinal surgery. *Ophthalmology*. 2003;110(12):2409-12.
40. De Juan E, McCuen BW II. Management of anterior vitreous traction in proliferative vitreoretinopathy. *Retina*. 1989;9:258-62.
41. Machemer R, McCuen B, de Juan E. Relaxing retinotomies and retinectomies. *Am J Ophthalmol*. 1986;2:7-12.
42. The Silicone Study Group. Relaxing retinotomy with silicone oil or long acting gas in eyes with severe proliferative vitreoretinopathy. Silicone Study report-5. *Am J Ophthalmol.* 1993;116:557-64.
43. Federman JL, Eagle RC. Extensive peripheral retinectomy combined with posterior 360° retinotomy for retinal reattachment in advanced proliferative vitreoretinopathy cases. *Ophthalmology.* 1990;97:1305-20.
44. Tan HS, Mura M, Oberstein SY, de Smet MD. Primary retinectomy in proliferative vitreoretinopathy. *Am J Ophthalmol*. 2010;149(3):447-52.
45. Tsui I, Schubert HD. Retinotomy and silicone oil for detachments complicated by anterior inferior proliferative vitreoretinopathy. *Br J Ophthalmol*. 2009; 93(9):1228-33.
46. Banaee T, Hosseini SM, Eslampoor A, Abrishami M, Moosavi M. Peripheral 360 degrees retinectomy in complex retinal detachment. Retina 2009; 29(6): 811-8.
47. Lim AK, Alexander SM, Lim KS. Combined large radial retinotomy and circumferential retinectomy in the management of advanced proliferative vitreoretinopathy. *Retina*. 2009;29(1):112-6.

48. Tseng JJ, Barile GR, Schiff WM, Akar Y, Vidne-Hay O, Chang S. Influence of relaxing retinotomy on surgical outcomes in proliferative vitreoretinopathy. *Am J Ophthalmol.* 2005;140(4):628-36.
49. Scott IU, Flynn Jr. HW, Murray TG, Fewer WJ. The perfluoron study group. Outcomes of surgery for retinal detachment associated with proliferative vitreoretinopathy using perfluoro-n-octane: A multicenter study. *Am J Ophthalmol.* 2003;136:454-63.
50. Chang S, Zimmerman NJ, Iwamoto J, et al. Experimental vitreous replacement with perfluoro-tributylamine. *Am J Ophthalmol.* 1987;103:29-37.
51. Chang S. Low viscosity liquid fluorochemicals in vitreous surgery. *Am J Ophthalmol.* 1987;103:38-43.
52. Chang S, Ozmert E, Zimmerman NJ. Intraoperative perfluoro carbon liquids in the management of proliferative vitreoretinopathy. *Am J Ophthalmol.* 1988; 106:668-74.
53. Sirimaharaj M, Balachandran C, Chan WC, et al. Vitrectomy with short term postoperative tamponade using perfluorocarbon liquid for giant retinal tears. *Br J Ophthalmol.* 2005;89(9):1176-9.
54. Norton EWD. Intraocular gas in the management of selected retinal detachment. *Trans Am Acd Ophthalmol otolaryngol.* 1973;77:85-98.
55. The silicone study group. The effects of silicone oil removal. Silicone study report 6. *Arch Ophthalmol.* 1994;112:778-85.
56. Silicone study group. Macular pucker after successful surgery for proliferative vitreoretinopathy. Silicone study report 8. *Ophthalmology* 1995; 102: 1884-91.
57. Lincoff IT, Coleman J, Kreissig I, et al. The perfluorocarbon gases in the treatment of retinal detachment. *Ophthalmology.* 1983;90:546-51.
58. Schwartz SG, Flynn HW Jr, Lee WH, Ssemanda E, Ervin AM. Tamponade in surgery for retinal detachment associated with proliferative vitreoretinopathy. *Cochrane Database Syst Rev.* 2009; (4): CD006126.
59. Rizzo S, Genovesi-Ebert F, Vento A, Cresti F, Di Bartolo E, Belting C. A new heavy silicone oil (HWS 46-3000) used as a prolonged internal tamponade agent in complicated vitreoretinal surgery: a pilot study. *Retina.* 2007;27(5):613-20.
60. Wong D, Van Meurs JC, Stappler T, et al. A pilot study on the use of a perfluorohexyloctane/silicone oil solution as a heavier than water internal tamponade agent. *Br J Ophthalmol.* 2005;89(6):662-5.
61. Tognetto D, Minutola D, Sanguinetti G, Ravalico G. Anatomical and functional outcomes after heavy silicone oil tamponade in vitreoretinal surgery for complicated retinal detachment: a pilot study. *Ophthalmology* 2005;112(9):1574.
62. Parke DW, Aaberg TM. Intraocular argon laser photocoagulation in the management of severe proliferative vitreoretinopathy. *Am J Ophthalmol.* 1984;97:434-43.
63. Wiedemann P, Hilgers RD, Bauer P, Heimann K. Daunomycin study group. Adjunctive daunorubicin in the treatment of proliferative vitreoretinopathy: Results of a multicenter clinical trial. *Am J Ophthalmol.* 1998;126:550-9.
64. Asaria RHY, Kon CH, Bunce C, et al. Adjuvant 5-fluorouracil and Heparin prevent proliferative vitreoretinopathy. Results from a randomized, double-blind, controlled clinical trial. *Ophthalmology.* 2001;108:1179-83.
65. Blumenkraz MS, Ophir A, Claflin AJ, Hajek A. Fluorouracil for the treatment of massive periretinal proliferation. *Am J Ophthalmol.* 1982;94:458-67.
66. Tano Y, Sugita G, Abrams G, Machemer R. Inhibition of intraocular proliferations with intra vitreal corticosteroids. *Am J Ophthalmol.* 1980;89:131-6.
67. Ahmadieh H, Moradian S, Faghihi H, et al. Pseudophakic and Aphakic Retinal Detachment (PARD) Study Group. Anatomic and visual outcomes

of scleral buckling versus primary vitrectomy in pseudophakic and aphakic retinal detachment: six-month follow-up results of a single operation—report no. 1. *Ophthalmology*. 2005;112(8):1421-9.

68. Martínez-Castillo V, Boixadera A, Verdugo A, García-Arumí J. Pars plana vitrectomy alone for the management of inferior breaks in pseudophakic retinal detachment without facedown position. *Ophthalmology*. 2005; 112(7):1222-6.
69. Mura M, Tan SH, De Smet MD. Use of 25-gauge vitrectomy in the management of primary rhegmatogenous retinal detachment. Retina 2009; 29(9): 1299-1304.
70. Horozoglu F, Yanyali A, Celik E, Aytug B, Nohutcu AF. Primary 25-gauge transconjunctival sutureless vitrectomy in pseudophakic retinal detachment. *Indian J Ophthalmol.* 2007;55(5):337-40.
71. Oyagi T, Emi K. Vitrectomy without scleral buckling for proliferative vitreoretinopathy. *Retina*. 2004;24(2):215-8.
72. Weichel ED, Martidis A, Fineman MS, et al. Pars plana vitrectomy versus combined pars plana vitrectomy-scleral buckle for primary repair of pseudophakic retinal detachment. *Ophthalmology*. 2006;113(11):2033-40.
73. The Silicone Study Group: Vitrectomy with silicone oil or perfluoropropane gas in eyes with severe proliferative vitreoretinopathy. Silicone study report 3. *Retina*. 1993;13:279-84.
74. The Silicone Study Group: Vitrectomy with silicone oil or perfluoropropane gas in eyes with severe proliferative vitreoretinopathy. Results of a randomized clinical trial. Silicone study report 2. *Arch Ophthalmol.* 1992;110:780-92.
75. The Silicone Study Group: Vitrectomy with silicone oil or sulfur hexafluoride gas in eyes with severe proliferative vitreoretinopathy. Results of a randomized clinical trial. Silicone study report 1. *Arch Ophthalmol.* 1992;110:770-79.
76. Alexander P, Prasad R, Ang A, Poulson AV, Scott JD, Snead MP. Prevention and control of proliferative vitreoretinopathy: primary retinal detachment surgery using silicone oil as a planned two-stage procedure in high-risk cases. Eye (Lond). 2008; 22(6):815-8.
77. Quiram PA, Gonzales CR, Hu W, et al. Outcomes of vitrectomy with inferior retinectomy in patients with recurrent rhegmatogenous retinal detachments and proliferative vitreoretinopathy. *Ophthalmology*. 2006;113(11):2041-7.
78. Yang CM, Hsieh YT, Yang CH, Liu KR. Irrigation-free vitreoretinal surgery for recurrent retinal detachment in silicone oil-filled eyes. Eye (Lond). 2006; 20(12): 1379-82.
79. Lesnoni G, Rossi T, Gelso A, Nistril A. Patient satisfaction and vision improvement after multiple surgery for recurrent retinal detachment. *Eur J Ophthalmol.* 2005;15(1):102-8.
80. Bourke RD, Cooling RJ. Vascular consequences of retinectomy. *Arch ophthalmol.* 1996;114:155-60.
81. Pastor JC, Fernández I, Rodríguez de la Rúa E, et al. Surgical outcomes for primary rhegmatogenous retinal detachments in phakic and pseudophakic patients: the Retina 1 Project—report 2. *Br J Ophthalmol.* 2008;92(3):378-82.
82. Lam RF, Cheung BT, Yuen CY, Wong D, Lam DS, Lai WW. Retinal redetachment after silicone oil removal in proliferative vitreoretinopathy: a prognostic factor analysis. *Am J Ophthalmol.* 2008;145(3):527-533.
83. Heimann H, Bartz-Schmidt KU, Bornfeld N, Weiss C, Hilgers RD, Foerster MH. Scleral buckling versus primary vitrectomy in rhegmatogenous retinal detachment: a prospective randomized multicenter clinical study. Scleral Buckling versus Primary Vitrectomy in Rhegmatogenous Retinal Detachment Study Group. *Ophthalmology.* 2007;114(12):2142-54.
84. Brazitikos PD, Androudi S, Christen WG, Stangos NT. Primary pars plana vitrectomy versus scleral buckle surgery for the treatment of pseudophakic retinal detachment: a randomized clinical trial. *Retina*. 2005;25(8):957-64.

85. James M, O'Doherty M, Beatty S. The prognostic influence of chronicity of rhegmatogenous retinal detachment on anatomic success after reattachment surgery. *Am J Ophthalmol.* 2007;143(6):1032-4.
86. Doyle E, Herbert EN, Bunce C, Williamson TH, Laidlaw DA. How effective is macula-off retinal detachment surgery. Might good outcome be predicted? *Eye (Lond).* 2007;21(4):534-40.
87. Glasser BM, Carter JB, Kuppermann BD, Michels RG. Perfluoro-Octane in the treatment of giant retinal tears with proliferative vitreoretinopathy. *Ophthalmology*. 1991;98:1613-21.
88. Ang GS, Townend J, Lois N. Epidemiology of giant retinal tears in the United Kingdom: the British Giant Retinal Tear Epidemiology Eye Study (BGEES). *Invest Ophthalmol Vis Sci.* 2010;51(9):4781-7.
89. Wolf S, Schon V, Meier P, Wiedemann P. Silicone oil-RMN 3 Mixture (Heavy silicone oil) as internal tamponade for complicated retinal detachment. *Retina*. 2003;23:335-42.
90. Joussen AM, Wong D. The concept of heavy tamponades-chances and limitations. Graefes Arch Clin Exp *Ophthalmol.* 2008;246(9):1217-24.
91. Heimann H, Stappler T, Wong D. Heavy tamponade 1: a review of indications, use, and complications. *Eye (Lond).* 2008;22(10):1342-59.
92. Sandner D, Herbrig E, Engelmann K. High-density silicone oil (Densiron) as a primary intraocular tamponade: 12-month follow up. Graefes Arch Clin Exp *Ophthalmol.* 2007;245(8):1097-105.
93. Scott IU, Flynn HW Jr, Murray TG, Feuer WJ. Outcomes of surgery for retinal detachment associated with proliferative vitreoretinopathy using perfluoro-n-octane: a multicenter study. Perfluoron study group. *Am J Ophthalmol.* 2003;136(3): 454-63.
94. Duan A, She H, Qi Y. Complications after heavy silicone oil tamponade in complicated retinal detachment. *Retina*. 2011;31(3):547-52.
95. Drury B, Bourke RD. Short-term intraocular tamponade with perfluorocarbon heavy liquid. *Br J Ophthalmol.* 2011;95(5):694-8.
96. Furino C, Ferrari TM, Boscia F, et al. Triamcinolone-assisted parsplana vitrectomy for proliferative vitreoretinopathy. *Retina.* 2003;23:771-6.
97. Ahmadieh H, Feghhi M, Tabatabaei H, Shoeibi N, Ramezani A, Mohebbi MR. Triamcinolone acetonide in silicone-filled eyes as adjunctive treatment for proliferative vitreoretinopathy: a randomized clinical trial. *Ophthalmology*. 2008;115(11):1938-43.
98. Sundaram V, Barsam A, Virgili G. Intravitreal low molecular weight heparin and 5-Fluorouracil for the prevention of proliferative vitreoretinopathy following retinal reattachment surgery. *Cochrane Database Syst Rev.* 2010;(7):CD006421.
99. Charteris DG, Aylward GW, Wong D, Groenewald C, Asaria RH, Bunce C. A randomized controlled trial of combined 5-fluorouracil and low-molecular-weight heparin in management of established proliferative vitreoretinopathy. PVR Study Group. *Ophthalmology.* 2004;111(12):2240-5.
100. Shinohara K, Tanaka M, Sakuma T, Kobayashi Y. Efficacy of daunorubicin encapsulated in liposome for the treatment of proliferative vitreoretinopathy. *Ophthalmic Surg Lasers Imaging*. 2003;34:299-305.
101. Sakamoto T, Kimura H, Scuric Z, et al. Inhibition of experimental proliferative vitreoretinopathy by retroviral vector mediated transfer of suicide gene. Can proliferative vitreoretinopathy be a target of gene therapy? *Ophthalmology.* 1995;102:1417-24.
102. Mori K, Gehlbach P, Ando A, et al. Intraocular adenoviral vector-mediated gene transfer in proliferative retinopathies. *Invest Ophthalmol Vis Sci.* 2002;43: 1610-5.

14

chapter

P Mahesh Shanmugam

Choroidal Melanoma

ABSTRACT

Choroidal melanoma is the most common intraocular malignancy in adults. It presents as a pigmented or amelanotic mass causing visual symptoms and secondary effects to the adjacent retina, retinal pigment epithelium, vitreous and lens. Important investigations include ultrasonography, magnetic resonance imaging, fundus fluorescein and indocyanine green angiography, and rarely fine needle aspiration cytology. Small melanomas can be observed or treated with transpupillary thermotherapy with or without brachytherapy. Eyes with medium melanomas can be salvaged with brachytherapy or proton beam irradiation. Mortality rate remains the same with brachytherapy or enucleation of medium melanomas. Large melanomas are usually treated with enucleation. Contemporary thought process suggests that melanomas with potential for metastasis have already metastasized by the time of diagnosis of ocular disease. Two distinct types of melanoma based on their metastatic potential seem to exist and can be identified by genetic analysis of the tumor. Age, size, cell type, extraocular extension and presence of chromosomal alterations in the tumor are associated with poor prognosis.

Introduction

Choroidal melanoma (Fig. 14.1) arises from neuroectodermal melanocytes within the choroid. Choroidal and ciliary body melanomas are usually detected in the fifth and sixth decades.[1] Uveal melanoma (includes melanoma of the iris, ciliary body and choroid) has an incidence rate of 1.7–8.3 per million in the Caucasian population and is seen less frequently in pigmented population.[2] Uveal melanomas are rare in Indian population and appear at a relatively younger age (mean age 45.7 ± 14.2 years, range 14–82 years).[3]

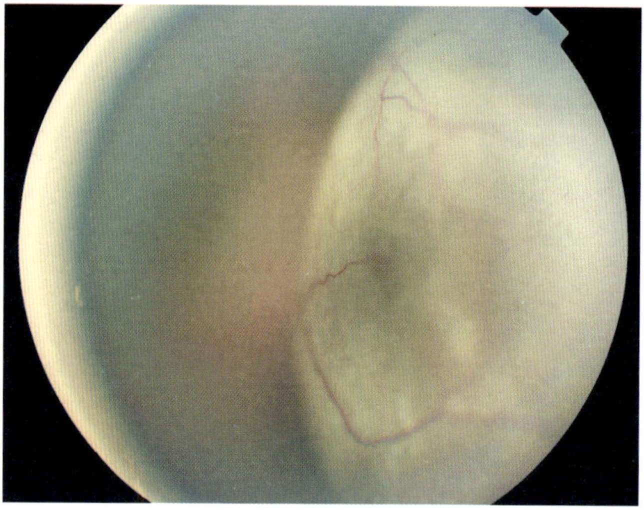

Fig. 14.1: Large choroidal melanoma

Predisposing factors for the development of uveal melanoma include:

1. Light colored skin or eyes
2. Oculodermal melanocytosis (Fig. 14.2)
3. Dysplastic nevus syndrome
4. Uveal nevus
5. Xeroderma pigmentosum
6. Family history of melanoma
7. Neurofibromatosis
8. Exposure to intense artificial ultraviolet light.

Clinical Features

Symptoms: Choroidal melanoma can cause visual symptoms due to:

a. Subfoveal location of the tumor
b. Cystoid macular edema
c. Exudative retinal detachment
d. Vitreous hemorrhage arising from the tumor due to tumor necrosis or erosion in to the choroid or overlying retina
e. Cataract
f. Tumor blocking the visual axis.

They may also present with floaters due to vitreous hemorrhage, pain and visual field loss (Fig. 14.3). A necrotic tumor may induce an inflammatory reaction. Few patients may present with a blind, painful eye without prior diagnosis of uveal melanoma underlining the need for an ultrasound examination in blind eyes wherein the fundus could not be seen. Rarely,

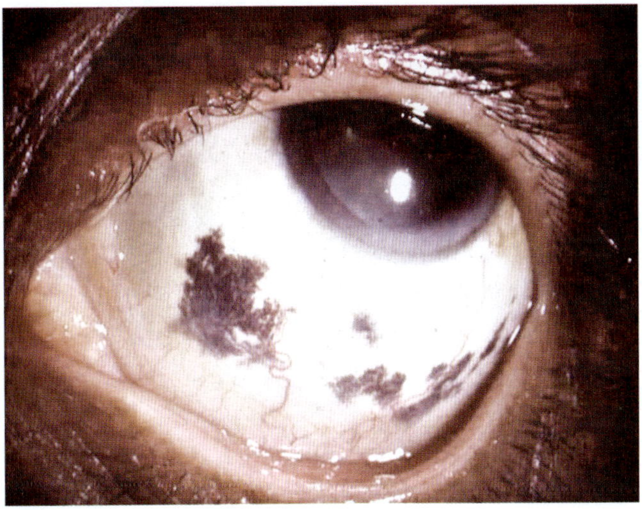

Fig. 14.2: Episcleral nevi

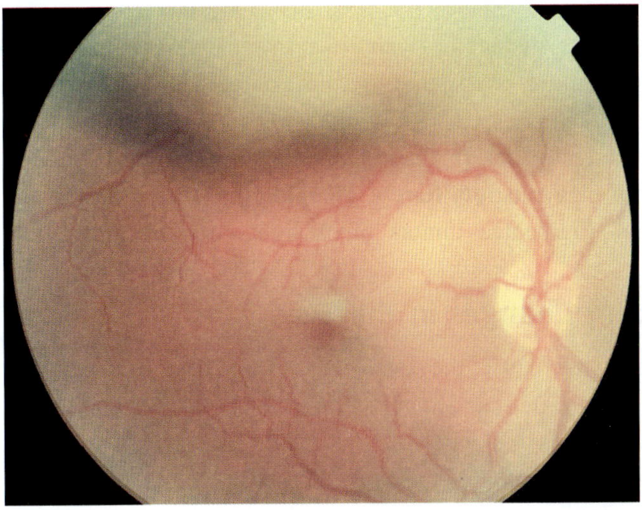

Fig. 14.3: Superior melanoma presenting as visual field deficit

the tumor may remain asymptomatic and be discovered on routine fundus examination.

The typical choroidal melanoma appears as a dark brown, dome-shaped, solid tumor. It can break through the overlying Bruch's membrane and form a dumb-bell or collar-button-shaped nodular mass under the retina. Diffuse melanoma (height <15% of the base; also defined as <5mm thick and covering >25% of the uveal tract) may present as an ill-defined thickening of the

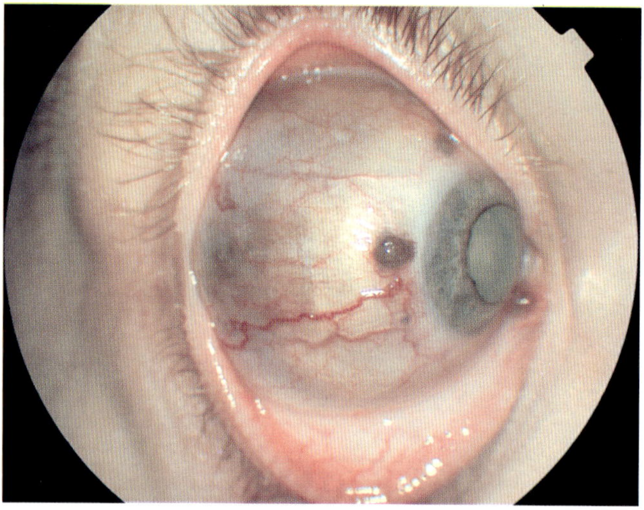

Fig. 14.4: Melanoma with multiple extraocular extension—a rare presentation

choroid. Diffuse melanomas carry the risk of early extrascleral extension (Fig. 14.4), more malignant cytologic features and worse systemic prognosis.[4]

The tumor may lack pigment and appear amelanotic or more commonly show dense pigmentation. Rarely, choroidal melanoma may be multicentric or bilateral. Pigmented tumors block light on transillumination.

Secondary Changes in the Eyes

The tumor may cause the following secondary effects in the eye:

1. Secondary retinal detachment is usually present (Fig. 14.5).
2. Overlying retinal pigment epithelium and photoreceptor atrophy.
3. Drusen formation (Fig. 14.6)
4. Retinal pigment epithelium detachment
5. Cystoid degeneration of the retina
6. Cystoid macular edema
7. Choroidal neovascularization
8. Severe ocular pain may occur when the tumor impinges on the posterior ciliary nerves.
9. Melanomas may exhibit orange colored lipofuschin pigment over their surface. Diffuse pigment indicates an active tumor while a localized pigment and drusen indicate a slow growing or a dormant tumor.
10. Rarely with subretinal exudation (Fig.14.7).

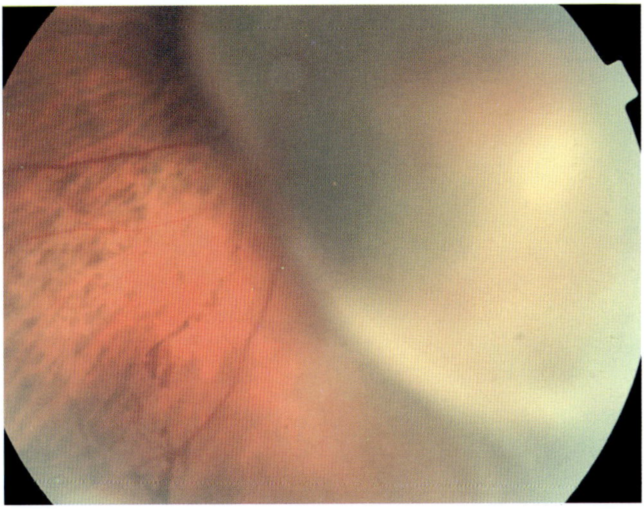

Fig. 14.5: Large choroidal melanoma with secondary retinal detachment inferiorly

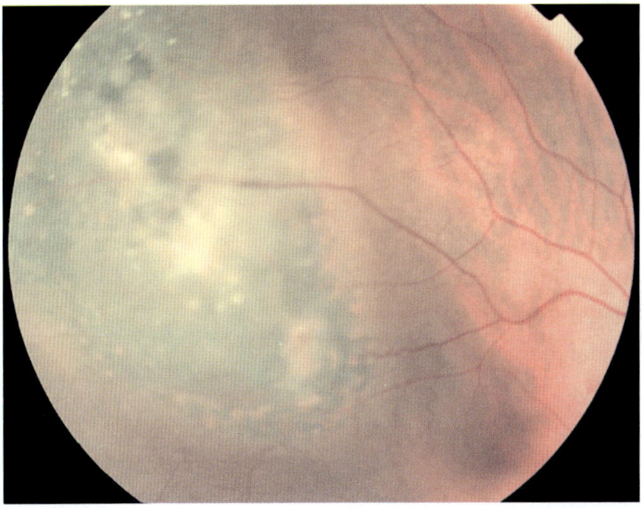

Fig. 14.6: Medium size melanoma with drusens and cryotherapy scars

The tumor may grow anteriorly to involve the ciliary body causing cataract, trabecular meshwork block causing glaucoma, erode blood vessels leading on to vitreous or anterior chamber hemorrhage. The tumor may also cause neovascular glaucoma secondary to rubeosis iridis and uveitis when undergoing necrosis. Subretinal hemorrhage and proptosis may occur due to posterior extrascleral extension of the tumor.

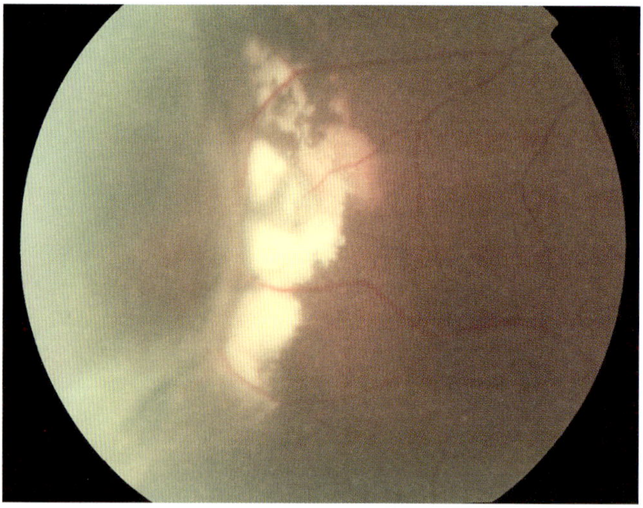

Fig. 14.7: Choroidal melanoma showing subretinal exudation—a rare presentation

Differential Diagnosis

The differential diagnosis of melanoma includes the following conditions:

1. Choroidal detachment
2. Choroidal nevus
3. Melanocytoma
4. Metastatic tumors
5. Medulloepithelioma (diktyoma)
6. Choroidal osteoma
7. Choroidal hemangioma
8. Adenoma
9. Adenocarcinoma
10. Combined hamartoma of the retina and pigment epithelium
11. Congenital hypertrophy and reactive hyperplasia of the retinal pigment epithelium
12. Leiomyoma
13. Tubercular granuloma.

Pathophysiology and Prognosis of Uveal Melanoma

Uveal melanoma arises from melanocytes in the uveal tract. Although uveal melanomas may grow *de novo*, most develop from preexisting melanocytic nevi. Three distinct cell types, spindle A, spindle B, and epithelioid cell type are found. Modified Callender classification divides uveal melanocytic tumors into spindle cell A and B melanomas, mixed cell and epithelioid cell melanomas. Presence of the latter two types is associated with more aggressive behavior and carries a poorer prognosis for the patient's survival.

Tumor features' such as larger size, anterior location, trans-scleral extension, proximity to the foveal avascular zone, advanced age of the patient, growth through Bruch's membrane, optic nerve extension, lack of pigmentation, and histologic characteristics such as mitotic activity, mean of 10 largest nucleoli, tumor infiltrating lymphocytes and cell type have been found to correlate with increased mortality.

Vascular networks, closed loops, parallel with cross linking microcirculation patterns noted on histopathological evaluation and chromosomal abnormalities appear to predict tumors that are likely to metastasize. Alterations in chromosome 3 (monosomy 3) and chromosome 8 (additional copies of long arm) are suggestive of poor prognosis (type II tumors). Tumor specimen is obtained using fine needle aspiration biopsy for chromosomal analysis that may allow prognostication. This would allow close follow-up of patients with type II tumors allowing prompt treatment of metastatic lesions.

Mutations of guanine nucleotide-binding protein G(q) subunit alpha (GNAQ, or G-alpha-q), which effectively turn it into a dominantly acting oncogene, have also been identified in approximately half of uveal melanoma[5]. Uveal melanomas tend to metastasize to the liver, lung, central nervous system, bone and skin. Less frequently, transcleral growth of the tumor through emissary channels can result in orbital and conjunctival metastasis. An overall mortality rate of approximately 30–50% occurs from uveal melanoma within 10 years from diagnosis and treatment. Silent hematogenous micrometstasis occurring prior to diagnosis of ocular disease is considered to be the cause for the high mortality rate. The collaborative ocular melanoma study (COMS) found a 5-year mortality rate of 6% for small (1–3 mm height/5–16 mm diameter), 18% for medium-sized tumors (2.5–10 mm height and <16 mm in diameter) and 30% for large (>10 mm height and or >16 mm diameter) tumors.[6-8]

Investigations

ULTRASONOGRAPHY

Choroidal melanomas appear as a solid mass with a biconvex or mushroom shape on B scan ultrasonography. A scan demonstrates high surface spike with low amplitude internal reflectivity, with a decremental reduction of spike height from the surface to the depth of the mass (angle kappa). Acoustic hollowing and choroidal excavation and rarely vascular pulsations may also be seen (Fig. 14.8).

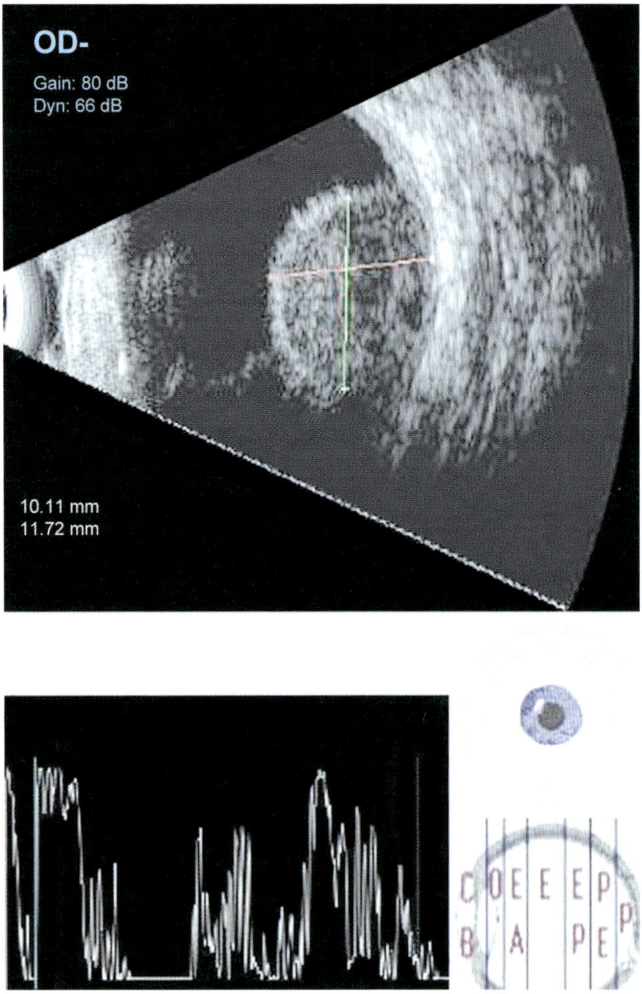

Fig. 14.8: B scan USG showing dome-shaped mass with choroidal excavation, mild to moderate internal reflectivity and acoustic hollowness

FUNDUS FLUORESCEIN ANGIOGRAPHY

Choroidal melanomas are predominantly hypofluorescent with pinpoint areas of hyperfluorescence due to retinal pigment epithelium loss in early frames and may show prominent intratumor blood vessels (double circulation). Leakage from the tumor and staining of the entire tumor with leakage into the subretinal fluid is seen in late phase of the angiogram (Figs 14.9 to 14.11).

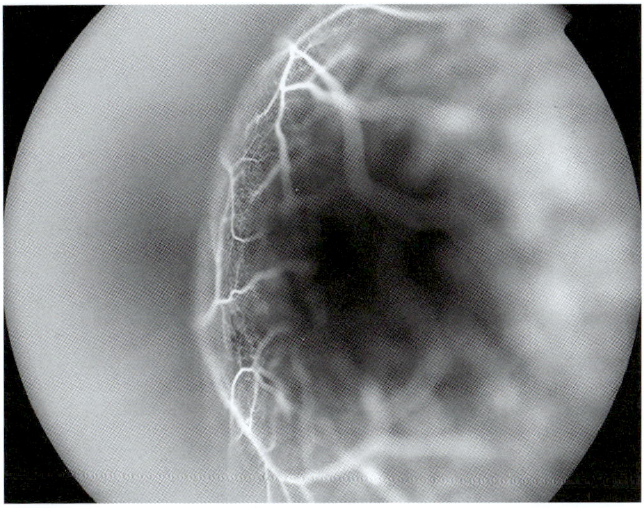

Fig. 14.9: Large choroidal melanoma FFA showing early phase double circulation

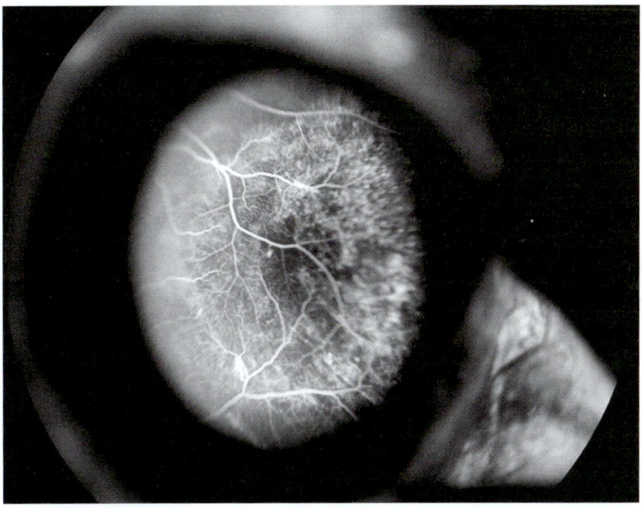

Fig. 14.10: FFA showing pin point hyperfluorescence during mid phase

INDOCYANINE GREEN ANGIOGRAPHY

Choroidal melanomas block choroidal filling on indocyanine green angiography (ICG); late phase pictures may demonstrate intratumor vessels and minimal late dye leakage. Confocal ICG angiograms may show complex microcirculation patterns that may indicate growth potential of the melanoma.[9]

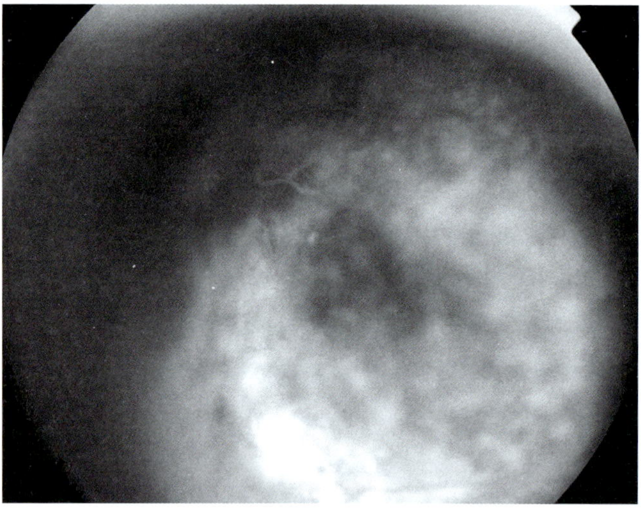

Fig. 14.11: FFA showing leakage during late phase

COMPUTERIZED TOMOGRAPHY

Computerized tomography (CT scan) can image most choroidal melanoma and a majority of them show enhancement on contrast CT.

MAGNETIC RESONANCE IMAGING

Choroidal melanoma appears bright (hyperintense) with respect to vitreous on T1 weighted images (Fig. 14.12) and dark (hypointense) with respect to vitreous in T2 weighted images on MRI scan (Fig. 14.13).

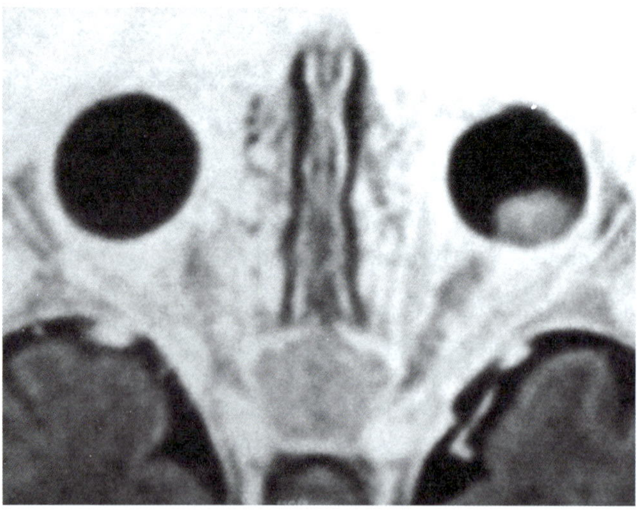

Fig. 14.12: Choroidal melanoma appears hyperintense in T1 weighted images on MRI

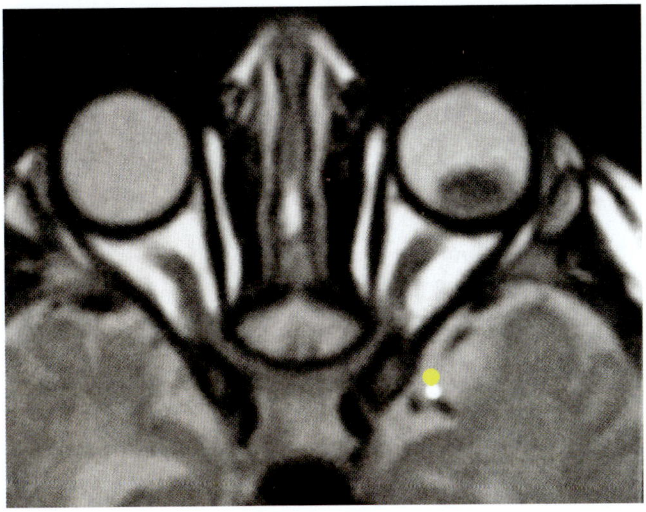

Fig. 14.13: Choroidal melanoma appears hypointense in T2 weighted images on MRI

FINE NEEDLE ASPIRATION BIOPSY

Rarely if the diagnosis cannot be made with reasonable certainty with non-invasive methods, a fine needle aspiration biopsy may be necessary to obtain tissue specimen.

METASTATIC WORK-UP

Premanagement evaluation of uveal melanoma includes complete physical examination with particular attention to the liver, lung, abdomen, skin and subcutaneous tissues, which are frequent sites of metastatic spread. Hepatic function tests (serum levels of gamma-glutamyl transpeptidase, lactic dehydrogenase, glutamic-oxaloacetic transaminase), ultrasound/CT scan examination of the abdomen are essential to rule out hepatic metastasis. However, the imaging studies do not exclude micrometastasis. CT/X-ray chest is also indicated to rule out lung metastasis. These investigations are to be repeated 6 monthly after treatment, for early diagnosis of metastatic disease. However, most patients do not have detectable metastasis at the time of presentation. Melanoma metastasis is associated with poor prognosis; a small percentage of patients with localized hepatic metastasis may benefit from local resection and chemoembolization.[10,11] Antitumor vaccines, systemic immune modulators, as well as chemotherapeutic agents, have been tried with limited success in treating extrahepatic metastasis. A promising new approach may involve broad activation of the immune system by blockade of cytotoxic T-lymphocyte antigen-4 (CTLA4).[12-14]

The validity of periodic metastatic surveillance has recently been questioned as available evidence from the peer-reviewed literature does not provide any compelling evidence of survival benefit for any metastatic treatment regimen or frequency of surveillance for metastasis relative to no such testing.[15]

MANAGEMENT OF CHOROIDAL MELANOMA

Small choroidal melanomas are observed or treated with laser photocoagulation, transpupillary thermotherapy, and rarely with brachytherapy.

Medium melanomas are treated with brachytherapy or charged particle radiation, rarely with enucleation, gamma knife or resection. Large melanomas usually necessitate enucleation of the eye. Uveal melanoma treatment does not seem to have a significant effect on patient survival and hence the management of uveal melanoma has shifted more towards eye-saving approach.[16]

OBSERVATIONS

Dormant, small and medium sized tumors, and slow growing small and medium tumors in sick and one eyed patients may generally be observed periodically after proper documentation with color fundus photograph and ultrasonography. Dormancy is indicated by (i) the absence of growth on follow-up, (ii) absence of subretinal fluid, and (iii) presence of drusen. Presence of subretinal fluid, growth, diffuse orange pigment, absence of drusen, proximity to the fovea/disk indicate the necessity for treatment. There is a shift towards obtaining tumor specimen of small-pigmented choroidal lesions for chromosomal anomalies, the presence of which prompt treatment.

LASER PHOTOCOAGULATION

Small nasal and temporal peripheral melanomas located away from macula and outside the arcade can be treated with laser photocoagulation. Less than 5% of melanomas meet the criteria laid down for use of photocoagulation. Multiple treatment sessions may be necessary before satisfactory regression of the tumor. Cystoid macular edema, branch retinal vein occlusion, and macular involvement with laser may occur as complications of laser treatment.[17]

TRANSPUPILLARY THERMOTHERAPY

Transpupillary thermotherapy (TTT) has found wide use in treating small melanomas (<3 mm in thickness) that are away from the disk and macula. With proper selection of tumors, 91–94% of treated small choroidal melanomas showed regression when treated with TTT.[18-20] In a series of 256 consecutive melanomas (mean 2.7 mm in height) treated only with mean 3 sessions of TTT, 91% of the tumors remained regressed at 3 years. More than 3 TTT sessions and tumor overhanging the optic disk were risk factors for recurrence. Risk factors for visual acuity <20/200 were documented tumor growth before treatment, mushroom tumor configuration, initial symptom of blurred vision, poor initial visual acuity, superior quadrant tumor location, underlying diabetes mellitus, and tumor overhanging the optic disk. Treating tumors larger than 3 mm in thickness increases the risk of recurrence.[21]

Though TTT results are good for short term regression of the tumor, local recurrence in 23–45% patients has been reported in other studies and enucleation in 8% of patients due to intrascleral and extrascleral involvement.[22-25] TTT is preferred in the treatment of small melanomas so that radiation induced complications can be avoided; however, a study comparing the visual results with TTT and brachytherapy found no difference in the visual outcome. There was an increased risk of recurrence of the tumor with TTT alone; suggesting that TTT is better used as an adjuvant treatment rather than a primary treatment.[26] Dense scotomas due to nerve fiber defects, epiretinal gliosis and macular abnormalities may also limit visual recovery after TTT.[27] ICG enhanced TTT is also effective in treating small and medium melanomas, particularly amelanotic tumors (100 mg ICG infused over 10 minutes, 2 minutes after starting TTT).[28,29]

PHOTODYNAMIC THERAPY

Photodynamic therapy (PDT) has rarely been used as a primary treatment or as an adjunct to treat tumor close to the posterior pole to avoid radiation related complications. A bolus dose of verteporfin and treatment at 1 minute with double the light dose for 166 seconds and multiple sessions have been employed. PDT may be particularly suitable to treat amelanotic melanomas that do not respond well to TTT.[30-32]

RADIATION

Role of External Beam Radiotherapy

Conventional external beam radiotherapy (EBRT) is not used in the management of choroidal melanoma as the large radiation dose involved will invariably cause radiation related complications leading to blindness. The COMS study failed to show any benefit of 2000 cGy radiation delivered to the eye prior to enucleation in decreasing mortality. Post enucleation irradiation may be useful in cases where extrascleral extension has been transected intraoperatively.[32]

Charged Particle Radiation

Large uveal melanomas up to 24 mm in diameter and 14 mm in height have been treated with charged particle irradiation with a recurrence rate of 33% and a metastatic rate of 10% at 2 years.[33] Tumors involving the fovea, optic nerve head, those with small extrascleral extension are also treatable with proton beam radiation. The five-year survival rate following proton beam radiation has been to be comparable with of plaque brachytherapy. The disadvantage of the current charged particle radiation systems is that they are expensive to install and maintain and hence are available in few centers in the world. Risk of radiation maculopathy is high after proton beam radiation of paramacular melanomas.[34]

Brachytherapy

Brachytherapy is the process of delivering radiation as precisely as possible to the tumor, the main advantage being the limited exposure of normal surrounding tissue to radiation. Brachytherapy is the mainstay in the conservative treatment of choroidal melanomas (Figs 14.14 and 14.15). Various radioisotopes, such as cobalt 60, iridium, ruthenium106, palladium 103 and Iodine 125/131 have all been used to treat intraocular tumors, but iodine 125 and ruthenium 106 remain the safe and effective isotopes of choice. Choroidal melanomas are treated with a dose of 8000–10000 cGy delivered to the apex of the tumor.

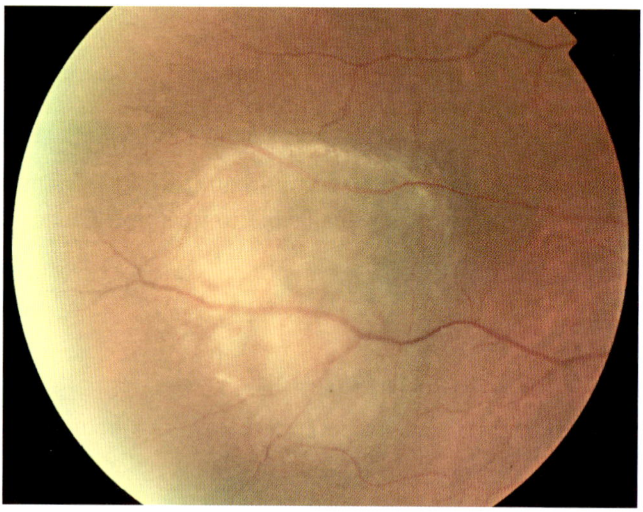

Fig. 14.14: Medium size melanoma—prebrachytherapy

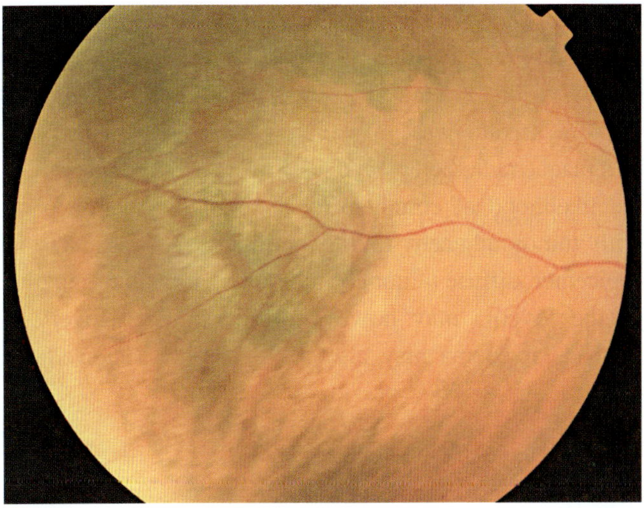

Fig. 14.15: Complete regression of melanoma—post-brachytherapy

The current relative indications of plaque brachytherapy for melanoma are:

i. Selected small melanomas that are documented to be growing or that show clear-cut signs of activity on the first visit.
ii. Most medium-sized and some large choroidal and ciliary body melanomas in an eye with potential salvageable vision.
iii. Almost all actively growing melanomas that occur in the patients' only useful eye.

The radioactive plaque is sutured directly on to the sclera overlying the tumor and retained in place until the desired dosage of radiation is delivered to the tumor and then removed surgically. COMS study found that brachytherapy offers the advantage of eye salvage as against enucleation in managing medium melanoma but same rate of mortality.[6]

Radiation induced complications can result in poor vision after brachytherapy. Forty-nine percent of the eyes with medium melanoma in COMS had lost more than 6 lines of vision 3 years after treatment. Patients with a history of diabetes and patients whose eyes had thicker tumors, tumors close to or beneath the foveal avascular zone, tumor-associated retinal detachment, or tumors that were not dome-shaped were those most likely to have a poor visual acuity.[35]

Large melanomas can also be treated with iodine-125 brachytherapy with 5-year and 10-year metastatic rate of 33 and 55%, respectively. Local tumor recurrence was only observed in 13% of eyes at 10 years [36]. Larger melanomas are associated with increased chances of visual morbidity and local recurrence of tumor with radiation therapy.[37] A study of brachytherapy for large melanomas found that 91% of the treated eyes had lost more than 6 lines of vision 3 years after treatment. Tumor height and location posterior to ora serrata were associated with poor visual results.[38]

Combined plaque radiotherapy and laser photocoagulation or thermotherapy increase the likelihood of complete local tumor destruction particularly in patients with tumor adjacent to the optic disk.[39,40] Macular location of the tumor epicenter, diffuse tumor configuration, and tumor margin extending underneath the foveola may however, limit visual recovery.[39]Epiretinal gliosis and macular edema may also result in poor vision after combined therapy.[40]

Surgery

RESECTION

Choroidal melanoma not greater than 15 mm in diameter, anterior to the equator can be considered for partial lamellar sclerouvectomy if the overlying retina is spared, and penetrating sclerochorioretinovitrectomy if the retina and sclera are involved.[41-43] The concerns are of residual tumor and recurrence, other than tumor dissemination during surgery. The current concept of combining brachytherapy prior to or following resection ensures eradication of the tumor more completely. Internal resection of melanoma after delimiting preoperative photocoagulation around the tumor followed by vitrectomy and internal removal of the tumor piecemeal has been attempted for posteriorly located melanomas that are not amenable to lamellar sclerouvectomy and also have an increased risk of radiation maculopathy.[44-45] Short-term results do not report increased metastatic or recurrence risk. Combining brachytherapy with resection and pre-enucleation radiation is preferable to reduce the risk of tumor recurrence and metastasis.

ENUCLEATION

Eyes with melanoma >10 mm in height or >16 mm in diameter are usually enucleated. Small or medium-sized tumors with optic nerve invasion, posterior uveal melanomas with total retinal detachment or severe glaucoma however, are also managed by enucleation.[43-48] Pre-enucleation radiation does not alter the mortality rate and hence not advised.[46] A "no touch technique" has been advocated to prevent hematogenous dissemination of the tumor.[47,48]

Conclusion

Choroidal melanoma appears to be a systemic disease with micrometastasis existing even when the ocular lesion is diagnosed resulting in the death of 50% of patients to metastatic disease. Newer insights in to genetic aberrations in the tumor impacting the prognosis will pave way for early diagnosis of patients at risk and better treatment of metastasis in the future.

References

1. Egon, KM, Seddon JM, Glynn RJ, et al. Epidemiologic aspects of uveal melanoma. *Surv Ophthalmol.* 1998;32:239-51.
2. Iscovich J, Abdulrazik M, Pe'Er J. Posterior uveal malignant melanoma: temporal stability and ethnic variation in rates in Israel. *Anticancer Res.* 2001;21: 1449-54.
3. Biswas J, Kabra S, Krishnakumar S, Shanmugam MP. Clinical and histopathological characteristics of uveal melanoma in asian indians. A study of 103 patients. *Ind J Ophthalmol.* 2004;52:41-4.
4. Ou JI, Wheeler SM, O'Brien JM.Posterior pole tumor update. Ophthalmol Clin North Am. 2002 Dec;15(4):489-501.
5. Sisley K, Doherty R, Cross NA. What hope for the future? GNAQ and uveal melanoma. *Br J Ophthalmol.* 2011;95:620-23.
6. The Collaborative Ocular Melanoma Study Group. Mortality in patients with small choroidal melanoma. COMS report no. 4. *Arch Ophthalmol.* 1997; 115:886-93.
7. The Collaborative Ocular Melanoma Study Group. The collaborative ocular melanoma study randomized trial of iodine 125 brachytherapy for choroidal melanoma, III: initial mortality findings. COMS report no. 18. *Arch Ophthalmol.* 2001;119:969-82.
8. The Collaborative Ocular Melanoma Study Group. The collaborative ocular melanoma study randomized trial of pre-enucleation radiation of large choroidal melanoma II: initial mortality findings. COMS report no. 10. *Am J Ophthalmol.* 1998;125:865-67.
9. Mueller AJ, Freeman WR, Schaller UC, Kampik A, Folberg R and Munic/San Diego/ Iowa city collaboration. Complex microcirculation patterns detected by confocal indocyanine green angiography predict time to growth of small choroidal melanocytic tumors. MuSIC report II. *Ophthalmology.* 2002;109:2207-14.
10. Augsburger JJ, Corre^a ZM, Shaikh AH. Effectiveness of treatments for metastatic uveal melanoma. *Am J Ophthalmol.* 2009;148:119-27.
11. Frenkel S, Nir I, Hendler K, et al. Long-term survival of uveal melanoma patients after surgery for liver metastases. *Br J Ophthalmol.* 2009;93:1042-6.
12. Sato T, Han F, Yamamoto A. The biology and management of uveal melanoma. *Curr Oncol Rep.* 2008;10:431-38.
13. Cranmer LD, Hersh E. The role of the CTLA4 blockade in the treatment of malignant melanoma. Cancer Invest 2007; 25:613-631.
14. Lens M, Ferrucci PF, Testori A. Anti-CTLA4 monoclonal antibody Ipilimumab in the treatment of metastatic melanoma: recent findings. *Recent Pat Anticancer Drug Discov.* 2008;3:105-13.
15. Augsburger JJ, Correa ZM, Trichopoulos N. Surveillance Testing for Metastasis From Primary Uveal Melanoma and Effect on Patient Survival. *Am J Ophthalmol.* 2011;152:5-7.

16. Yevgeniy Shildkrot Y, Wilson MW. Update on posterior uveal melanoma: treatment of the eye and emerging strategies in the prognosis and treatment of metastatic disease. *Curr Opin Ophthalmol.* 2009;20:504-10.
17. Qiang Z, Cairns JD. Laser photocoagulation treatment of choroidal melanoma. *Aust N Z J Ophthalmol.* 1993;21(2):87-92.
18. Oosterhuis JA, Journee-de Korver HG, Kakebeeke-Kemme HM, et al. Transpupillary thermotherapy in choroidal melanomas. *Arch Ophthalmol.* 1995;113:315-21.
19. Shields CL, Shields JA. Transpupillary thermotherapy for choroidal melanoma. *Curr Opin Ophthalmol.* 1999;10:197-203.
20. Shields CL, Shields JA, Perez N, Singh AD, Cater J. Primary transpupillary thermotherapy for small choroidal melanoma in 256 consecutive cases: outcomes and limitations. *Ophthalmology.* 2002;109(2):225-34.
21. Stoffelns BM. Primary transpupillary thermotherapy (TTT) for malignant choroidal melanoma. *Acta Ophthalmol Scand.* 2002;80(1):25-31.
22. Stoffelns BM. Tumor regression and visual outcome after transpupillary thermotherapy (TTT) for malignant choroidal melanoma Klin Monatsbl Augenheilkd. 2006 Jan;223(1):74-80.
23. Robertson DM, Buettner H, Bennett SR. Transpupillary thermotherapy as primary treatment for small choroidal melanomas. *Trans Am Ophthalmol Soc* 1999;97:407-27.
24. Aaberg TM Jr, Bergstrom CS, Hickner ZJ, Lynn MJ. Long-term results of primary transpupillary thermal therapy for the treatment of choroidal malignant melanoma. *Br J Ophthalmol.* 2008;92:741-6.
25. Singh AD, Kivela T, Seregard S, et al. Primary transpupillary thermotherapy of 'small' choroidal melanoma: is it safe? *Br J Ophthalmol.* 2008; 92:727-8.
26. Harbour JW, Meredith TA, Thompson PA, Gordon ME. Transpupillary thermotherapy versus plaque radiotherapy for suspected choroidal melanomas. *Ophthalmology*. 2003 Nov;110(11):2207-14.
27. Liggett PE, Lavaque AJ, Chaudhry NA, Jablon EP, Quiroz-Mercado H. Preliminary results of combined simultaneous transpupillary thermotherapy and ICG-based photodynamic therapy for choroidal melanoma. *Ophthalmic Surg Lasers Imaging*. 2005 Nov-Dec;36(6):463-70.
28. Stoffelns BM. Kinetics of indocyanine green (ICG) and clinical use for enhancement of transpupillary thermotherapy (TTT) in hypopigmented small choroidal melanomas Klin Monatsbl Augenheilkd. 2004;221(5):374-8.
29. Kim RY, Hu LK, Foster BS, Gragoudas ES, Young LH. Photodynamic therapy of pigmented choroidal melanomas of greater than 3-mm thickness. *Ophthalmology.* 1996;103:2029-36.
30. Barbazetto IA, Lee TC, Rollins IS, Chang S, Abramson DH. Treatment of choroidal melanoma using photodynamic therapy. *Am J Ophthalmol.* 2003; 135:898-9.
31. Donaldson MJ, Lim L, Harper CA, Mackenzie J, G Campbell W. Primary treatment of choroidal amelanotic melanoma with photodynamic therapy. *Clin Experiment Ophthalmol.* 2005;33(5):548-9.
32. Robertson DM. Changing concepts in the management of choroidal melanoma. *Am J Ophthalmol*. 2003;136:161-70.
33. Conway RM, Poothullil AM, Daftari IK, et al. Estimates of ocular and visual retention following treatment of extra-large uveal melanomas by proton beam radiotherapy. *Arch Ophthalmol*. 2006; 124:838-43.
34. Guyer DR, Mukai S, Egan KM, Seddon JM, Walsh SM, Gragoudas ES. Radiation maculopathy after proton beam irradiation for choroidal

melanoma. *Ophthalmology*. 1992;99(8):1278-85.

35. Melia BM, Abramson DH, Albert DM, Boldt HC, Earle JD, Hanson WF, Montague P, Moy CS, Schachat AP, Simpson ER, Straatsma BR, Vine AK, Weingeist TA; Collaborative Ocular Melanoma Study Group. Collaborative ocular melanoma study (COMS) randomized trial of I-125 brachytherapy for medium choroidal melanoma. I. Visual acuity after 3 years COMS report no. 16. *Ophthalmology*. 2001;108(2):348-66.
36. Shields CL, Naseripour M, Cater J, et al. Plaque radiotherapy for large posterior uveal melanomas (> or ¼8-mm thick) in 354 consecutive patients. *Ophthalmology*. 2002;109:1838-49.
37. Jampol LM, Moy CS, Murray TG, et al. The collaborative ocular melanoma study randomized trial of I-125 brachytherapy for choroidal melanoma. IV. Local treatment failure and enucleation in the first five years after brachytherapy. COMS Report No.19. *Ophthalmology.* 2002;109:2197-2206.
38. Puusaari I, Heikkonen J, Summanen P, Tarkkanen A, Kivela T. Iodine brachytherapy as an alternative to enucleation for large uveal melanomas. *Ophthalmology.* 2003;110(11):2223-34.
39. Shields CL, Cater J, Shields JA, Chao A, Krema H, Materin M, Brady LW. Combined plaque radiotherapy and transpupillary thermotherapy for choroidal melanoma: tumor control and treatment complications in 270 consecutive patients. *Arch Ophthalmol.* 2002;120(7):933-40.
40. Stoffelns BM, Kutzner J, Schopfer K, Frising M.Prospective nonrandomised analysis of "Sandwich Therapy" for malignant melanoma of the choroid] Klin Monatsbl Augenheilkd. 2002;219(4):211-5.
41. Damato BE, Foulds WS. Surgical resection of choroidal melanoma. In: Ryan SJ. Editor. *Retina*. St. Louis, CV Mosby, 2001, pp 762-72.
42. Shields JA, Shields CL. Surgical approach to lamellar sclerouvectomy for posterior uveal melanomas: The Schoenberg lecture. *Ophthalmic Surg.* 1988;19: 774-780.
43. Peyman GA, Juarez CP, Diamond JG, Raichand M. Ten years experience with eye wall resection of uveal melanomas. *Ophthalmology.* 1984;91: 1720-24.
44. Peyman GA, Charles H. Internal eyewall resection in the management of uveal melanoma. *Can J Ophthalmol.* 1988;23:219-23.
45. Garcia-Arumi J, Sararols L, Martinez V, Corcostegui BF. Vitreoretinal surgery and endoresection in high posterior choroidal melanomas *Retina*. 2001;21: 445-52.
46. The Collaborative Ocular Melanoma Study Group. The collaborative ocular melanoma study randomized trial of pre-enucleation radiation of large choroidal melanoma II: initial mortality findings. COMS report no. 10. *Am J Ophthalmol.* 1998;125:865-67.
47. Fraunfelder FT, Boozman FW, Wilson RS, et al. No touch technique for intraocular malignant tumors. *Arch Ophthalmol.* 1977;95:1616-20.
48. Midgal C. Effect of the method of enucleation on the prognosis of choroidal melanoma. *Br J Ophthalmol.* 1983;67:385-8.

15

chapter

AK Grover
Shaloo Bageja

Fracture of the Orbital Floor: Management

ABSTRACT

Orbital fractures secondary to blunt trauma are not uncommon. The most common orbital walls affected are the floor and the medial wall. The orbital floor fractures may occur alone or may be associated with other facial fractures. Clinical presentation may vary. The floor fractures may present with proptosis, restriction of motility, diplopia and enophthalmos. Clinical indications for repair have been categorized into emergent, semi-emergent and delayed. Goals of repair are restoration of the prolapsed orbital contents and cover the bony defect with an implant to prevent prolapse. The ideal implant should be easy to insert and manipulate, inert, not prone to infection or extrusion, easily anchored to surrounding structures, and should not induce fibrosis. Most orbital floor defects can be repaired with hydroxyapatite or synthetic implants composed of porous polyethylene, silicone, metallic rigid mini plates, vicryl mesh, or metallic mesh. Autogenous bone from the maxillary wall or the calvarium may be used. Results of repair are gratifying with few complications.

Introduction

The bony orbit and its soft tissues are frequently involved in facial trauma occasionally resulting in orbital floor fracture. The isolated orbital floor fracture known as a *blow-out fracture* is a common presentation following blunt trauma. The floor fractures may also occur in combination with zygomatic arch fractures, Le Fort II or III or with fracture of other orbital bones.

The goal of the treatment is reduction of the fracture fragments to restore the orbital anatomy and to restore the physiologic functions and the esthetic appearance of an individual. Recent advances have made it possible to early diagnose and manage orbital fracture and prevent its troublesome sequelae. The differences between the 'active' and the 'conservative' schools of management have narrowed down with newer diagnostic modalities making the indications and timing of repair well defined.[1]

Mechanism of Blow-out Fracture

The two theories which are proposed to explain development of blow-out fractures are 'hydraulic' and 'buckling'. Smith and Regan[2] hypothesized the hydraulic theory. According to this theory when an object larger than the orbital entrance impacts the globe and the upper eyelid, it transmits the kinetic energy to the periocular tissue. To relieve the increased intraorbital pressure, the floor blows out into the maxillary sinus. Most fractures occur in the postero-medial region of the orbit that is comprised of the thinnest bone.

The alternative buckling force theory proposed by Fujino[3] suggests that when infraorbital rim is displaced posteriorly, the force is transmitted to the orbital floor which buckles and fractures while the rim returns to its normal position without fracturing. This concept was supported by an experimental model. The two theories are, however, not mutually exclusive and variable degrees of each may be applicable in a given patient of blow-out fracture.

Clinical Assessment

A patient presenting with orbital trauma needs a comprehensive assessment of associated ocular injuries and injuries to other parts of the body.[4-6] Examination of the globe is essential. The possibility of globe rupture should always be ruled out. Management of these take precedence over diagnosis and treatment of orbital fracture. Assessment of pupil is essential as pupillary dysfunction along with decreased visual acuity, may be due to traumatic optic neuropathy. Suspicion of an orbital floor fracture is based on clinical features and is usually confirmed radiologically.

Forced duction test is a very important part of assessment and contributes significantly to the decision making.

Clinical Presentation

The clinical features of the patient with orbital fracture may vary according to the time of presentation. Common features include eyelid ecchymosis/ hematoama, subcutaneous emphysema, infraorbital hypoesthesia, restriction of ocular motility with diplopia, initial proptosis followed by enophthalmos/ hyphothalmos.

EYELID ECCHYMOSIS/HEMATOMA AND PROPTOSIS

Periorbital ecchymosis and hematoma with proptosis are usually seen after the acute trauma (Figs 15.1A and B). However, these signs may be absent in 'white eyed' fracture inspite of presence of other signs of blow-out fracture.

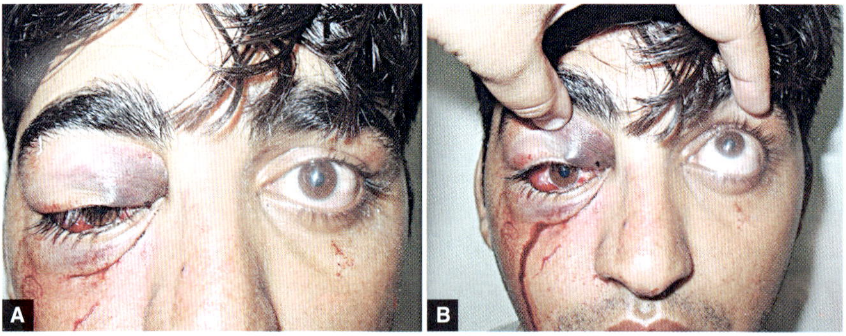

Figs 15.1A and B: (A) Periorbital ecchymosis and hematoma of RE and (B) RE showing gross restriction in up gaze

SUBCUTANEOUS EMPHYSEMA

Emphysema occurs due to the communication of the periorbital soft tissue with air filled sinuses. It usually occurs with medial wall fractures and results in palpable crepitus.

INFRAORBITAL HYPOESTHESIA

Infraorbital hypoesthesia is almost pathognomic of an orbital floor fracture. This occurs as the fracture extends along the infraorbital groove injuring the nerve. These sensory defects tend to resolve spontaneously over a period of months.

RESTRICTION OF OCULAR MOTILITY WITH DIPLOPIA

Limitation of ocular motility associated with diplopia is one of the hallmarks of orbital floor fracture (Figs 15.2A to C). Vertical diplopia is more common than the horizontal diplopia. Ocular motility is usually restricted either due to entrapment of the subcutaneous tissue or an extraocular muscle or due to hematoma or edema within the orbit or due to the neuronal damage. It is important to assess the patient 7–10 days after the injury to assess the improvement in motility due to resolution of hematoma or edema.

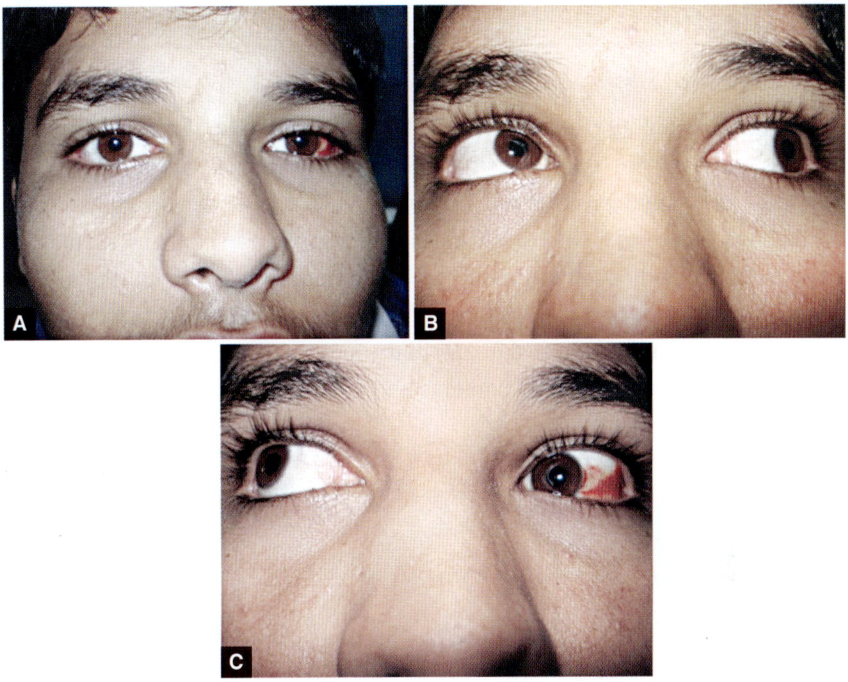

Figs 15.2A to C: A. 12-year-old boy with left orbital floor fracture showing restriction of ocular motility in dextroelevation

ENOPHTHALMOS/HYPOPHTHALMOS

Enophthalmos is due to increased orbital volume. Hypoglobus is seen in cases of large floor fracture where globe displaces downward in the orbit due to floor fracture or into the maxillary antrum (Figs 15.3A and B).

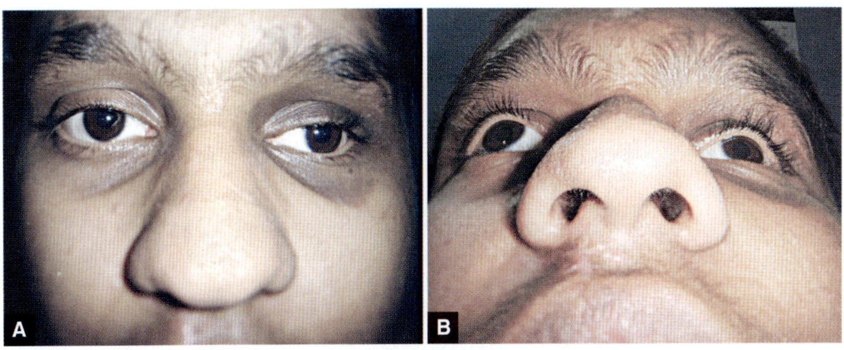

Figs 15.3A and B: 16-year-old boy with (A) enophthalmos LE and (B) hypophthalmos LE

Investigations

X-RAYS

X-ray has limited usefulness due to lack of ability to detect differences of less than 10% in tissue densities. However, Caldwell and Water's view are commonly used projections. Caldwell view allows the visualization of orbital rim, floor and sinuses. A classical 'trap door' sign was earlier the only modality indicative of tissue incarceration in fracture of the orbital floor. Water's view provides more information as X-ray trajectory places the petrous pyramid below the maxillary sinus, allowing visualization of orbital floor, prolapsed orbital contents and air-fluid levels in maxillary sinus (Fig. 15.4).

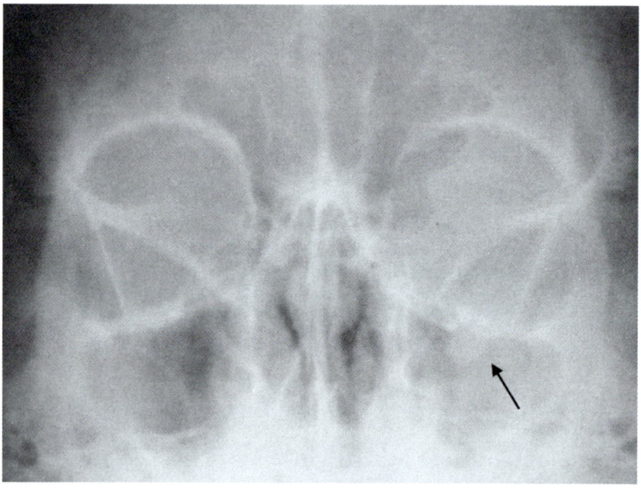

Fig. 15.4: Water's view showing hanging drop sign in left orbital floor

COMPUTED TOMOGRAPHY (CT SCAN)

CT scan has become the gold standard modality for evaluation of orbital fractures.[7] CT scan without contrast provides views of high-density bone. Both axial and coronal 1.5 to 2.0 mm cuts should be ordered to properly evaluate the orbit and the floor (Fig. 15.5). It has the advantage of delineating soft tissue of eye, orbit and adnexae. A 3-dimensional scan provides more detailed evaluation (Fig. 15.6).

MAGNETIC RESONANCE IMAGING (MRI)

MRI scan is not the first line diagnostic modality. However, it can be done in cases of suspected intracranial injuries or optic nerve pathology.[8]

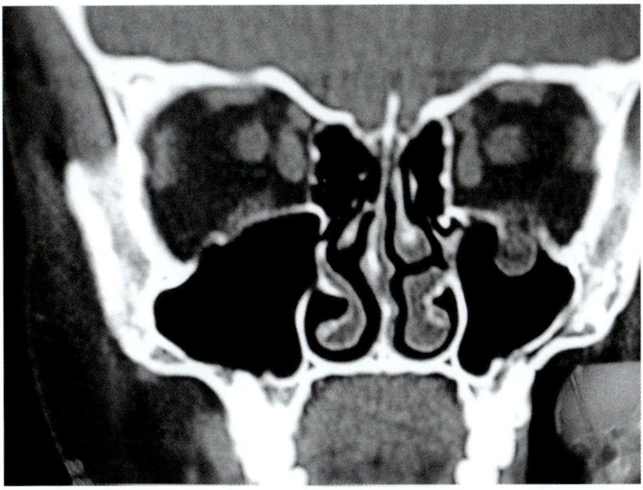

Fig. 15.5: CT scan showing fracture in left orbital floor with incarceration of the orbital contents

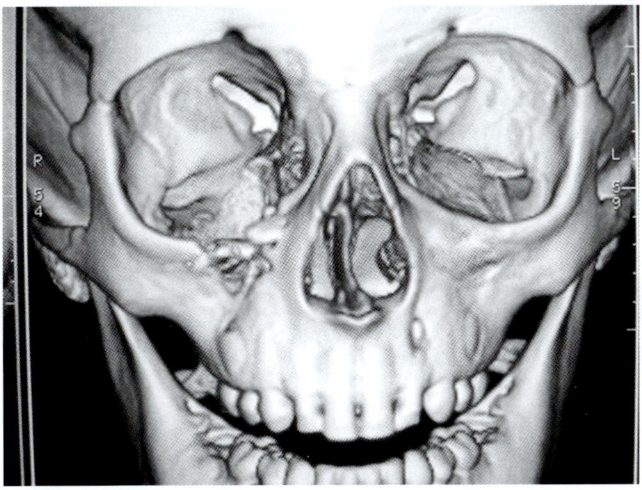

Fig. 15.6: 3D CT scan showing the right orbital floor fracture

Indications of Repair

Indications and timing of repair of orbital fractures are debatable. Not all fractures need to be repaired. Whenever in doubt, the patient must be revaluated every 2–3 days during the first 2 weeks. Orbital hemorrhage and edema will resolve rapidly over the first week. CT has become a widely accepted and reliable adjunct to help determine the need for early surgical intervention.

Currently, the indications for the repair of the fracture of orbit have been divided into three groups: immediate repair, repair within 2 weeks and observation.[9]

Immediate Repair

1. Nonresolving oculocardiac reflex with entrapment causing nausea, vomiting, syncope, bradycardia, and heart block.
2. Early enophthalmos or hypoglobus causing facial asymmetry
3. 'White-eyed'floor fracture with entrapment

Repair Within 2 Weeks

1. Symptomatic diplopia with positive forced duction test
2. Large floor fracture causing enophthalmos
3. Significant hypoglobus
4. Progressive infraorbital hypoanesthesia

Observation

1. Minimal diplopia but not present in the primary gaze
2. Good ocular motility
3. No significant enophthalmos
4. No significant hypoglobus

Surgical Management

The surgical approach is same, whether performed immediately or within 2 weeks.The repair done during the first two weeks offers good chances of recovery for the restoration of ocular motility. Beyond this period, adhesions between bone fragments and orbital soft tissue may develop and render the repair more difficult. A residual diplopia may persist because of the fibrotic changes.

Preoperative Management

In the preoperative phase, the patient is advised to avoid blowing the nose to prevent orbital emphysema. Prophylactic antibiotic, antihistaminic and decongestantare prescribed. Some surgeons advocate initial high dose steroids to reduce inflammation. During the preoperative phase an estimation of extent of the fracture as well as of enophthalmos helps the surgeon to plan the shape and size of the implant to correct the deformity.

Surgical Approaches

The orbital floor can be repaired through following 3 approaches:

1. Transconjunctival incision
2. Transcutaneous-subciliary or over the inferior orbital rim incision
3. Caldwell-Luc approach.

The transconjunctival incision approach is most preferred one, however, due to lack of access it is combined with lateral canthotomy and cantholysis (swinging eyelid approach).[10] Some surgeons prefer subciliary transcutaneous incision. The only drawback of this approach is that postoperatively patients may develop ectropion or inferior scleral show.

Anesthesia

Surgery can be performed under general anesthesia or local anesthesia with sedation. Local anesthetic 2% xylocaine with adrenaline 1:100000 with 0.5% bupivacaine is infiltrated along the inferior orbital rim and lateral canthus.

TRANSCONJUNCTIVAL APPROACH—SWINGING EYELID APPROACH

Three traction sutures are placed with 4'0 silk sutures in the lower eyelid (Fig.15.7A). A bridle suture is also passed through the inferior rectus muscle, to assess the muscle. It also helps in rotating the globe upwards intraoperatively. A forced duction test is performed before commencing the surgery to assess mechanical restriction (Fig.15.7B). A subtarsal or inferior fornix incision is given which is combined with lateral canthotomy and inferior cantholysis. This detaches the lid from the lateral orbital rim and facilitates exposure. Subcutaneous dissection is carried out till the inferior orbital rim is exposed. The orbital septum is maintained intact to avoid prolapse of orbital fat and prevent postoperative eyelid retraction.

Periosteum is incised about 2 mm below the inferior orbital rim (Fig.15.7C). It is then elevated with periosteal elevator lifting the periorbita as well. The fracture site is exposed (Fig.15.7D). Majority of the orbital floor fractures involve the posteromedial aspect of the floor, which is adjacent to infraorbital canal. All margins of the floor fracture should be exposed. The prolapsed contents are repositioned into the orbit by making them free by hand-over-hand technique. However, one should avoid aggressive dissection posteriorly as it may risk damage to the optic nerve and other orbital apical structures.

Once the prolapsed contents are released, forced duction test is performed to assess that all entrapment has been released. An implant is placed over

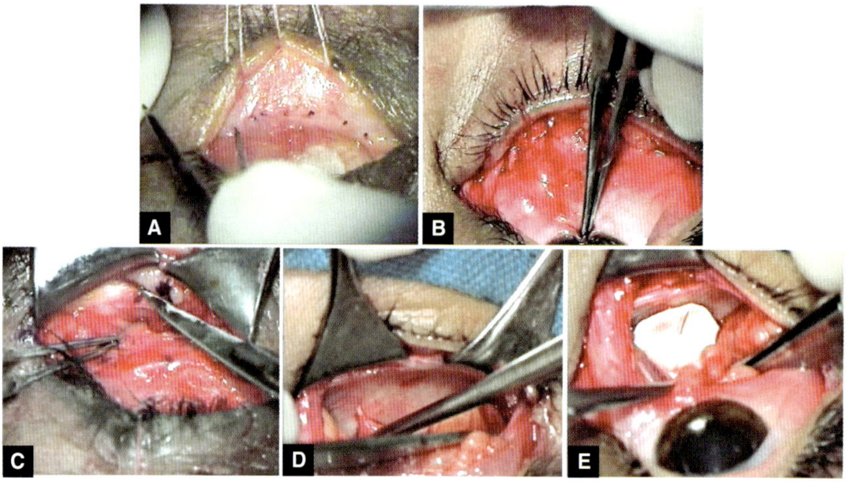

Figs 15.7A to E: (A) Showing marking for transconjunctival incision. (B) Forced duction test being performed to assess restriction. (C) Periosteum is incised 2 mm below the inferior orbital margin. (D) Periorbita lifted up, fracture site exposed and incarcerated contents released. (E) ePTFE implant placed over the fracture site

the fracture site (Fig. 15.7E) ensuring that all margins are covered and that no tissue is herniating into the sinus. The forced duction test is repeated again to ensure that no tissue is entrapped below the implant.

The implant should be of an adequate size and shape to fulfill this objective. The implant should not be more than 20–22 mm anteroposteriorly, to avoid compression of apical structures. The fixation of the implant is not necessary. However, one can make a tongue of the implant which can be engaged in the orbital rim and thus provides good support.

In case, orbital rim is fractured, microplating of the orbital rim can be performed prior to placement of an implant (Fig. 15.8).

The edges of the periosteum may or may not be closed with 5'0 vicryl sutures. After closure of the subcutaneous tissue and conjunctiva with 5'0 vicryl, the lateral canthal tendon is reattached. The marginal skin sutures and skin sutures for closure of lateral canthotomy are applied with 6'0 nylon or 6'0 silk suture.

A four-year-old boy sustained injury and developed marked restriction of ocular motility in levoelevation due to small fracture of orbit (Figs. 15.9A to C). Coronal cut section revealed a small fracture of left orbit with incarceration of orbital content (Figs 15.9D and E).

He was operated by transconjunctival approach and incarceration of orbital tissue was released. The postoperatively the child's appearance in the primary position is improved and the ocular movements are restored to almost normal (Figs 15.10A to D).

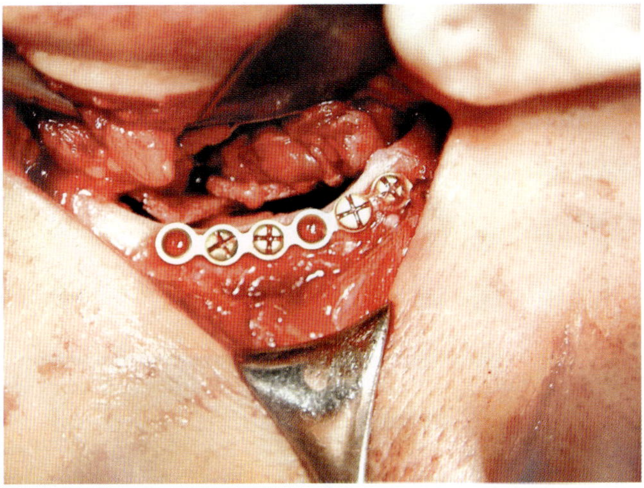

Fig. 15.8: Showing microplating of inferior orbital rim through the wound

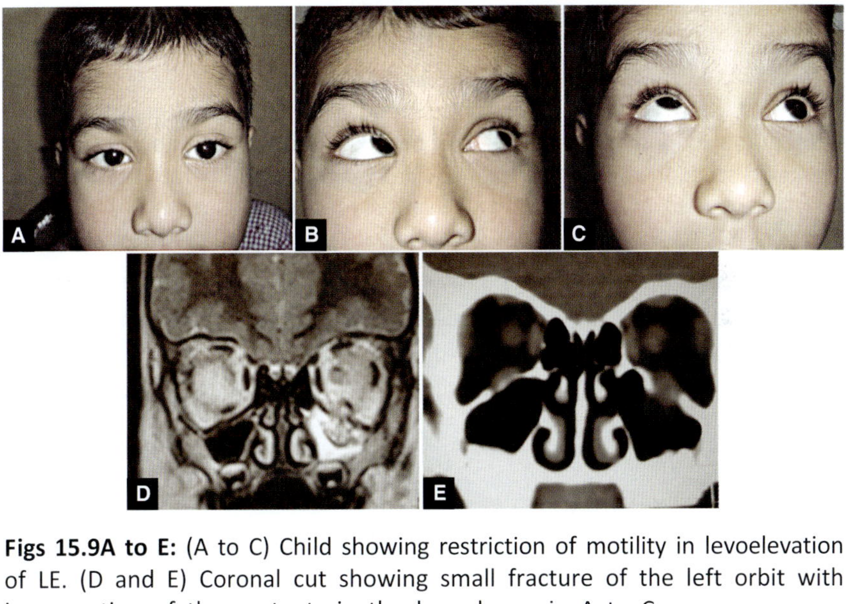

Figs 15.9A to E: (A to C) Child showing restriction of motility in levoelevation of LE. (D and E) Coronal cut showing small fracture of the left orbit with incarceration of the contents in the boy shown in A to C

TRANSCUTANEOUS APPROACH

The subciliary incision is preferred. The orbital rim incision is not commonly used as it leads to scarring and is associated with postoperative eyelid lymphedema. Traction sutures are passed through the lower lid. These are used to keep lower eyelid under tension and assist in dissection. The

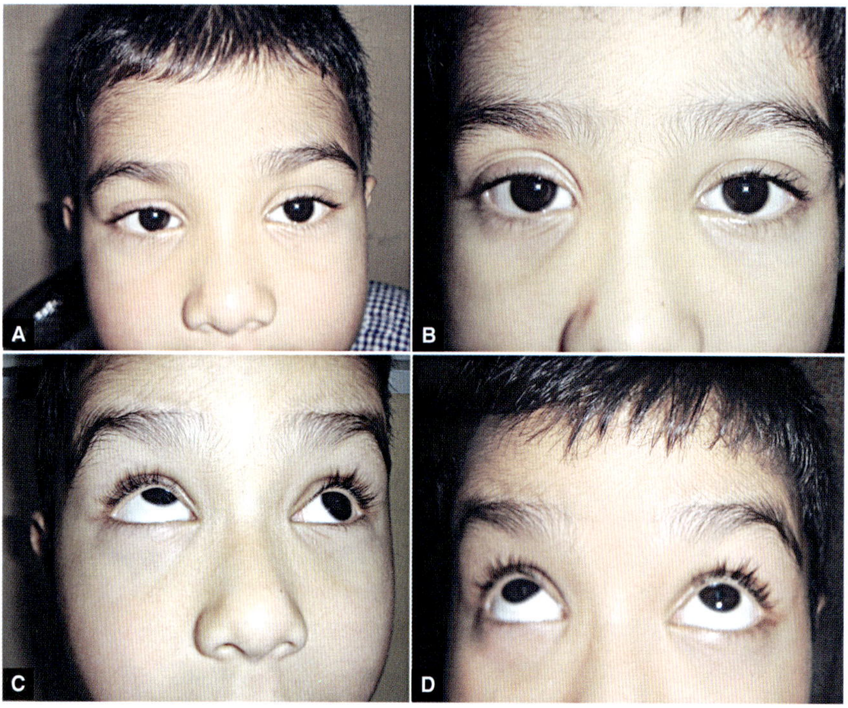

Figs 15.10A to D: (A) Preoperative photograph in primary gaze. (B) Postoperative photograph in primary gaze. (C) Preoperative photograph showing showing marked restriction of elevation LE in upward gaze. (D) Postoperative photograph showing marked improvement in elevation in upward gaze

skin is incised just below the lashes (Fig. 15.11A). Dissection is carried out between the skin and the orbicularis muscle till the orbital rim is reached (Fig. 15.11B). The orbicularis and the periosteum are incised about 2 mm beyond the orbital rim (Fig. 15.11C). The dissection then proceeds as described above (Figs 15.11D to G).

CALDWELL-LUC APPROACH

This approach is rarely used. In this an opening is made into maxillary sinus in the area of the superior gingiva.

Orbital Implant Materials

There is no consensus on the material that should be used in the reconstruction of the orbit. Both biological (autologous/homologous) and alloplastic materials have been used, each having its advantages and disadvantages.[11-14]

The characteristics of an ideal alloplastic implant material are that it is readily sized during surgery, and sterilizable. It should have adequate

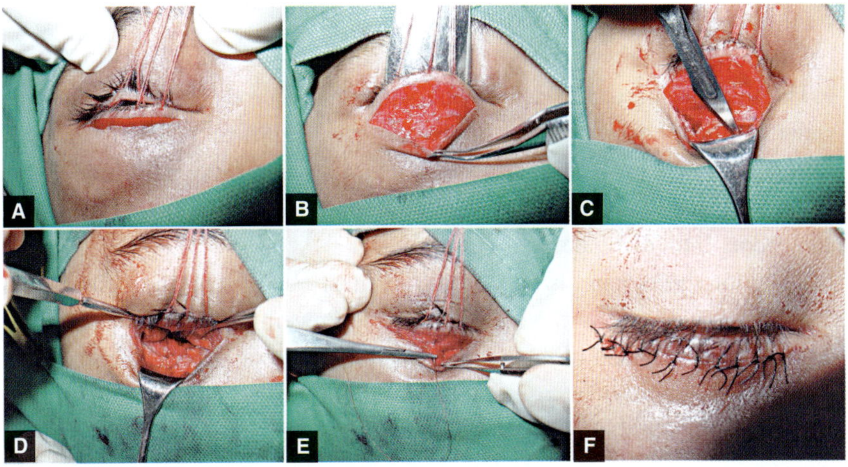

Figs 15.11A to G: (A) Subciliary incision given. (B) Dissection between skin and orbicularis till the orbital rim is reached. (C) Periosteum is incised 2 mm to the orbital rim. (D) Orbital contents being lifted. (E) ePTFE implant being placed overbridging the fracture site. (F) Subcutaneous closure being done with 5'0 vicryl. (G) Skin closure with 6'0 silk

strength and possess physical, chemical and biological inertness. It must be durable, noncarcinogenic, stable, easily manipulable and allows single stage reconstruction.

The biological materials available for reconstruction include: bone graft from the iliac crest and ribs, autogenous or banked fascia lata, irradiated coastal cartilage and calvarium. The advantages of autogenous materials are their incorporation into the tissues with no extrusion and less postoperative discomfort.

The disadvantages are that a separate surgical incision is necessary, and assistance from an orthopedic or plastic surgeon may be required. They may show unpredictable resorption and cause deformities due to scarring.

Alloplastic materials include both absorbable and unabsorbable materials. Absorbable materials are:

1. Polymerized polyactide
2. Gelatin film
3. Polyglactin mesh

Unabsorbable materials are:

1. Expanded polytetrafuoro-ethylene (e-PTFE)
2. Silastic implants
3. Teflon implants
4. Metallic alloys
5. Hydroxyapatite

6. Porous polyethylene (Medpore)
7. Titanium sheets.

The material used is based on the surgeon's choice and on whether the ocular motility or enophthalmos can be corrected significantly with it. Initially, silastic implants or Teflon plates were used. They were stiff, thick, less pliable and lead to complications like migration and extrusion, and therefore, have gone into disrepute.

Titanium sheets can also be used, but must be fixed to the surrounding stable bone with screws. A new device has recently become available, a titanium sheet covered on both sides by thin sheets of porous polyethylene. The new design provides a smooth surface on both the superior and inferior aspects of the implant, and when cut, hides the sharp edges of the cut titanium, eliminating the need to burr down the edges.

Nowadays, our preferred choice is porous polyethyelene (medpore) or e-PTFE implants, as they are thin and get incorporated into the local tissues, and the incidence of migration is remarkably less. They have a decreased bacterial adherence because of the hydrophobic nature and show minimal encapsulation and inflammation.

Management of Late Sequelae

LATE PERSISTENT DIPLOPIA

Late persistent diplopia can be due to patient's refusal for the primary surgery or in patients who were showing improvement initially in diplopia following trauma but did not show full resolution or as a result of inadequate release of entrapped muscle or adjacent orbital tissue or paresis of inferior rectus muscle. Putterman et al[15] recommended extraocular muscle surgery after stabilization of the ocular motility and diplopia measurement.

The most common ocular motility problem causing visual handicap in untreated blow-out fractures is double vision in down gaze. In these cases if eye moves upward normally and forced duction test is negative, reverse Knapp procedure is performed. In this procedure medial and lateral rectus muscles are placed at or several millimetres behind the inferior rectus insertion. If forced duction test is positive and eye does not move upward, an inferior rectus recession is performed.

LATE ENOPHTHALMOS

Late enophthalmos is often associated with downward sinking of the eyeball (hypophthalmos), narrowed palpebral aperture and supratarsal sulcus deformity.

For correction of enophthalmos, implants should be positioned behind the equator of the globe. Either silastic or cortical and cancellous bone taken from the crest may be used for correction of enophthalmos. An implant is placed in a subperiosteal pocket along the floor of the orbit through a subciliary or transconjunctival approach. Methog et al[16] prefer to carry out additional bone implantation in subperiosteal pockets along the posterior superolateral and medial walls of the orbit through two different incisions. The inferior pocket helps correct hypophthalmos, the superotemporal one helps in projecting the globe and the medial pocket offsets the medial projection caused by the superotemporal implant.

Injection of fat in retrorbital intramuscular cone[17] or free fat injection in the eyelid has provided promising results. Deep orbital sub-Q Rstalyne injection (non-animal stabilized hyaluronic acid) have also shown encouraging results.[18]

The cosmetic appearance of the patients with narrowed palpebral aperture may be significantly improved by Muller's muscle-conjunctival resection or Fasanella-Servat procedure. Patients with deep supratarsal sulcus are cosmetically benefitted by excision of skin and orbital fat with elevation of the contralateral upper lid crease to restore symmetry. The correction of enophthalmos is a difficult proposition and results of the surgery are often less than perfect.

Postoperative Complications

Postoperative complications can be minimized by good surgical technique. However, due to severe injuries or damage to adjacent soft tissue, complications do occur.[10] Some of the complications are:

1. Loss of vision
2. Persistence of ocular motility restriction and diplopia
3. Lower eyelid retraction
4. Infraorbital nerve damage
5. Persistence of enophthalmos
6. Symblepharon
7. Implant extrusion
8. Orbital infection.

LOSS OF VISION

Postoperative loss of vision or blindness is rare but dreaded complication. It may be caused by orbital hemorrhage or due to compression of the optic nerve by malpositioning or placement of a large implant. Adequate hemostasis should be achieved before closure. Patients' visual acuity should be monitored in the recovery-room in the early post operative period. The orbital implant should be of appropriate size and shape and should not be pushed posteriorly.

OCULAR MOTILITY RESTRICTION AND PERSISTENCE OF DIPLOPIA

Patients should be explained that diplopia may be worse in early postoperative period (Figs 15.12A to C). It usually resolves over a period of 4–6 weeks postoperatively. It is important to perform forced duction test after placement of the implant to assess any residual tissue entrapment as well as the motility of the globe.

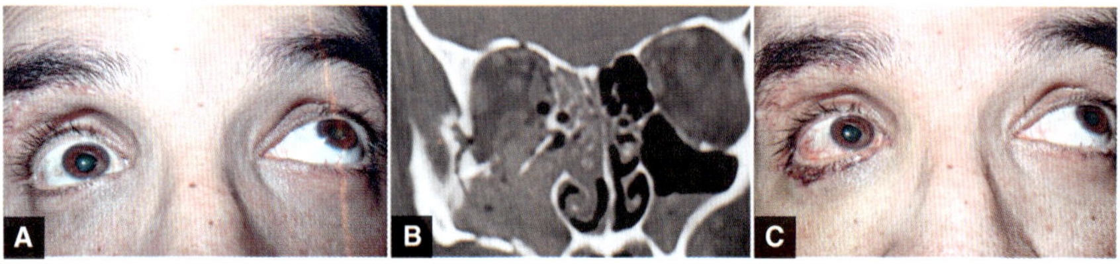

Figs 15.12A to C: (A) Showing enophthalmos RE with gross restriction of motility. (B) CT scan showing large fracture of the right orbital floor. (C) Showing restriction of motility in levoelevation

LOWER EYELID RETRACTION

Lower eyelid retraction is most commonly seen with subciliary incision. It is either due to incorrect closure of periosteum with inclusion of orbital septum within the sutures or due to adhesions of the orbital septum to the infraorbital rim. This can be prevented by meticulous dissection between the orbicularis and orbital septum and proper closure.

INFRAORBITAL NERVE DAMAGE

Patient should be explained prior to surgery about the potential for permanent sensory loss in the distribution of the infraorbital nerve or it may take several months for its recovery. However, care should be taken not to cause any trauma to inraorbital nerve intraoperatively.

PERSISTENCE OF ENOPHTHALMOS

Residual enophthalmos is either due to placement of smaller implant or of failure to treat medial wall fractures (Fig. 15.13). Enophthalmos may also occur due to delayed orbital fat atrophy. However, there is a gradual improvement in the cosmet appearance of the patiet (Fig. 15.14).

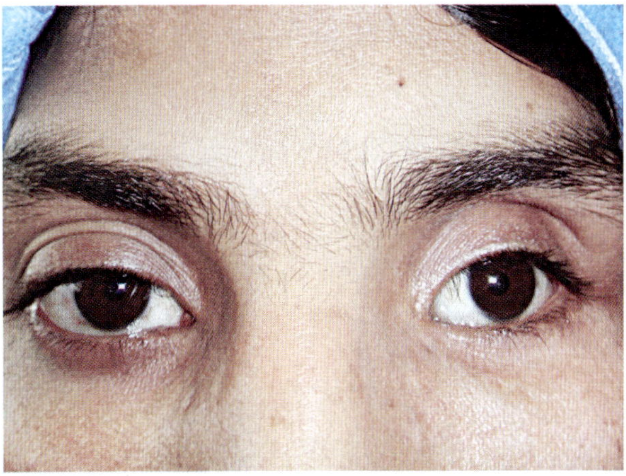

Fig. 15.13: Showing residual enophthalmos LE

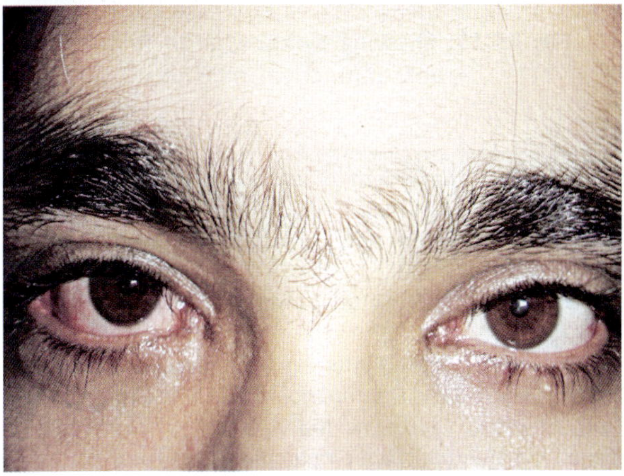

Fig. 15.14: Showing improvement in enophthalmos

SYMBLEPHARON

Symblepharon is seen following a transconjunctival incision, usually more common with forniceal incision than subtarsal incision (Fig. 15.15).

IMPLANT EXTRUSION

The extrusion of implant may occur either due to infection, oversized implant or inadequate closure of the periosteum to the inferior orbital rim.

ORBITAL INFECTION

Orbital infection is managed by intravenous antibiotics but may sometimes require explantation of the implant.

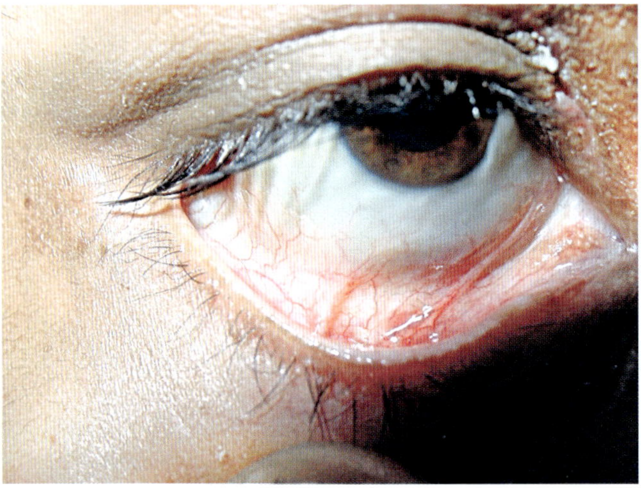

Fig. 15.15: Showing symblepharon following transconjunctival incision

References

1. Jonathan Dutton: Management of blow out fractures of the orbital floor. Surv Ophthalmol. 1991;35(4):279-98.
2. Smith B et al: Mechanism and correction of internal orbit fracture. *Am J Ophthalmol.* 1957;44:733-9.
3. Fujino T: Mechanism of orbital blow out fracture—Experimental study. *Orbit.* 1987;6:237-40.
4. Dutton JJ, Manson PN, Iliff N, Putterman AM: Management of blow-out fractures of the orbital floor. *Surv Ophthalmol.* 35:279,1990.
5. Rubin PAD, Bilyk JR, Shore JW: Management of orbital trauma: fractures, hemorrhage, and traumatic optic neuropathy. In: Focal Points, Vol XXI(7). San Francisco, American Academy of Ophthalmology, 1994.
6. Nunery WR: Diagnosis and management of blunt orbital trauma. In: Focal Points, Vol IV(11). San Francisco, American Academy of Ophthalmology, 1986.
7. Chu C, Young N,Soo M: Imaging of orbital floor fractures. *Australas Radiol.* 1996;40(3):264-8.
8. Ilankovan V,Hadley D, Moss K, et al. A comparison of imaging techniques with surgical experience in orbital injuries. A prospective study. *J Craniomaxillofac Surg.* 1991;19(8):348-52.
9. Burnstine MA. Clinical Recommendations for Repair of Isolated Orbital Floor Fractures. An Evidence- based Analysis. *Ophthalmology.* 2002;109:1207-10.
10. Westfall CT, Shore JW, Nunery WR, et al. Operative complications of the transconjunctival inferior fornix approach. *Ophthalmology.* 1991;98:1525.
11. Meyer DR. Orbital fractures. In: Tasman W, Jaeger EA, eds. *Duane's Clinical Ophthalmology*, Philadelphia, Pa: Lipincott-Raven;1996.
12. Meyer DR. Alloplastic materials for orbital surgery. *Curr Opin Ophthalmol.* 1995;6:43.
13. Johnson L et al: Experimental evaluation of expanded polytetrafluoroethylene for reconstruction of orbital floor defects. *J Oral Maxillfac Surg.* 1994;52: 1050-55.

14. Gupta AK, Grover AK, Kumar S et al: Silicone support in the management of fracture floor of orbit. Proceedings of the 47th Annual conference of the All India Ophthalmological Society, Madras, 1989;401-5.
15. Putterman AM, Smith BC: Blow out fractures. In Della Rocca RC, Nesi FA and Lisman, RD (eds) Ophthalmic plastic and Reconstructive surgery, St. Louis, CV Mosby vol. 1 1987;477-490.
16. Mathog RH: Traumatic enophthalmos. In Della Rocca RC, Nesi FA and Lisman, RD (eds) Ophthalmic plastic and Reconstructive surgery, St. Louis, CV Mosby vol. 1 1987;491-505.
17. Hunter PD, Baker SS.The Treatment of Enophthalmos by Orbital Injection of Fat Autograft. *Arch Otolaryngol Head Neck Surg.* 1994;120(8):835-9.
18. Malhotra Raman. Deep Orbital Sub-Q Restylane (Nonanimal Stabilized Hyaluronic Acid) for Orbital Volume Enhancement in Sighted and Anophthalmic Orbits. *Arch Ophthalmol.* 2007;125(12):1623-9.

16

chapter

Kalpana Narendran
Sandra C Ganesh

Restrictive Strabismus

ABSTRACT

Restrictive strabismus is often encountered in the ophthalmic clinical practice. The characteristic feature of restrictive strabismus is abnormal limitation of ocular motility. In this chapter etiology, classification, clinical features and diagnostic criteria of different types of ocular restriction and management are described.

Introduction

Restrictive strabismus should incorporate all strabismus caused by abnormal relationships between the orbital structures and the eye resulting in restriction of eye movements. Classically, the term ocular restriction describes a mechanical tether or a leash that limits ocular rotations.[1]

Etiology

The conditions that can result in restriction to eye movements include adhesions, a tight or inelastic extra-ocular muscle or an orbital mass. The causes for restrictive adhesions in turn would include scarring of the conjunctiva or Tenon's capsule, congenital fibrotic bands and orbital fat adherence. Inelastic or fibrosed muscle can be seen in thyroid myopathy, congenital fibrosis syndrome, inferior rectus muscle in monocular elevation deficit and local anesthesia myotoxicity. An orbital mass, such as tumors or glaucoma implants can cause restriction either directly or by pressure effect on extraocular muscle. Restriction can also occur due to misdirected muscle force vectors in conjunction with aberrant innervations of antagonistic muscle as seen in Duane's retraction syndrome. Sometimes restriction and muscle paresis can coexist as seen in long-standing lateral rectus paresis with secondary contracture of medial rectus muscle.[1]

Classification

Passive restriction seen in patients can be classified in 3 groups:

1. Relative restriction: It is seen in incipient muscle contracture.
2. Absolute restriction: It is often found in Brown's syndrome and orbital floor fracture.
3. Mixed restriction: It develops in long-standing cases of paralytic strabismus

Difference between Restriction and Paresis

Failure of ability of the eye to perform a duction fully can occur because of paresis of extraocular muscle and mechanical restriction or a combination of the two. The differences between the two conditions are presented in follow Flowchart 16.1.

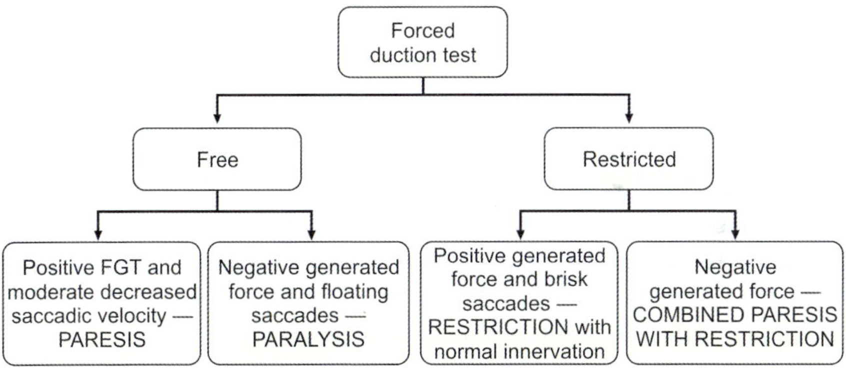

Flowchart 16.1: The difference between restriction and paresis

In addition to positive forced duction test and active force generation test, the other points which help differentiate between muscle paresis and restriction include rise of intraocular pressure when eye attempts to look in the field of limited movement and a brisk saccade which abruptly stops on reaching the area of restriction. A restriction also causes eyeball retraction and lid fissure narrowing as the agonist muscle pulls the eye backward against the restrictive leash.[1]

Specific Types of Restrictive Strabismus

THYROID OPHTHALMOPATHY

This is an autoimmune disease associated with inflammation of the extra ocular muscles and is seen more frequently in middle aged women. The natural course of the disease typically shows an *acute phase* during which there is lymphocytic infiltration of the extra ocular muscles resulting in muscle enlargement and proptosis. It is followed by a *cicatricial phase* with secondary muscle contracture resulting in the development of strabismus. The ocular myopathy does not necessarily reflect the state of thyroid activity. Inferior rectus and medial rectus muscles are most commonly affected. A restrictive hypotropia due to tight inferior rectus is the most commonly seen type of strabismus followed by esotropia with tight medial rectus.[2]

Management

The goal of surgery is to align eyes in the primary gaze and reading position with some increase in the range of rotation and diplopia-free field. The surgery is performed only after active phase has subsided and strabismus measurements have stabilized. Orbital decompression, if needed should be performed prior to strabismus surgery. Use of adjustable sutures is recommended because results are often unpredictable.[2,3]

Principles of Surgical Treatment

- Intraoperative forced duction test must be performed in every case
- Rectus muscle recession is the procedure of choice
- Care must be taken while hooking as well as while disinserting the tight inferior rectus to avoid perforating the sclera
- Conjunctival recession may be needed in long-standing cases to relieve the restriction.

Postoperative Complications

- **Late over correction**
  Late overcorrection has been reported in about 50% cases following inferior rectus recession. It may be due to stretched scar at the insertion site. The use of nonabsorbable suture seems to reduce this problem.
- **Lower lid retraction**
  The lower lid retraction (Fig. 16.1) occurs due to attachments between inferior rectus, inferior oblique and the lower lid retractors. Careful dissection of the muscle from its tarsal attachments can reduce this problem.[2]

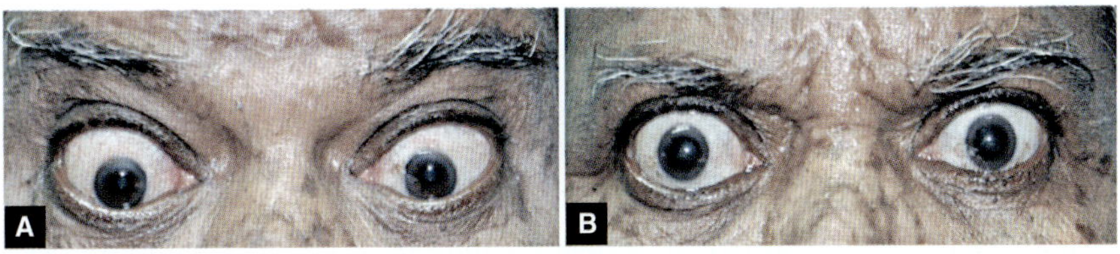

Figs 16.1A and B: (A) Preoperative appearance of a 60-year-old man with thyroid ophthalmopathy. He had severe restricted ocular motility with chin up. (B) Postoperative appearance of same patient after 7 mm recession of inferior rectus muscle on right and 6 mm position on the left. Note lower lid retraction in right eye

CONGENITAL FIBROSIS OF EXTRAOCULAR MUSCLES

Congenital fibrosis of extraocular muscles (CFEOM) is a predominantly autosomal dominant inherited condition characterized by generalized fibrosis of the extraocular muscles resulting in bilateral ptosis and external ophthalmoplegia. This condition has been classified by Harley and coworkers in following 5 groups:[2]

1. Generalized fibrosis
2. Fibrosis of inferior rectus with blepharoptosis
3. Strabismus fixus
4. Vertical retraction syndrome
5. Congenial unilateral fibrosis.

Clinical Features

The characteristic clinical features of congenital fibrosis of the extraocular muscles are:

- Blepharoptosis (Fig. 16.2) and chin elevation
- Absence of elevation or depression with eyes fixed 20 to 30 degrees below the horizontal line
- Little or no horizontal movement

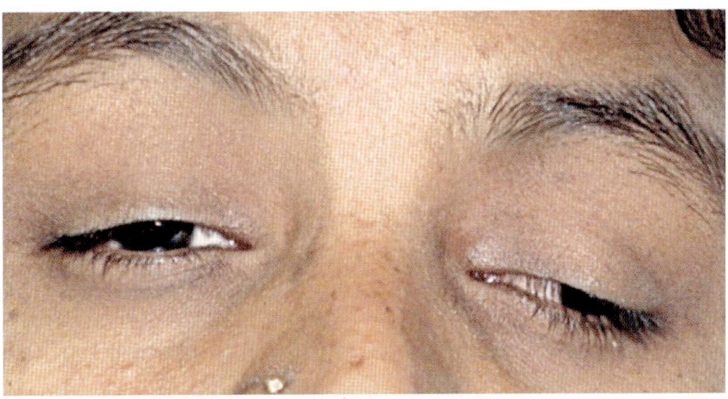

Fig. 16.2: Classical appearance of patient with congenital fibrosis syndrome

The diagnosis can be confirmed on histopathologic evidence of fibrosis of extraocular muscles.

Associated Ocular Findings

A number of congenital ocular anomalies may be associated with CFEOM. They include bilateral optic nerve hypoplasia, chorioretinal coloboma, microophthalmos, oculocutaneous albinism, globe retraction, Marcus Gunn-Jaw winking phenomenon, and enophthalmus.

Treatment

Nonsurgical: Optical correction of refractive errors and treatment of amblyopia must be done.

Surgical: Attempts should be made to obtain following surgical goals:
1. Alleviate chin up procedure
2. Align eye in primary position
3. Strabismus is corrected first followed by
4. Ptosis correction.

Procedure

Pre- and intraoperative forced duction test and a large recession or free tenotomy of the involved muscles should be performed. A conjunctival recession may be needed in some cases.

BROWN SYNDROME

Brown syndrome is also known as superior oblique sheath syndrome. The syndrome is characterized by bilateral ptosis with associated backward tilt of the head. There is marked restriction of the eye movements in the direction of the action of the superior oblique muscle. It may be associated with under action of the inferior oblique muscle.

Clinical Features

The limitation of elevation is maximal in adduction. The eye dips down on adduction and widening of palpebral fissure occurs. There is no or minimal superior oblique muscle action. However, near normal elevation is found in abduction (Fig. 16.3). Limitation of elevation is restrictive on forced duction test.

Occasionally, V pattern with XT may be seen in upward gaze. The patient may have head turn or chin-elevation to achieve fusion (Fig. 16.4).

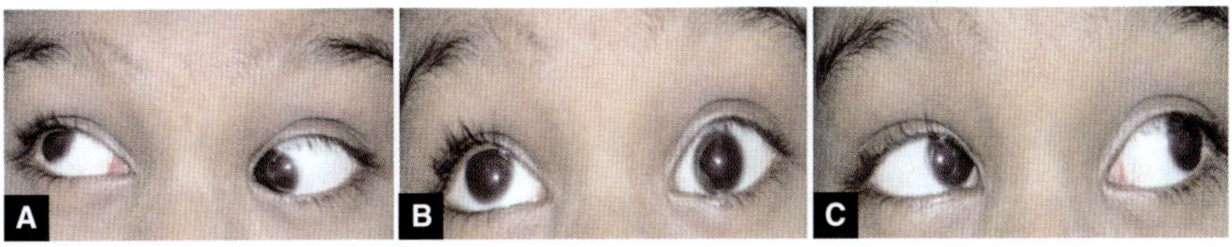

Figs 16.3A to C: (A) Limitation of elevation of left eye in adduction. (B) Normal in primary position. (C) Normal elevation in abduction

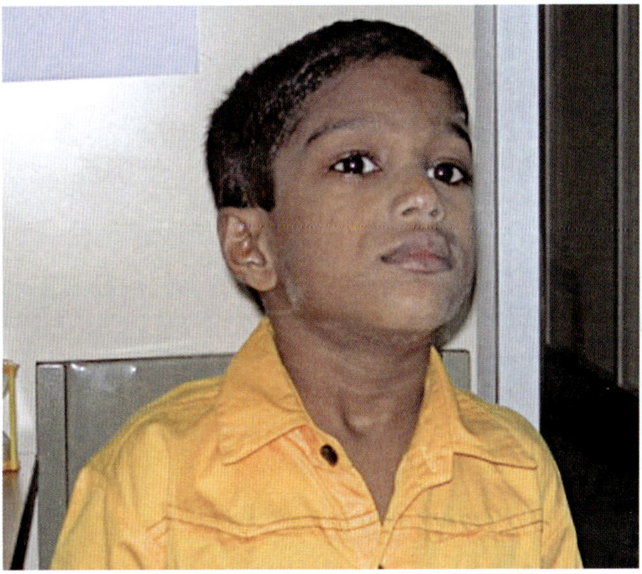

Fig. 16.4: A child with Browns syndrome is showing face turn and chin elevation

Etiology

Brown syndrome has an obscured etiology and affects both sexes equally. It can present in two forms: congenital or acquired.

Congenital Brown syndrome

Congenital Brown syndrome may occur due to:

- Sheath anomalies
- Short or inelastic tendon
- Trochlear or Tendon-trochlear-complex anomalies

Acquired Brown syndrome

Acquired Brown syndrome has multiple etiologies.

- Iatrogenic
  - Superior oblique surgery (e.g., Tuck)
  - Scleral buckling
  - Glaucoma valve surgery
  - Sinus surgery

- Infectious
  - Sinusitis
- Traumatic
  - Blunt trauma
  - Direct trauma
- Inflammatory
  - Rheumatoid arthritis
  - Systemic lupus erythomatosus
  - Sjögren's syndrome
  - Hurler-Scheie syndrome
  - Hypogammaglobulinemia
  - Graves' disease
  - Enteropathic arthropathy

Management

Spontaneous resolution has been reported in some cases of congenital Brown syndrome. It occurs more commonly in acquired cases. Surgery in patients with acquired or intermittent Brown syndrome should be avoided until the underlying disease has been controlled medically and the syndrome persists and meets the criteria as outlined below.

Indications for surgery are absolute or relative

Absolute indications

Severe and constant strabismus that may cause the loss of binocularity if not corrected is considered as an absolute indication.

Relative indications

Following conditions are relative indications of surgery:

- Hypotropia in primary position
- Cosmetically significant head posture
- Significant down shoot of the eye
- To expand the binocular diplopia-free fields.

Surgical techniques

1. Initially tenotomy and tenectomy of superior oblique tendon were the procedure of choice. This was done using a superonasal conjunctival approach, isolating the superior oblique tendon and cutting it in tenotomy or cutting a length of it in tenectomy.
2. To reduce the risk of iatrogenic superior oblique palsy (commonly encountered in free tenotomy), Wright introduced a controlled weakening procedure in which a segment of silicone band is sutured between the cut ends of the tenotomized muscle.[4]

3. Variations of the above includes tendon lengthening with fascia lata/ chicken suture
4. Z-tenotomy of superior oblique.[5]

DUANE'S RETRACTION SYNDROME

Duane's syndrome is a congenital form of strabismus characterized by horizontal eye movement limitation, globe retraction and palpebral fissure narrowing on attempted abduction (Fig. 16.5).

Etiology

Agenesis of the sixth cranial nerve with inferior division of the third cranial nerve splitting to innervate both the medical and lateral rectus muscles.

Huber's Classification

- Type I—limited adduction
- Type II—limited abduction
- Type III—both adduction and abduction restricted.

Associations

Duane's syndrome is often associated with other ocular and systemic anomalies. The ocular anomalies include heterochromia, iris dyspalsia, coloboma of iris and choroid, Marcus-Gunn phenomena, microphthalmos and morning glory syndrome.

Duane's syndrome may be associated with other syndromes or systemic abnormalities such as Goldenhar syndrome, Klippel Feil syndrome, Rubinston-Taybi syndrome, and Dandi-Walker syndrome. Sensory neural hearing loss may be found.

Indications for Surgery

Surgery is recommended in Duane's syndrome in following situations:
1. Significant head posture
2. Significant misalignment
3. Narrowing of palpebral fissure due to retraction
4. Significant up shoot or down shoot.

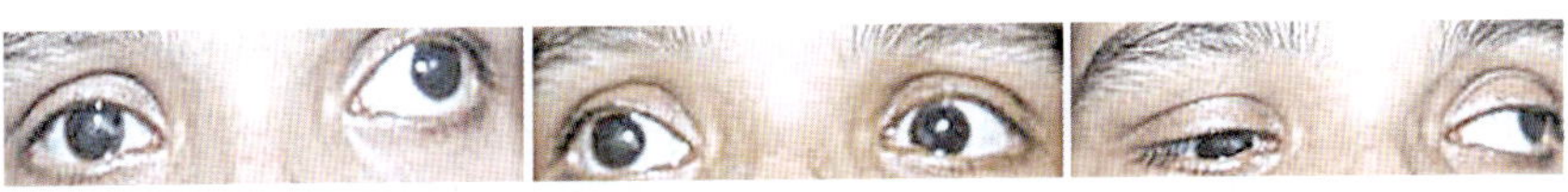

Fig. 16.5: Left exotropic Duane's with narrowing on adduction and widening on abduction

The efficacy of rectus transposition has been described in the surgery of the syndrome by Rosenbaum.[6] The surgical procedures for the correction of Duane's syndrome are diagrammatically presented in Figure 16.6.

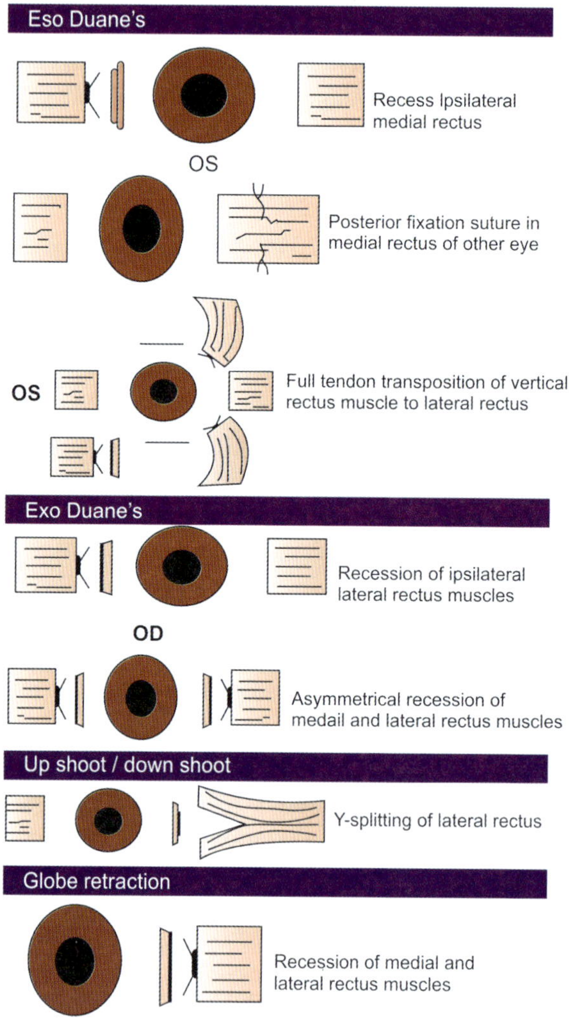

Fig. 16.6: Surgical procedures for the correction of Duane's syndrome

MONOCULAR ELEVATION DEFICIT SYNDROME

Patients with monocular elevation deficit syndrome (MED) present with hypotropia, chin elevation and ipsilateral ptosis. Studies using saccadic velocity measurements and forced ductions have shown that almost 70% of patients diagnosed with this syndrome have up gaze limitation due to a tight inferior rectus, and hence is included under restrictive strabismus. About 25% of cases have true ptosis (Fig. 16.7). The cause for the tight inferior rectus could be abnormal development of cranial nerves with secondary muscle fibrosis.

MANAGEMENT

Nonsurgical

Initially an optical correction of refractive errors and treatment of amblyopia are recommended. The surgical correction is indicated if there are significant hypotropia in primary position, and when deficit is associated with chin elevation.

Surgical Procedures

1. Tight inferior rectus muscle with good superior rectus function (primary IR restriction)
   Recession of ipsilateral inferior rectus (5 to 6 mm)
2. True double elevator palsy
   Knapps (full tendon) / split tendon transposition of medial and lateral rectus muscles to superior rectus
3. Secondary inferior rectus restriction
   Recession of ipsilateral inferior rectus (5 to 6 mm) with Knapps (full tendon) / split tendon transposition of medial and lateral rectus muscles to superior rectus

STRABISMUS FOLLOWING ORBITAL FRACTURE

Orbital fracture may occur at different sites but blow-out fracture is most common. Classification of orbital fracture is given below:

Classification

- Blow-out fracture
- Orbital floor fractures not associated with orbital rim fracture

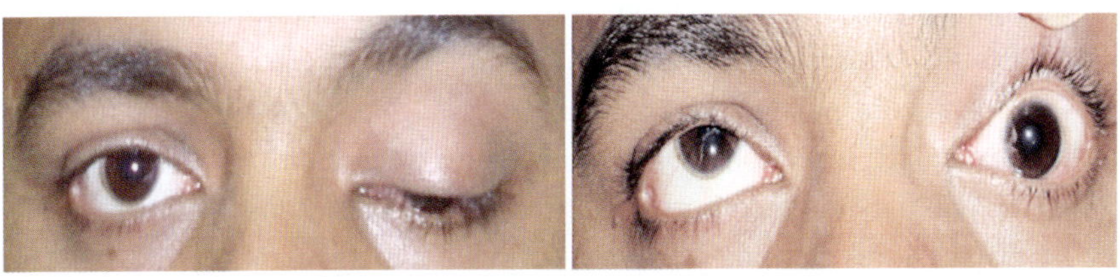

Fig. 16.7: Monocular elevation deficit syndrome left eye showing true ptosis and hypotropia and restriction of elevation

- Medial orbital wall fracture
- Lateral orbital wall fracture
- Orbital roof fractures (blow-in)

Clinical Features

The important clinical features of fracture of orbit are diplopia, enophthalmos, infraorbital nerve anesthesia and hypotropia with limited elevation or depression. The cause of ocular motility disturbance and diplopia following orbital trauma could be due to soft tissue swelling, muscle entrapment or nerve palsy.

Mechanisms of Strabismus following Orbital Fracture

- True entrapment of IR:
  If it occurs posterior to equator, causes depression restriction
  If it occurs anterior to equator it causes elevation restriction
- Entrapment of fibrous orbital septa: It results in movement restriction
- Injury to an extra ocular muscle or its innervations: It results in paresis without restriction.

Treatment of Strabismus

Strabismus surgery should be performed after reconstructive orbital surgery. If orbital surgery is not indicated and patient has persistent diplopia 4 to 8 weeks following injury, then strabismus surgery can be performed.

Conservative Management

- Keep the patient in observation; diplopia resolves in 76% patients without surgery
- Prisms may relieve diplopia
- Botulinum toxin can provide temporary relief.

Surgical Management

- Inferior rectus (IR) restriction with hypotropia: IR recession with (±) adjustable sutures
- Inferior rectus palsy:
  If partial: IR resection or superior rectus recession
  If IR palsy complete: horizontal rectus muscles transposition
- IR palsy + restriction: complex surgical management
- MR entrapment: as for isolated IR restriction.

Surgical plan can also be based on the presence of hypo or hypertropia in primary position.

- Tight inferior rectus muscle (hypo in primary position)
- Small angle-recession of ipsilateral IR
- Large angle - recession of ipsilateral IR + contralateral superior rectus recession
- Pseudoinferior rectus palsy (hyper in primary position)
- Placation of ipsilateral IR + contralateral IR recession.

STRABISMUS FOLLOWING RETINAL DETACHMENT SURGERY

Persistent strabismus occurs in approximately 7% of individuals following sclera buckling procedures. It may develop due to many factors.

Etiology

Mechanical factors

- Adhesions
- Buckle effect

Anatomical factor

- Nerve damage
- Macular ectopia or gliosis

Sensory factors

- Break down in fusion
- Sensory deprivation
- Anisokonia
- Anisometropia

Muscle factors

- Muscle ischemia
- Direct trauma
- Disinsertion
- Muscle slip/lost muscles/displaced muscle/split muscle.

Management

Nonsurgical

Observation of the patient, prescription of prisms and chemodenervation can provide relief.

Surgery

Before posting the patient for surgery following points should be taken into consideration:

1. FDT/FGT/saccadic velocity analysis
2. Type of deviation and muscles involved
3. Degree of scarring
4. Contribution of buckle/need for exoplant removal
5. Use of adjustable technique.

Surgical Approach

Intraoperative forced duction test allows one to gauge if the restriction has been adequately relieved. A limbal conjunctival incision is preferred for better exposure. Adhesions are meticulously released. Based on the preoperative evaluation, surgery is planned (e.g. suspect anterior displacement of superior oblique if there is hypertropia, limited down gaze and positive FDT for down gaze, as superior oblique now functions as an elevator). The insertion of the muscle in scar tissue around the buckle is taken as the effective insertion. Adjustable sutures may be used. Conjunctival recession can be done if significant restriction is present.

GLAUCOMA EXPLANTS AND STRABISMUS

Most commonly, strabismus following glaucoma explants is due to the formation of a larger conjunctival bleb. This can cause strabismus due to orbital mass displacing the eye, mass directly under a muscle or tendon and scarring and adhesions. Newer valve implants have reduced the size of the filtering blebs and hence produced the lowest incidence of strabismus.

Reducing the size of the bleb by suturing the bleb wall to the explants and replacing old explants with newer valve explants are effective.

MYOTOXIC EFFECT OF LOCAL ANESTHETIC

Any of the extraocular muscles can be infiltrated following retro- or peribulbar injection of local anesthetic agent. For example inferior rectus muscle can be infiltrated with anesthetic agent which results in a initial transient period of muscle paresis resulting in hypertropia followed by muscle fibrosis and restriction resulting in hypotropia. Treatment consists of recession of the tight or overacting muscle[7].

References

1. Wright KW, Spiegel PH. Pediatric Ophthalmology and Strabismus. 2nd ed, New York, 2003; pp 250-62.
2. Rosenbaum AL, Santiago AP. Clinical strabismus management Principles and Surgical Techniques. 1ST edi, WB Saunders;1999. pp 272-363 .
3. Pratt-Johnson A, Tillson G. Management of Strabismus and Amblyopia A Practical Guide . 2nd ed, New York, Thieme; 2001. pp 187-202.

4. Wright KW, Min BM, Park C. Comparison of superior oblique tendon expander to superior oblique tenotomy for the management of superior oblique overaction and Brown syndrome. 1992;29(2):92-7.
5. Ron Y, Snir M, Axer-Seigel R, Friling R. Z-tenotomy of the superior oblique tendon and horizontal rectus muscle surgery for A-pattern horizontal strabismus. *J AAPOS*. 2009;13(1):27-30.
6. Rosenbaum AL. Costenbader Lecture. The efficacy of rectus muscle transposition surgery in esotropic Duane syndrome and VI nerve palsy. *J AAPOS*. 2004;8(5):409-19.
7. Walimbe P. Step by Step Squint Surgery. 1st ed, New Delhi, Jaypee Brothers Medical Publishers, 2011; pp 143-67.

17

chapter

Alay Banker
Deepa Banker

HIV and Opportunistic Infections of Eye

ABSTRACT

Ocular manifestations can occur in about 50% of patients with acquired immune deficiency syndrome (AIDS), particularly if they are not on highly active antiretroviral therapy (HAART). They can lead to severe visual loss affecting the quality of life of the patient. Common lesions include relatively benign conditions, such as blepharitis and dry eye, to severe infections, such as herpes-zoster ophthalmicus and molluscum contagiosum, and malignancies like squamous cell carcinoma and Kaposi's sarcoma. The posterior segment manifestations include retinal vasculopathy, opportunistic infections, malignancies and neuro-ophthalmologic abnormalities, and CMV retinitis. Effective antiretroviral therapy and improved prophylaxis and treatment of opportunistic infections have led to an increase in the survival of individuals afflicted with AIDS and decrease in the occurrence of the opportunistic infections. Immune recovery uveitis is a new cause of vision loss in patients on HAART. Diagnosis and treatment are guided by associated conditions and immune status of the patient.

Introduction

Numerous ophthalmic manifestations of HIV infection may involve the anterior or posterior segment of the eye. Anterior segment findings include tumors of the periocular tissues and a variety of external infections. Posterior segment changes include an HIV-associated retinopathy and a number of opportunistic infections (OIs) of the retina and choroid. The increasing longevity of individuals with HIV disease may result in greater numbers of patients with opportunistic infections of the retina. Fortunately, many of these infections are now treatable with therapeutic agents. It is important to recognize these infections early so that an appropriate therapy can be instituted. Partial immune system recovery following initiation of effective antiretroviral therapy (ART) may modify clinical presentation of ophthalmic opportunistic infections and can affect response to treatment. In addition, in one eye, several infections may occur at the same time, rendering diagnosis and therapeutic intervention more difficult.

Due to the potentially devastating and rapid course of retinal opportunistic infections, all persons with HIV disease should undergo routine ophthalmologic evaluations. Any HIV-infected person who experiences ocular symptoms also should receive prompt and competent ophthalmologic care. In patients with early-stage HIV disease (CD4 count >300 cells/μL), ocular syndromes associated with immunosuppression are uncommon. Nonetheless, eye infections associated with sexually-transmitted diseases (STDs), such as herpes simplex virus, gonorrhea, and Chlamydia may be more frequent in HIV-infected persons; therefore, clinicians should screen patients for HIV in the presence of these infections.

It was estimated that by 2007, more than one million people were living with HIV infection in the United States, and an estimated 33.2 million people were infected with HIV worldwide.[1] Women all around the world now account for one quarter of HIV infections, and HIV disease disproportionately affects racial and ethnic minorities. Most HIV-infected individuals are in sub-Saharan Africa, but the number of new cases is increasing rapidly in other areas of the world, including India[1] and Southeast Asia. In the vast majority of cases worldwide, HIV transmission occurs through heterosexual contact. Infections attributed to perinatal transmission from mother to child and from transfusion of blood and blood products have dropped markedly.[2] There has also been a steady decline in new HIV/AIDS diagnoses among injection-drug users.[1]

In spite of the widespread use of highly active antiretroviral therapy (HAART), ocular manifestations of AIDS at some point affect 50–75% of infected patients.[2] Opportunistic infections develop when there is a deterioration of the immune status of the individual which can be measured with the help of CD4 cell counts. Posterior segment lesions, especially cytomegalovirus (CMV) retinitis, can be associated with severe visual morbidity. Corneal and anterior segment lesions affect more than 50% of all HIV patients.[3] Ocular adnexal complications, seen in about 25% of patients an be a sign of severe systemic immunosuppression.[3] Also, the spectrum of ocular manifestations of AIDS in the developing world differs from that of developed nations.[4]

Treatment of HIV infection with HAART seeks to inhibit progression to AIDS (defined by a CD4 cell count of <200 cells/mm^3) or death. This is achieved by reducing plasma HIV RNA to permanently low levels, reduction in the viral load and a rise in CD4 cell counts which help in improvement in the immune status of the individual.[2] With the advent of HAART, HIV and AIDS-related morbidity and mortality have drastically decreased in the developed world, but since more patients live longer and there are more HIV-positive patients, the overall population based prevalence would be expected to creep up. However, the situation in the developing countries is still grim even with advent of HAART. While the clinical immune recovery is, in general, of great benefit to the patient, about 10–25% of people initiated on HAART, experience "immune recovery" or immune reconstitution inflammatory problems, including those occurring in the eye leading to severe visual loss.

Goldberg et al showed that in the pre-HAART era, CMV retinitis was the most common HIV-associated retinopathy, occurring in 20–40% of patients and retinal detachment in 24–50% of patients annually. Herpetic retinopathy and toxoplasmosis retinochoroiditis were seen in 1–3% of patients and *Pneumocystis carinii* choroiditis, syphilitic retinitis, tuberculous choroiditis, cryptococcal choroiditis, and intraocular lymphoma were found infrequently. As compared to that, in the HAART era, there was 80% decline in the incidence of CMV retinitis. The incidence, visual morbidity, and mortality of CMV retinitis and other HIV-associated retinopathies have significantly decreased in the era of HAART.[5] A study from Croatia found that the mortality had decreased to 59.3%, vascular changes had reduced to 54.3% and incidence of CMV retinitis reduced from 57.2 to 7.6% from pre-HAART to post-HAART era.[6]

The chapter provides a comprehensive update of the ocular manifestations of the HIV-positive patients.

Ophthalmic Manifestations of AIDS

Ophthalmic manifestations of AIDS can be categorized under following 5 groups:

1. ***Opportunistic infections***
   i. Retina
      a. CMV retinitis
      b. Immune recovery uveitis: complication of treatment
      C. Other retinal infections by VZV, and *Toxoplasma gondii*
   ii. Choroid
      Choroiditis by fungi and mycobacteria—being most common
   iii. Ocular surface and adnexa
      Infection by varicella-zoster virus, microsporidia, molluscum contagiousum

2. ***Vascular abnormalities***
   i. Microvasculopathy
      HIV retinopathy—cotton-wool spots, retinal hemorrhages
   ii. Retinal arteriolar and venular occlusions (uncommon)
3. ***Neoplasia***
   i. Kaposi sarcoma (conjunctiva, eyelids)
   ii. Lymphoma (intraocular)
   iii. Squamous cell carcinoma (conjunctiva)
4. ***Other disorders of uncertain pathogenesis***
   i. Intraocular inflammation
      a. Chronic anterior uveitis (uncommon)
      b. Chronic multifocal retinal infiltrates (uncommon)
      c. Iatrogenic uveitis (drug related: cidofovir; rifabutin)
   ii. Blepharitis
   iii. Dry eye
5. ***Neuroophthalmic disorders associated with orbital or intracranial Diseases***

The spectrum of AIDS-related eye diseases differs in various parts of the world. Squamous cell carcinoma of the conjunctiva and ocular tuberculosis have been greater problems in Africa than CMV retinitis, attributed to the fact that patients die of other complications before reaching levels of immunodeficiency associated with CMV disease. During the early years of the epidemic in the United States, the prevalence of CMV retinitis increased as treatment of other life-threatening opportunistic infections improved, and patients survived longer. As was feared, the same phenomenon is now being seen in the developing world. As treatment for HIV-associated opportunistic infections and neoplasms improves worldwide, CMV retinitis may emerge as a global problem.

Cytomegalovirus retinitis

Cytomegalovirus retinitis is the most common AIDS-related ocular opportunistic infection and was found in about 40 to 50% of AIDS patients prior to HAART.[7,8] Although its incidence has declined markedly since the advent of HAART in the western world, it still remains the leading cause of ocular morbidity in the developing countries.[9] In India, CMV retinitis remains the most common ocular manifestation in patients with AIDS.[10,11] In our series of 2,356 cases, the incidence of CMV retinitis remains high even in the era of HAART. It was unilateral to start with, but eventually became bilateral in 52% of patients.[12]

Clinical Features

There are three clinical forms of CMV retinitis. The *classical form* (pizza pie retinopathy or cottage cheese with ketchup) is characterized by confluent retinal necrosis with hemorrhage that develops mostly in the posterior retina (Fig. 17.1A). The advancing edge of these lesions is usually very sharp and spreads contiguously. In contrast, the *indolent form* is recognized as a granular lesion in the peripheral retina, often with little or no hemorrhage. A third uncommon presentation is *frosted branch angitis*. Because approximately 15% of patients with active CMV retinitis are asymptomatic, routine screening with dilated indirect ophthalmoscopy has been recommended at three months intervals in patients with CD4+ counts less than 50 cells/μl.[13] Cytomegalovirus retinitis may result in either serous or rhegmatogenous retinal detachment, although the latter is much more common. The rhegmatogenous retinal detachment has been reported in 13–29% of patients with CMV retinitis and may occur during the active or healed phase of the disease. However, since the advent of HAART, incidence of retinal detachment has decreased by approximately 60–77% in the western world.[14] In contrast, the incidence of CMV-related retinal detachment was found to have increased in our series. It may be due to higher number of patients taking inappropriate HAART, and/or people taking HAART have larger areas of healed CMV retinitis which eventually develop necrotic holes leading to detachment.[15,16]

Treatment

Treatment of CMV retinitis is individualized and depends on the location of the active retinitis, and the immune status of the patient. Currently, available

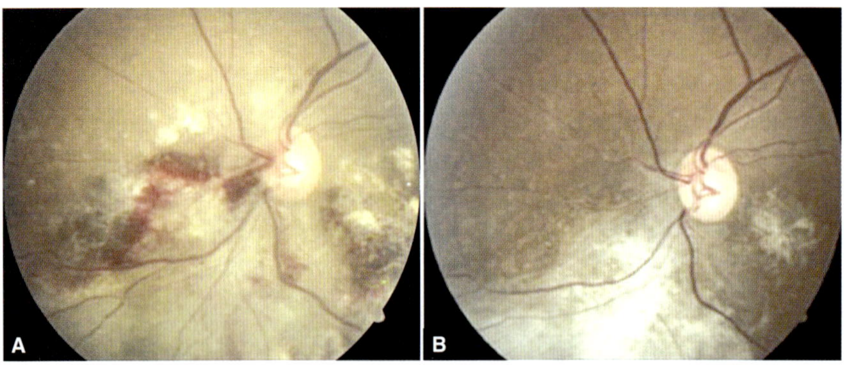

Figs 17.1A and B: (A) Active CMV retinitis and (B) Healed CMV retinitis after intravitreal cidofovir

anti-CMV agents include ganciclovir and its prodrug valganciclovir, foscarnet, cidofovir, fomivirsen, ganciclovir implant and oral valganciclovir. These drugs are listed in Table 17.1.

TABLE 17.1: Treatment for CMV retinitis

Medication	Route	Induction dose	Maintenance dose	Adverse effects
Ganciclovir	Intravenous	5 mg/kg bid for 2–3 weeks	5–10 mg/kg/day	Neutropenia, anemia, thrombocytopenia, liver toicity
	Oral	–	1 gm tid	Same as intravenous ganciclovir
	Intravitreal	400–2000 μg twice/week	400–2000 μg once/week	Vitreous hemorrhage, retinal detachment, endophthalmitis
	Intraocular sustained-release implant	4–6 mg pellet implanted through pars plana	Replaced every 6–8 months	Vitreous hemorrhage, retinal detachment, cataract, endophthalmitis, extraocular CMV, fellow-eye CMV, dislocated implants
Foscarnet	Intravenous	90 mg/kg bid for 2–3 weeks	90–120 mg/kg/d	Elevated creatinine, decreased Ca, Mg, K; tetany
	Intravitreal	2400 μg twice/week	2400 μg once/week	Vitreous hemorrhage, retinal detachment
Cidofovir	Intravenous	5 mg/kg weekly for 2 weeks	5 mg/kg every other week	Proteinuria, renal failure, neutropenia, uveitis
	Intravitreal	15 μg/0.1 ml	15 μg/0.1 ml every 6 weekly	Uveitis, ocular hypotony, vitreous hemorrhage, retinal detachment, IRU
Valganciclovir	Oral	900 mg bid for 3 weeks	900 mg/d	Neutropenia, anemia, thrombocytopenia
Fomivirsen	Intravitreal	330 μg on days 1 and 15	330 μg monthly	Vitreous hemorrhage, retinal detachment, endophthalmitis, iritis

INITIAL DRUG TREATMENT

The most important therapeutic maneuvre for the initial treatment of newly diagnosed CMV retinitis is to start HAART (for patients not taking antiretroviral drugs) or to reestablish immune recovery (for HAART-failure patients, by changing antiretroviral medications, if possible); however, it is a common practice among HIV specialists to delay the start of HAART for patients with systemic infectious diseases, such as tuberculosis, until treatments for the infections are started, to reduce the risk of systemic inflammatory reactions against the pathogens. The same may be true for reducing the risk of immune recovery uveitis. After the start of HAART, immune recovery is not achieved immediately; therefore, anti-CMV drugs should be given until certain immunologic (and possibly virologic) parameters are achieved. The induction treatment should be continued until CMV retinitis is inactive, to limit the size of lesions (Fig. 17.1B). Doing so presumably reduces the risk of retinal detachment and vision loss in individuals who have the prospect of prolonged survival.

DISCONTINUATION OF ANTICYTOMEGALOVIRUS TREATMENT

Immune recovery allows eventual discontinuation of specific anti-CMV therapy without reactivation of infection. A decision to discontinue anti-CMV drugs usually is based on several factors: a sustained rise in CD4+ T-lymphocyte count; a drop in HIV blood level; duration of HAART that is sufficient to affect immune recovery; and inactivity of CMV retinitis lesions. Patients receiving HAART should have CD4+T-lymphocyte counts of more than 100–150 cells/μl for three to six months.[17] Moreover HIV blood levels should have dropped by 2 log10 units, to fewer than 200 copies/ml. HIV blood levels can be a useful marker for eventual reactivation.

Monitoring Patients

CMV retinitis eventually can reactivate after anti-CMV drugs are stopped. The risk of recurrence is approximately, 0.02 events per year. Thus, continued monitoring of patients is critical. CD4+T-lymphocyte count is the laboratory measure followed most commonly, but a rising or very high HIV blood level may be an additional important indicator of risk for new CMV retinitis lesions or reactivation of the disease after discontinuation of anti-CMV drugs.

Screening Strategies

Serial ophthalmic examinations and patient education about symptoms of CMV retinitis are additional components of effective monitoring programs. Periodic screening examinations of patients with CMV retinitis for reactivation (and of people at risk for new disease) is a well-accepted practice, although there is little evidence to support the common recommendation that examinations can be performed at three-month intervals. The percentage of asymptomatic patients seems to be higher among those who are experienced with HAART, possibly because of reduced disease activity; this observation highlights the need for screening programs. Because the incidence of CMV retinitis is decreased, screening will need to be targeted to those at greatest risk, and because the infection can occur in patients with good parameters on current laboratory tests, better markers of impaired CMV immunity are needed.

NECROTIZING HERPETIC RETINOPATHY

Necrotizing herpetic retinopathy (NHR) is a continuous spectrum of posterior segment inflammation induced by herpes viruses, most commonly varicella zoster virus (VZV). Its two most recognizable clinical patterns are ARN and PORN.[18] The former usually occurs in healthy persons and AIDS patients with only mild immune dysfunction and elevated CD4+ counts, whereas the latter usually develops in those who are severely immunosuppressed. In addition to varicella zoster virus, herpes simplex virus and CMV have been isolated in patients with ARN, and herpes simplex in eyes with PORN.[11] The differential features between ARN, PORN and CMV retinitis are given in Table 17.2.

TOXOPLASMOSIS

In the majority of AIDS cases, toxoplasmosis is a primary infection rather than a reactivation. Ocular toxoplasmosis in AIDS, in contrast to toxoplasmosis in immunocompetent individuals, can be bilateral, multifocal, and not

TABLE 17.2: Differentiating features of viral retinitis in AIDS patients

Features	ARN	PORN	CMV retinitis
Immune status	Immunocompetent	Immunosuppressed	Immunosuppressed
Laterality	Unilateral/bilateral	Bilateral	Unilateral/bilateral
Visual loss	Severe	Early loss of vision	Variable
Anterior segment	Mild-moderate anterior uveitis	Nonganulomatous uveitis	Usually normal
Vitreous reaction	Significant vitritis	Minimum/no vitritis	Minimum/no vitritis
Retinal involvement	Full thickness	Deep retinal involvement	Full thickness with granular border
Vasculitis	Common	Uncommon	Seen
Retinal hemorrhage	Common	Uncommon	Common
Retinal detachment	Common	Common	Less common
Progression	Rapid	Rapid	Slow

associated with chorioretinal scars. It may cause a variety of ocular abnormalities including iritis, vitritis, choroiditis, multifocal or diffuse necrotizing retinitis, papillitis or retrobulbar neuritis, or outer retinal toxoplasmosis.[19] *Toxoplasma* retinitis may resemble CMV retinitis; however, intraocular inflammation is usually more severe and hemorrhages are fewer (Fig. 17.2). Treatment with standard antiparasitic drugs (pyrimethamine, clindamycin, sulfonamides) is successful in controlling ocular toxoplasmosis in most cases. Recently, intravitreal clindamycin has also been used effectively to treat active toxoplasmic retinochoroiditis.

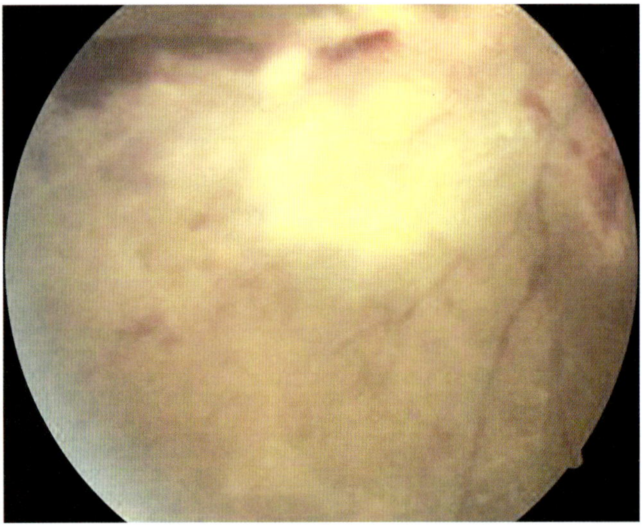

Fig. 17.2: Toxoplasmosis infections (resembling CMV retinitis)

Choroiditis

PNEUMOCYSTIS

Ocular manifestations of *P. carinii* include conjunctivitis, orbital mass, optic neuropathy, and choroiditis.[20] It is seen as classically bilateral and multifocal yellowish, well-demarcated, choroidal lesions located in the posterior pole not associated with vitritis, iritis, or vasculitis.[21] Ocular lesions respond in most cases to induction and subsequent maintenance treatment with systemic pentamidine, trimethoprim and sulfamethoxazole, or dapsone.

MYCOBACTERIAL DISEASE

Tuberculosis (TB) implies the presence of active disease from infection with the acid-fast bacillus.[22] *Mycobacterium tuberculosis* is the most common systemic opportunistic infection associated with AIDS even though ocular TB is not as common.[23]It is important to consider it as a differential diagnosis, especially in developing countries like India.

Clinical Features

Clinical manifestations include ulcers, tubercles, granular masses or pedunculated polypoid tumours. Patients may present with localized nodule in the eyelid simulating chalazion. Orbital and lacrimal gland involvement by *M. tuberculosis* leads to localized granuloma though they can present as a conjunctival mass. Infection of the iris can present either with or without iris nodules. TB is also a known cause of uveitis, although it is uncommon, even among those with systemic TB.[24] TB may cause interstitial keratitis with stromal infiltration. Interstitial keratitis secondary to TB is associated with uveitis. It may occur as an isolated finding or in association with scleritis. Sclerokeratitis can be seen with peripheral stromal inflammation in a triangular fashion associated with localized scleritis. Localized lesions are focal elevated nodules of the sclera that may undergo necrosis leading to scleromalacia and scleral perforation if untreated. Diffuse scleritis is less common than localized nodular scleritis. *M. tuberculosis* infection of the conjunctiva may involve the palpebral, bulbar, or forniceal conjunctiva. Tuberculous conjunctivitis is a very rare condition in the developed world. In recalcitrant cases of chronic red eye,[25] a definitive diagnosis requires the identification of *M. tuberculosis* organisms in conjunctival biopsy specimens, either through microscopic detection of acid-fast bacilli or through more sensitive culture techniques. Keratoconjunctivitis may occur in

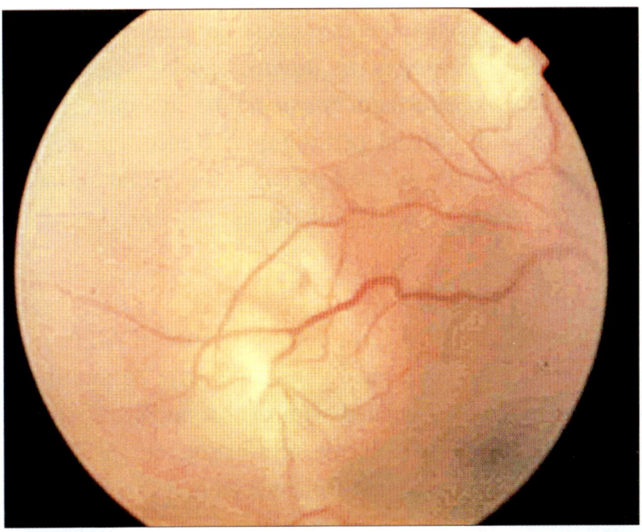

Fig. 17.3: Ocular tuberculosis with multiple tubercles

association with cutaneous TB.[26] While the intraocular disease is mostly a secondary infection, the cutaneous TB is almost always primary.[27] Commonest posterior segment manifestations include discrete choroidal tubercles (Fig. 17.3) or solitary mass-like lesion at the posterior pole. Rarely, endogenous endophthalmitis may occur.

Treatment

Systemic antituberculous therapy (ATT) with drugs such as isoniazid, rifampin, pyrazinamide and ethambutol is important as pulmonary or other foci of disease may coexist. Modified DOTS regimen (Directly Observed Treatment Short course) is the recommended regime in India. Specific ocular treatment should be instituted along with ATT. There have been reports of scleral TB responding favorably to additional topical drops (every 2 hourly) and subconjunctival injections (every three days) streptomycin sulfate along with ATT with healing of the lesion. In individuals with HIV infection, therapy may require longer duration and additional drugs. Newer drugs have also been incorporated in the ATT group of drugs, especially in the newer setting of multidrug-resistant TB, particularly in case of HIV-infected individuals.[3] These include quinolones, newer rifamycins like rifabutin and macrolides antibiotics.

FUNGAL INFECTIONS

In the general population, fungal corneal ulcers are rare in the absence of preceding trauma, ocular surface disease or corticosteroid therapy while HIV/AIDS patients can develop spontaneous fungal infections. Candida causes anterior segment keratitis. Cryptococci commonly triggers posterior segment pathology although they can sometimes cause conjunctivitis, limbal infection and iris granulomas.[2,8] *Cryptococcus albidus* causing scleral ulceration has been reported.[29] *Histoplasma* and *Pneumocystis* are more likely to result in bilateral disease with corneal perforation.[30] Hence, culture or biopsy of lesions is important for HIV-infected patients with ocular surface infections, to differentiate between bacterial and fungal etiology.

Cryptococcus

Cryptococcus meningitis is the most common cause of AIDS-related neuro-ophthalmolgic lesions. Cryptococcal choroiditis may be multifocal, solitary, or confluent and may be associated with eyelid nodule, conjunctival mass, granulomatous iritis, iris nodule, vitritis, necrotizing retinitis, endophthalmitis, and optic neuritis.[28] Fluconazole maintenance therapy 200 mg/day is currently recommended in all patients even in the era of HAART.

SPIROCHAETAL INFECTIONS

Treponema Pallidum

Ocular syphilis caused by *Treponema pallidum* tends to present with more aggressive, severe and relapsing manifestations in HIV-positive hosts as compared with immunocompetent hosts.[32-34] All patients with syphilis should be evaluated for HIV and *vice versa*. Anterior segment manifestations of syphilis include chancres of the conjunctiva (primary syphilis), conjunctivitis (secondary syphilis) and gummata (late syphilis).[32] Conjunctivitis can be granulomatous and histologically similar to sarcoidosis. The diagnosis of syphilis is done by serologic screening and confirmatory tests, such as the rapid plasma reagin or fluorescent treponemal antibody absorbent tests, respectively. Direct examination using darkfield microscopy or biopsy of suspicious lesions can be performed, if results are uncertain. Isolated episcleritis and scleritis are uncommon during any stage of the disease, but when present, are usually features of secondary or late syphilis.

Treatment of ocular syphilis is similar to that of neurosyphilis. The most effective treatment involves high-dose IV penicillin G 12–24 million units/day for 14 days.[34,35] Because of the high rate of relapse, HIV-positive patients are recommended to have extensive follow-up subsequently at least for two years.[36]

BACTERIAL INFECTIONS

Bacterial Keratitis

The risk of infection with normal bacterial flora may be greater for severely immunosuppressed individuals.[37] *Staphylococcus aureus, Staphylococcus epidermidis* and *Pseudomonas aeruginosa* are most frequently implicated.[37] Some cases of recalcitrant infection may require keratoplasty and even evisceration of the globe.[38-40] Other risk factors predisposing to epithelial defects include the use of crack cocaine by HIV-infected individuals.[41]

The clinical presentation of bacterial keratitis in HIV-infected individuals differs from that in the general population. In immunosuppressed individuals, they are usually bilateral, involve multiple pathogens and carry a higher risk of perforation. There have been reports of eyes having to be eventually enucleated despite having been treated with intensive antibiotic therapy, based on in vitro sensitivities, for more than two weeks. Paucity of inflammation in immunosuppressed patients also contributes to delay in diagnosis and treatment. Gram staining and culture helps in the identification of the etiological agent. Systemic treatment with ceftriaxone or other appropriate antibiotics must be used to treat gonococcal conjunctivitis. Topical therapy alone will be ineffective.

PROTOZOAL INFECTIONS

Microsporidial Keratitis

Microsporidia are spore-forming, obligate intracellular, protozoan parasites. Infection occurs when the CD4 + counts drop to about 100cells/cu.mm; 39 to 44% of HIV-infected individuals with diarrhea are infected with microsporidia, in comparison to only 2.3% of HIV-infected individuals without diarrhea.[42] AIDS-associated microsporidial keratoconjunctivitis is characterized by bilateral superficial punctate epithelial keratitis, white intraepithelial infiltrates, mild anterior chamber reactions, and conjunctivitis in the form of mild conjunctival follicular hypertrophy.[42,43] Patients may complain of photophobia and grittiness. Vision loss is secondary to keratitis. Diagnosis is by Gram or Giemsa stain and spores from conjunctival scrapings or corneal biopsies can be easily seen with Masson trichrome or Giemsa stain. Immunofluorescence and electron microscopy can help confirm the diagnosis.

Treatment

Fumagillin 70 mg/ml eye drops are used indefinitely in HIV-positive individuals.[44] Albendazole 400 mg twice daily orally should be used as an adjunct for the management of systemic infection.

VIRAL KERATITIS

Cytomegalovirus Keratitis

Cytomegalovirus (CMV) can be transmitted by blood, saliva, breast milk, and mucous membrane contact is usually asymptomatic in immunocompetent individuals, but can sometimes produce transient conjunctivitis. CMV rarely involves the anterior segment tissues. The infection of the iris has been reported in a patient with CMV retinitis.[45] CMV has been reported to be associated with both epithelial and/or stromal keratitis, although both conditions are probably uncommon.[46] Corneal endothelial deposits have been described in about 80% of eyes with CMV retinitis. These asymptomatic lesions are seen in up to 81% of cases of HIV/AIDS-related CMV retinitis, they appear as linear or stellate lesions and form a reticular pattern. Best visualized on retroillumination, they are commonly found in the inferior cornea. These deposits are known to be composed of fibrin and macrophages, with no active CMV infection. CMV has been proven, with the help of aqueous humor analysis to be the causative agent of endothelitis and anterior uveitis in immunocompetent patients.

Herpes-zoster Ophthalmicus

Herpes-zoster ophthalmicus (HZO) is caused by varicella-zoster virus (VZV) which causes varicella (chickenpox) and herpes zoster (shingles). Over 90% of the population develops clinical or serologic evidence of infection with VZV by adolescence, and the prevalence is almost 100% by age 60 years.[46]The virus usually remains latent in sensory neurons. Herpes zoster eventually occurs in 10–20% of all individuals and reactivation in the ophthalmic division of the trigeminal nerve gives rise to HZO. Incidence of HZO is greater in HIV-infected individuals than in noninfected, age-adjusted populations. Approximately 5–15% of HIV-positive patients are co-infected with herpes zoster, but only half of these individuals are at risk of ocular involvement.[47] It can even be an initial manifestation of HIV. In immunosuppressed individuals, herpes zoster is more likely to be severe, prolonged, and can lead to viremia, which may result in visceral or neurologic infection, leading to increased morbidity and mortality. It is characterized by vesiculobullous rash over the distribution of the ophthalmic branch of the trigeminal nerve (Fig. 17.4) and may be associated with dendritiform and stromal keratitis, conjunctivitis, blepharitis, uveitis (with secondary glaucoma), hemorrhagic hypopyon[48] scleritis, retinitis[49] or encephalitis. Herpes zoster presenting in any apparently healthy young individual (<45 years) with these characteristics and without any obvious cause of immuno-

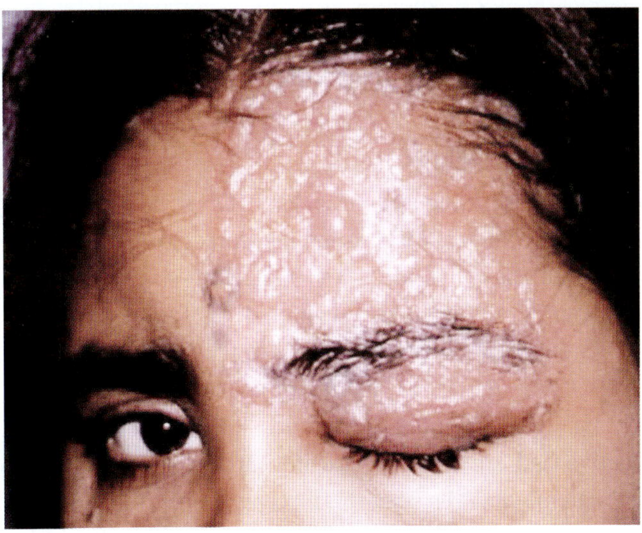

Fig. 17.4: Herpes-zoster ophthalmicus

suppression should be investigated for HIV. Tissue damage can be mediated through a necrotizing vasculitis. Diagnosis of HZO is mainly clinical. To confirm a clinical diagnosis, however, various tests are available, including virus cultures, Tzanck smears, polymerase chain reaction (PCR), techniques for VZV DNA, fluorescent antibody testing, and antigen detection by direct immunofluoresence.

Treatment

HZO in individuals with HIV disease requires aggressive initial treatment, with intravenous acyclovir, followed by a prolonged course of oral antivirals as maintenance therapy, to prevent recurrence. The regime is intravenous acyclovir (10 mg/kg of body weight, eight-hourly for seven days followed by an oral maintenance regimen of 800 mg five times a day for at least three to six weeks).[11]Recently, oral valganciclovir has shown equal efficacy as intravenous acyclovir. Early initiation of systemic antiviral therapy can reduce the duration of skin lesions and ocular complications by about 50%.

Herpetic Keratitis

Herpes simplex virus (HSV) and VZV are the most common etiologic agents of infectious keratitis. Herpetic keratitis can cause painful and often recurrent corneal ulcerations with a characteristic branching or dendritic pattern on slit-lamp examination. Epithelial keratitis typically appears in conjunction with follicular conjunctivitis[11] and vesicular eyelid lesions; stromal and interstitial keratitis present less frequently. HSV keratitis is usually associated with corneal scarring, iritis and raised intraocular pressure and is known to recur frequently. VZV keratitis may be accompanied by herpes-zoster ophthalmicus in 65% of individuals with HZO, dendritiform lesions occur in up to 51% cases.

Molluscum Contagiosum

Molluscum contagiosum, caused by a large DNA pox virus, affects up to 5% of HIV-infected patients and is highly contagious. It is transmitted by direct contact and has an incubation period of six to eight weeks.[46] In immunocompetent children, it is transmitted via fomites, infected clothing, bed linen, and towels.[50] They are usually fewer in number, smaller in size and are found to be unilateral. In young adults, it is typically transmitted sexually. In HIV-positive individuals, such lesions can occur in the eyelid and conjunctiva and are characteristically larger in number and size, often confluent, bilateral and resistant to therapy. Face (Fig. 17.5), trunk and genitalia are commonly affected. A distribution in the chin-strap region is

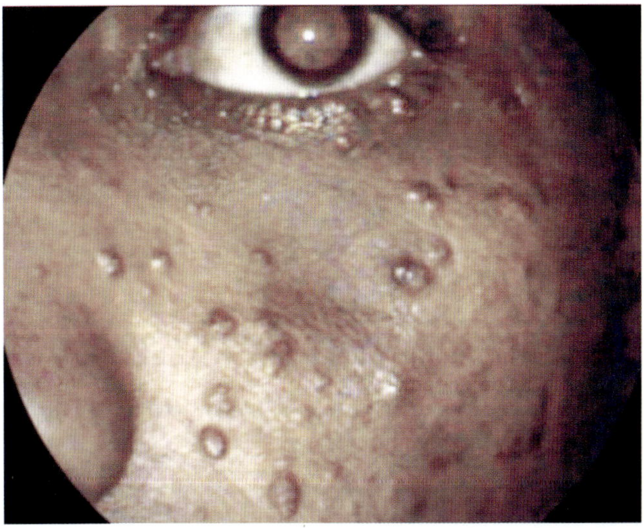

Fig. 17.5: Mollscum contagiosum (near eye)

common in HIV-positive patients. The lash line should be examined carefully in all patients with chronic conjunctivitis so as not to miss a molluscum lesion. It is characterized by pink or pearly white wart-like nodules on the skin. Sections of the lesions show large (20–30 microns) eosinophilic hyaline inclusion bodies which displace the nuclei to the margin. These bodies are composed of large numbers of virus particles, embedded in a protein matrix. Rarely, conjunctival involvement in AIDS patients can also result in nodular pink lesions.

Treatment

Typically these lesions regress on their own in immunocompetent individuals. Treatment options include usage of topical agents like phenol and trichloroacetic acid or serial applications of liquid nitrogen. Incision with or without curettage, excision, and cryotherapy are equally effective. Despite treatment, eyelid lesions will commonly recur. Administration of HAART with restoration of immunity leads to complete resolution of disseminated molluscum contagiosum and limitation of infection.

VASCULOPATHY

Microvasculopathy is the most common ocular manifestation of AIDS, seen in about 40–60% of HIV-positive patients.[7]Clinically, it manifests as cotton-wool spots located in the posterior pole and may simulate small patches of cytomegalovirus (CMV) retinitis. However, unlike CMV retinitis, cotton-wool spots are not associated with large amounts of hemorrhages, subtle iritis, or mild posterior vitritis. They have more rounded borders, and are usually oriented along the vascular arcades, and represent focal areas of ischemia in the nerve fiber layer. Most patients with retinal microvasculopathy are asymptomatic. Treatment is not indicated in most cases. The prevalence of microvasculopathy is inversely proportional to CD4+ count.

Large Vessel Disease

Large vessel occlusions, including central and branch retinal vein occlusions and branch retinal artery occlusions are uncommon and usually occur in association with viral retinitis, infiltrative lymphomatous optic neuropathy,[51-53] and as isolated abnormalities. Usually visual prognosis is very poor once there is central vein occlusion. Frosted branch vasculitis has been associated with CMV retinitis in AIDS.[54]

Conjunctival Microvasculopathy

Seventy to eighty percent patients have some form of asymptomatic conjunctival microvascular changes. These include segmental vascular dilatation and narrowing, microaneurysm formation, comma-shaped vascular fragment and visible granularity to the flowing blood column (sludging).[2]The cause is not known. It is postulated to be due to increased plasma viscosity, endothelitis or immune-complex deposition. No treatment is required.

NEOPLASMS

Kaposi's Sarcoma of Eyelid and Conjunctiva

Kaposi's sarcoma (KS) is a highly vascular mesenchymal tumor that appears as multiple purple-to-red nodules on the skin and mucous membranes. It occurs in 30% of all AIDS patients in the US. In approximately 10–20% of individuals, the tumor involves the eyelids, conjunctiva and in rare cases, the orbit. Kaposi's sarcoma of the eyelid and conjunctiva is rare in the Indian subcontinent possibly due to the rarity of the probable causative agent, human herpes virus.[8] The appearance of KS on the eyelids is similar to the lesions elsewhere on the skin. It can mimic a chalazion and can be seen in the upper or lower lids. Conjunctival lesions may be seen in any part of the palpebral or bulbar conjunctiva but are usually more common in the inferior fornix.[55] Kaposi's sarcoma in the conjunctiva can be mistaken for a subconjunctival hemorrhage or pyogenic granuloma. Histologically, it can resemble an angioma, hemangioma, lymphangioma or granulation. It has a complex arrangement of capillary channels and vascular spaces ("slits") without endothelium. Malignant spindle cells are arranged around these incomplete vascular spaces. The spindle-shaped interstitial cells are of vascular endothelial origin, with vacuolated cytoplasm which may demonstrate mitotic activity.

Treatment

Kaposi's sarcoma does not invade the eye and treatment is not necessary if it is asymptomatic and is cosmetically acceptable. The principal goal of therapy is palliation when disease is disfiguring, painful, or interfering with function. It may be treated by cryotherapy, surgical excision (if the lesion is small), radiation and/or chemotherapy. Radiation therapy is effective in treating the eyelid and conjunctival lesions but can lead to loss of lashes, irritation, conjunctivitis, conjunctival keratinization, cicatricial ectropion and retinopathy. Systemic agents are warranted for patients with advanced disease such as extensive cutaneous disease, visceral disease or lymphedema. Intralesional vinblastin or interferon-alpha have known to produce good results.

Cutaneous and Conjunctival Lymphoma

Non-Hodgkin's lymphoma (NHL) accounts for 3.5–5% of AIDS-defining illnesses and tends to be of a higher grade of malignancy in HIV patients and can affect eyelids and conjunctiva.[56] Involvement of the optic nerve in patient with AIDS may be recognized as perineuritis, papilledema, papillitis, retrobulbar neuritis, and optic atrophy.[56] NHL should be suspected in all HIV patients of any age who have prominent vitreous cells, with or without subretinal exudation. Intraocular lymphoma usually is seen with CD4 cell counts of less than 50 cells/ml.

Treatment

Radiotherapy and/or chemotherapy, such as vinblastin and interferon alpha have been used as part of treatment modality.

Squamous Cell Carcinoma of Conjunctiva

Squamous cell carcinoma of conjunctiva (SCC) is one of the most common neoplasm associated with HIV.[57] The eyelid or conjunctiva is seldom a site of initial presentation in the developed world though they can be the first presenting sign of AIDS in up to 50% of African patients though it is not as common in the Indian population.[58-60] The exact etiological role of HIV in ocular surface squamous cell neoplasia (OSSN) in Africa remains unclear. Important cofactors in HIV associated OSSN may be UV-light induced DNA damage and HPV-infection. Sun-light related mutations of p53 - a protein that has a crucial role, in tumor suppression and cell-cycle control, have been identified with high frequency in OSSN in HIV positive patients. The prevalence of HPV in Africa is not very different from South-East-Asia or Europe and newer studies found a rather weak association of HPV with OSSN. Most commonly noted clinical characteristics of conjunctival SCC are corneal overriding (90%), fast growth rates (with a rate of 1mm in 83%), tumors larger than 1 cm (17%), change of conjunctival color (66%), and nasal locations (66%). When the tumor is found at the limbus, gonioscopy has to be performed to rule out intraocular extension.

Treatment

A wide excision with frozen section monitoring of the margins of the lesion is recommended. HAART has been known to cause complete regression of invasive conjunctival SCC in an HIV-positive patient, which raises the possibility of antiviral therapy from topical interferon[61] as an alternative to radical surgery.[62]

OTHER MANIFESTATIONS

Keratoconjunctivitis Sicca

Keratoconjunctivitis sicca (KCS) or dry eye occurs in 20–38.8% of HIV-positive hosts in the later stages of AIDS.[47] It is thought to be due to lymphocytic infiltration of the lacrimal gland.[63,64] It has multifactorial etiology. The virus is also postulated to play a significant role in spontaneous corneal thinning and perforation which is observed in some infected patients.[37,65,66] Contrary to its effect on many other HIV/AIDS-related ocular diseases, HAART has not played a part in significantly reducing the prevalence of KCS.[47]

Management options include artificial tears, long-acting lubricants and punctal occlusion.

Conjunctivitis

Nonspecific, culture-negative conjunctivitis[2] has been reported to be seen in less than 1% of patients with HIV. Rarely, cytomegalovirus or cryptococcus can be the causative organism. Grams stain and culture need to be done before labeling it as noninfective. Biopsy is indicated in unresponsive cases.

Trichomegaly

Acquired trichomegaly or hypertrichosis has been described, especially in the late stages. The cause is not known although drug toxicity,[67]and elevated viral load have been suggested to play a role. It has to be treated if annoying or if cosmetically unacceptable.

Atopic Dermatitis and Blepharitis

Atopic dermatitis has a prevalence of approximately 10% in the general population and can be the first ocular manifestation in some individuals after HIV infection.[46] The atopic eyelid disease in both HIV-infected and non infected patients is treated by topical corticosteroids.

IATROGENIC AND POST-TREATMENT MANIFESTATIONS

Immune Recovery Uveitis

The introduction of HAART brought with it the new ophthalmic problem of immune recovery uveitis (IRU), which can be devastating for patients whose health has otherwise improved, because it can result in vision loss. It is well accepted that IRU is caused by a response to CMV antigens, which is made possible by immune recovery. The same phenomenon can occur in patients with other intraocular infections, such as toxoplasmosis or tuberculosis. The reported incidence of IRU has varied from 0.1 to 0.8/PY on follow-up.[68] Risk factors for IRU include larger lesions and previous use of cidofovir, presumably because it also is associated with intraocular inflammation.[69]There may be immunologic factors unique to those in whom IRU develops that explain its occurrence in only a subset of patients; this issue is under study, but it is not yet possible to identify *at-risk* patients on the basis of laboratory tests of immune function. IRU generally is recognized by the presence of complications of inflammation, including anterior chamber or vitreous reaction (Fig. 17.6), such as panuveitis with hypopon, optic disk and cystoid macular edema, epiretinal membrane formation, cataract, vitreomacular traction syndrome, and proliferative vitreoretinopathy. Treatment of IRU-associated macular edema has been difficult. Treatment with corticosteroids (sub-Tenon or systemic or intravitreal) is effective in controlling inflammation and improving vision in some cases. However, vitrectomy may be required in patients with vitreomacular traction syndrome, epiretinal membrane formation, and proliferative vitreoretinopathy.

Retinal Detachment

In the pre-HAART era, retinal detachments occurred in more than one-third of patients with CMV retinitis who survived one year or longer. Vitrectomy with silicone oil tamponade became the standard method for repair of these detachments. Since removal of silicone oil is difficult in these patients, it is preferable to use 5000 CST oil. However, with the increasing longivity of these patients due to use of HAART treatment this may become an issue in the future. In the western countries, the risk of

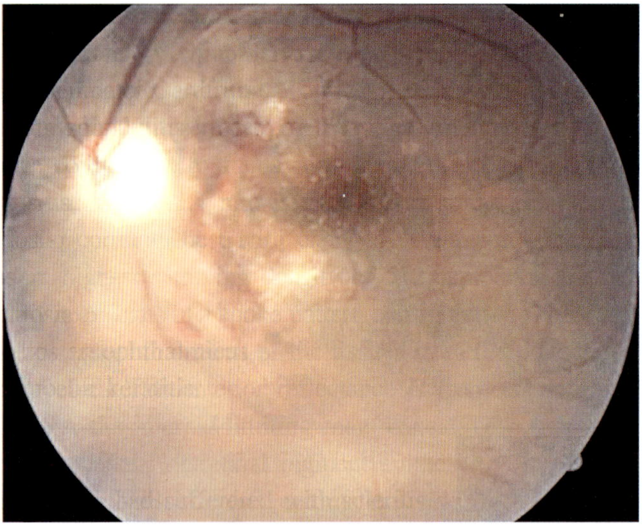

Fig. 17.6: Severe vitritis due to immune recovery uveitis

detachment is substantially less among patients receiving HAART,[31] which has been attributed to better control of infection, resulting in smaller, inactive lesions, and therefore, better healed and more adherent scars. However, in our series we found an increase in incidence of retinal detachment in patients on HAART. It may be due to a higher incidence of IRU and also larger areas of CMV retinitis which was untreated prior to starting the HAART. In eyes with PORN and ARN, the area of retinal necrosis is more extensive and the surgical results are very disappointing. Where feasible, the principles of surgery remain the same.

Drug-induced Uveitis

Another group of new diseases has been attributed to the toxic effects of of Rifabutin[70] and Cidofovir.[71] In both instances, a predominantly anterior form of uveitis develops, which is characterized by a discrepancy between clinical symptoms and morphological changes; the former condition is distinguished by severe pain and the latter by marked inflammation.

Stevens-Johnson Syndrome

HIV-infected individuals are frequently exposed to many medications, especially drugs, such as nevirapine, that are capable of causing hypersensitivity or toxic reactions. Altered cell-mediated immunity may also lead to increased risk of Stevens-Johnson syndrome (SJS)[46] as a response to infectious agents as well. Associated dry eye may aggravate the problems associated with SJS in HIV-infected individuals (Fig. 17.7).

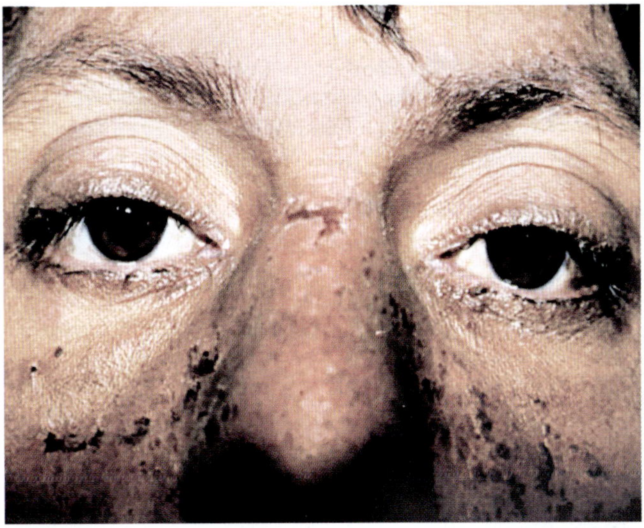

Fig. 17.7: Steven-Johnson syndrome

Corneal Phospholipidoses

Vortex keratopathy or corneal phospholipidosis[72] can be caused by antivirals such as ganciclovir, acyclovir or atovaquone, a drug used in the treatment of toxoplasmosis.

Summary

Though ocular opportunistic infections are becoming much less common in the era of HAART, they still remain as common ocular complications of AIDS in the developing countries like India unlike the western world. CMV retinitis remains the leading cause of vision loss in HIV positive individuals. HAART has been shown to cause regression of CMV retinitis, increase time to relapse of CMV retinitis, reduce the incidence of CMV-related retinal detachments, and prolong patient survival. Anterior segment manifestations in the eye in HIV-infected individuals are varied. They can affect the quality of life, which ultimately hampers the rehabilitation of the individual, which is the ultimate goal of the treating ophthalmologist. Multiple pathogens can be found in the same individual. Patients on HAART can develop severe inflammatory reaction due to immune recovery phenomenon, which can cause severe ocular morbidity. Hence, it is important that ophthalmologists should be aware of this new emerging phenomenon so that it is managed appropriately.

References

1. Sudarshan S, Biswas J. Introduction and immunopathogenesis of AIDS and Anterior segment manifestation of HIV/AIDS. *Ind J Ophthalmol.* 2008;56:357-62.
2. Kestelyn PG, Cunningham Jr. ET. HIV/AIDS and blindness. *Bull World Health Organ. 2001;*79:208-13.
3. Holland GN. Acquired immunodeficiency syndrome and ophthalmology: the first decade. *Am J Ophthalmol.* 1992;114:86-95.
4. Vrabec TR. Posterior segment manifestations of HIV/AIDS. *Survey of Ophthalmology.* 2004;49:131-57.
5. Goldberg DE, Smithen LM, Angelilli A, Freeman WR. HIV-associated retinopathy in the HAART era. *Retina.* 2005;Jul-Aug;25(5):633-49.
6. Mesariæ B, Lisiæ M, Kniewald T, Ugrinoviæ N, Begovac J. Ocular manifestations in patients with human immunodeficiency virus infection before and after the introduction of highly active antiretroviral therapy. *Lijec Vjesn.* 2005;127 (5-6):123-8.
7. Jabs DA. Ocular manifestations of HIV infection. *Trans Am Ophthalmol Soc. 1995;*93:623-83.
8. Banker AS and Patel A. Effect Of Combination Antiretroviral Therapy on Cytomegalovirus Retinitis. *Ind J Ophth*almol. 2002;50:29-33.
9. Holbrook JT, Jabs DA, Weinberg DV, et al. Visual loss in patients with cytomegalovirus retinitis and acquired immunodeficiency syndrome before widespread availability of highly active antiretiroviral therapy. *Arch Ophthalmol.* 2003;121:99-107.
10. Biswas J, Madhavan HN, George AE, Kumarasamy N, Solomon S. Ocular lesions associated with HIV infection in India: A series of 100 consecutive patients evaluated at a referral center. *Am J Ophthalmol* 2000;129 (1): 9-15.
11. Biswas J, Fogla R, Gopal L, Narayana KM, Banker AS, Kumarsamy N, Madhavan HN. Current Approaches to Diagnosis and Management of Ocular Lesions in Human Immunodeficiency Virus Positive patients. *Ind J Ophth*almol. 2002;50: 83-96.
12. Kuppermann BD, Petty JG, Richman DD, et al. Correlation between CD4+ counts and prevalence of cytomegalovirus retinitis and human immunodeficiency virus-related noninfectious retinal vasculopathy in patients with acquired immunodeficiency syndrome. *Am J Ophthalmol. 1993;*115:575-82.
13. Baldassano VF, Dunn JP, Feinberg J, et al. Cytomegalovirus retinitis and low CD 4+ T-lymphocyte counts. *N Engl J Med.* 1995;333:670.
14. Cassoux N, Bodaghi B, Lautier-Frau M, et al. Current status of retinal detachment in AIDS patients. *J Fr Ophtalmol. 2000;*23:1031-4.
15. Freeman WR, Quiceno JI, Crapotta JA, Listhaus A, Munguia D, Aguilar MF. Surgical repair of rhegmatogenous retinal detachment in immunosuppressed patients with cytomegalovirus retinitis. *Ophthalmology.* 1992;99:466-74.
16. Reed JB, Schwab IR, Gordon J, Morse LS. Regression of cytomegalovirus retinitis associated with protease-inhibitor treatment in patients with AIDS. *Am J Ophthalmol. 1997;*124:199-205.
17. Holland GN. Discussion of MacDonald JC, Karavellas MP, Torriani FJ, et al (Highly active antiretroviral therapy-related immune recovery in AIDS patients with cytomegalovirus retinitis). *Ophthalmology.* 2000;107:877-83.
18. Ormerod LD, Larkin JA, Margo CA, et al. Rapidly progressive herpetic retinal necrosis: a blinding disease characteristic of advanced AIDS. *Clin Infect Dis.* 1998;26: 34-45.

19. Cano-Parra JL, Diaz-LLopis ML, Cordoba JL, Gobernado ML, Navea AL, Menezo JL. Acute iridocyclitis in a patient with AIDS diagnosed as toxoplasmosis by PCR. *Ocul Immunol Inflamm.* 2000;8:127-30.
20. Freeman WR, Gross JG, Labelle J, et al. Pneumocystis carinii choroidopathy. A new clinical entity. *Arch Ophthalmol.* 1989;107:863-7.
21. Shami MJ, Freeman W, Friedberg D, et al. A multicenter study of pneumocystis choroidopathy. *Am J Ophthalmol.* 1991;112:15-22.
22. Helm CJ, Holland GN. Ocular tuberculosis. *Surv Ophthalmol.* 1993;38:229-56.
23. Babu RB, Sudharshan S, Kumarasamy N, Therese KL, Biswas J. Ocular tuberculosis in acquired immunodeficiency syndrome. *Am J Ophthalmol.* 226;142: 413-8.
24. Bouza E, Merino P, Munoz P, Sanchez-Carrillo C, Yopez J, Cortés C. Ocular tuberculosis: A prospective study in a general hospital. *Medicine (Baltimore).* 1997;76:53-61.
25. Jennings A, Bilous M, Asimakis P, Maloof AJ. Mycobacterium tuberculosis presenting as chronic red eye. *Cornea.* 2006;25:1118-20.
26. Singal A, Aggarwal P, Pandhi D, Rohatgi J. Cutaneous tuberculosis and phlyctenular keratoconjunctivitis: A forgotten association. *Indian J Dermatol Venereol Leprol.* 2006;72:290-2.
27. Dinning WJ, Marston S. Cutaneous and ocular tuberculosis: A review. *J Royal Soc Med.* 1985;78:576-81.
28. Muccioli C, Belfort Junior R, Neves R, Rao N. Limbal and choroidal Cryptococcus infection in the acquired immunodeficiency syndrome. *Am J Ophthalmol.* 1995;120:539-40.
29. Garelick JM, Khodabakhsh AJ, Lopez Y, Bamji M, Lister M. Scleral ulceration caused by cryptococcus albidus in a patient with acquired immune deficiency syndrome. *Cornea.* 2004;23:730-1.
30. Acharya NR, Cunningham ET Jr. Corneal, anterior segment, and adnexal manifestations of human immunodeficiency virus. *Int Ophthalmol Clin.* 1998;38:161-77.
31. Jabs DA, van Natta ML, Thorne JE, et al. Course of cytomegalovirus retinitis in the era of highly active antiretroviral therapy: 2 (Second eye involvement and retinal detachment). *Ophthalmology.* 2004;111:2232-9.
32. McLeish WM, Pulido JS, Holland S, Culbertson WW, Winward K. The ocular manifestations of syphilis in the human immunodeficiency virus type 1-infected host. *Ophthalmology.* 1990;97:196-203.
33. Becerra LI, Ksiazek SM, Savino PJ, Marcus DK, Buckley RM, Sergott RC, et al. Syphilitic uveitis in human immunodeficiency virus-infected and non infected patients. *Ophthalmology. 1989;*96:1727-30.
34. Musher DM, Hamill RJ, Baughn RE. Effect of human immunodeficiency virus (HIV) infection on the course of syphilis and on the response to treatment. *Ann Intern Med.* 1990;113:872-81.
35. Rosberger DF, Heinemann MH, Friedberg DN, Holland GN, Uveitis associated with human immunodeficiency virus infection. *Am J Ophthalmol.* 1998;125: 301-5.
36. Moloney G, Branley M, Kotsiou G, Rhodes D. Syphilis presenting as scleritis in an HIV-positive man undergoing immune reconstitution. *Clin Experiment Ophthalmol.* 2004;32:526-8.
37. Moraes HV Jr. Ocular manifestations of HIV-AIDS. *Curr Opin Ophthalmol.* 2002;13:397-403.
38. Aristimuno B, Nirankari VS, Hemady RK, Rodrigues MM. Spontaneous ulcerative keratitis in immunocompromised patients. *Am J Ophthalmol.* 1993;115: 202-8.

39. Hansen B, Kronborg G. Acanthamoeba keratitis in a non-contact lens wearer with human immunodeficiency virus. *Scand J Infect Dis.* 2003;35: 207-9.
40. Tandon R, Vajpayee RB, Gupta V, Vajpayee M, Satpathy G, Dada T. Polymicrobial keratitis in an HIV-positive patient. *Indian J Ophthalmol.* 2003;51:87-8.
41. Kestelyn PG, Cunningham ET Jr. HIV-AIDS and blindness. *Bull World Health Organ.* 2001;79:208-13.
42. Friedberg DN, Stenson SM, Orenstein JM, Tierno PM, Charles NC. Microsporidial keratoconjunctivitis in acquired immunodeficiency syndrome. *Arch Ophthalmol.* 1990;108:504-8.
43. Lowder CY, McMahon JT, Meisler DM, Dodds EM, Calabrese LH, Didier ES, et al. Microsporidial keratoconjunctivitis caused by septata intestinalis in a patient with acquired immunodeficiency syndrome. *Am J Ophthalmol.* 1996;121:715-7.
44. Benson CA, Kaplan JE, Masur H, Pau A, Holmes KK; CDC; et al. Treating opportunistic infections among HIV-infected adults and adolescents: Recommendations from CDC, the National Institutes of Health, and the HIV Medicine Association. *MMWR Recomm Rep.* 2004;53:1-112.
45. Cheng L, Rao NA, Keefe KS, Avila CP Jr, Macdonald JC, Freeman WR. Cytomegalovirus iritis. *Ophthalmic Surg Lasers.* 1998;29:930-2.
46. Jeng BH, Holland GN, Lowder CY, Deegan WF 3rd, Raizman MB, Meisler DM. Anterior segment and external ocular disorders associated with human immunodeficiency virus disease. *Surv Ophthalmol.* 2007;52:329-68.
47. Liesegang TJ. Varicella-zoster virus eye disease. *Cornea.* 1999;18:511-31.
48. Adnexal and anterior segment manifestations of HIV-AIDS. *Int Ophthalmol Clin.* 2007;47:15-32.
49. Biswas J, Samanta TK, Madhavan HN, Kumarasamy N, Solomon S. Acute panuveitis with haemorrhagic hypopyon as a presenting feature of acquired immunodeficiency syndrome (AIDS). *Indian J Ophthalmol.* 2000;48:311-2.
50. Sellitti TP, Huang AJ, Schiffman J, Davis JL. Association of herpes zoster ophthalmicus with acquired immunodeficiency syndrome and acute retinal necrosis. *Am J Ophthalmol. 1993;*116:297-301.
51. Pannell RS, Fleming DM, Cross KW. The incidence of molluscum contagiosum, scabies and lichen planus. *Epidemiol Infect.* 2005;133:985-91.
52. Conway MD, Tong P, Olk RJ. Branch retinal artery occlusion (BRAO) combined with branch retinal vein occlusion (BRVO) and optic disc neovascularization associated with HIV and CMV retinitis. *Int Ophthalmol.* 1995;19:249-52.
53. Friedman SM, Margo CE. Bilateral central retinal vein occlusions in a patient with acquired immunodeficiency syndrome. Clinico-pathologic correlations. *Arch Ophthalmol.* 1995;113:1184-88.
54. Park KL, Marx JL, Lopez PF, Rao NA. Noninfectious branch retinal vein occlusion in HIV-positive patients. *Retina.* 1997;17:162-4.
55. Mansour AM, Li HK. Frosted retinal periphlebitis in the acquired immunodeficiency syndrome. *Ophthalmologica.* 1993;207:182-6.
56. Corti M, Solari R, de Carolis L, Corraro R. Eye involvement in AIDS-related Kaposi sarcoma. *Enferm Infect Microbiol Clin.* 2001;19:3-6.
57. Mansour AM. Neuro-ophthalmic findings in acquired immunodeficiency syndrome. *J Clin Neuroophthalmol.* 1990;10:167-174.
58. Guech energy et. al Elevated risk for squamous cell carcinoma among the adults with AIDS in US. *Int J Cancer.* 2008;122(11):2590-3.

59. Muccioli C. Belfort R, Burnier M, Rao N. Squamous cell carcinoma of the conjunctiva in a patient with the acquired immune deficiency syndrome. *Am J Ophthalmol.* 1996;121:94-6.
60. Fogla R, Biswas J, Krishnakumar S, Madhavan HN, Kumarasamy N, Solomon S. Squamous cell carcinoma of the conjunctiva as initial presenting sign in a patient with acquired immunodeficiency syndrome (AIDS) due to human immunodeficiency virus type-2. *Eye.* 2000;14:246-7.
61. Porges Y, Groisman GM. Prevalence of HIV with conjunctival squamous cell neoplasia in an African provincial hospital. *Cornea.* 2003;22:1-4.
62. Amber Struges. Topical interferon or surgical excision for the primary management of primary ocular surface neoplasia, *Ophthalmology.* 2008;115:1297-1302.
63. Holkar S, Mudhar HS, Jain A, Gupta M, Rogstad KE, Parsons MA, *et al.* Regression of invasive conjunctival Squamous carcinoma in an HIV-positive patient on antiretroviral therapy. *Int J STD AIDS.* 2005;16:782-3.
64. Ormerod LD, Dailey JP. Ocular manifestations of cat-scratch disease. Curr Opin *Ophthalmol.* 1999;10:209-16.
65. Matui R, Nussenblatt R, de Smet MD. Prevalance of tear hyposecretion and vitamin A deficiency in patients with AIDS. *Invest Ophthalmol Vis Sci.* 1995;35:1308.
66. Akpek EK, Haddad RS,Winkelstein JA, Gottsch JD. Bilateral consecutive central corneal perforations associated with hypogammaglobulinemia. *Ophthalmology.* 2000;107:123-6.
67. Raina UK, Sharma V, Jain S, Arora R, Mehta DK. Peripheral corneal thinning and silent corneal perforation in an HIV seropositive case. *Acta Ophthalmol Scand.* 2004;82:246-7.
68. Graham DA, Sires BS. Acquired trichomegaly associated with acquired immunodeficiency syndrome. *Arch Ophthalmol.* 1997;115:557-8.
69. Kuppermann BD, Holland GN. Immune recovery uveitis. *Am J Ophthalmol* 130: 103-106.
70. Kempen JH, Min YI, Freeman WR, et al. Risk of immune recovery uveitis in patients with AIDS and cytomegalovirus retinitis. *Ophthalmology. 2006;*113:684-694.
71. Tseng AL, Walmsley. Rifabutin-associated uveitis. *Ann Pharmacother.* 1995;29:1149-55.
72. Davis JL, Taskintuna I, Freeman WR, Weinberg DV, Feuer WJ, Leonard RE. Iritis and hypotony after treatment with intravenous cidofovir for cytomegalovirus retinitis. *Arch Ophthalmol.* 1997;115:733-7.

Website References

1. UNAIDS. AIDS epidemic update: December 2007. http://data. unaids. org/ pub/EPISlides/2007/2007_epiupdate_en. pdf .
2. AAO Statement, "Minimizing Transmission of Bloodborne Pathogens and Surface Infectious Agents in Ophthalmic Offices and Operating Rooms" http://aao. org/ education/statements which summarizes universal precautions, identifies resources for management of occupation exposure, and provides a list of relevant publications.
3. Rathinam SR, Lalitha P. Paradoxical worsening of ocular tuberculosis in HIV patients after antiretroviral therapy. *Eye advance online publication.* 1 December 2006.

18

chapter

Parthopratim Dutta Majumder
A Ramanan
Jyotirmay Biswas

Ocular Involvement in Systemic Rheumatic Diseases

ABSTRACT

Systemic rheumatic diseases are a heterogenous group of immune mediated, multisystem disorders often associated with various ocular manifestations like uveitis, episcleritis, scleritis, corneal disease, retinal vascular disease and vasculitis. Ocular involvement is usually seen as a complication of systemic collagen vascular disease. It may range from a mild to a very severe form resulting in loss of vision. In this chapter some of the common rheumatic diseases are described with their ocular manifestations.

Introduction

Systemic rheumatic diseases are a heterogenous collection of immune mediated, multisystem disorders. Ocular involvement is common, and varies with the type of rheumatic disease. The various ocular manifestations include uveitis, episcleritis, scleritis, corneal disease, retinal vasculitis, etc. Ocular involvement is usually seen as a complication of systemic collagen vascular disease. Ocular complications associated with systemic rheumatic disorders can range from mild to severe with significant outcomes including loss of vision. In this chapter we have tried to summarize the ocular manifestations of following systemic rheumatic disorders:

- Rheumatoid arthritis (RA)
- Systemic lupus erythematosus (SLE)
- Polyarteritis nodosa (PAN)
- Wegener's granulomatosis (WG)
- Systemic sclerosis (SSc)
- Ankylosing spondylitis (AS).

Rheumatoid Arthritis

Rheumatoid arthritis (RA) is the most common inflammatory arthritis, affecting about one percent of the population worldwide. It has a wide spectrum of disease manifestations and extra-articular involvement. Females are affected three times more frequently than men. The common age of involvement is mostly between 40 and 60 years.[1-4]

There is some genetic predisposition conferred by a handful of specific HLA-DQ and HLA-DR alleles. Morning stiffness of the joints is the hallmark of the disease and probably the most widely noted presenting symptom. The swan neck deformity (Fig. 18.1) is often found.

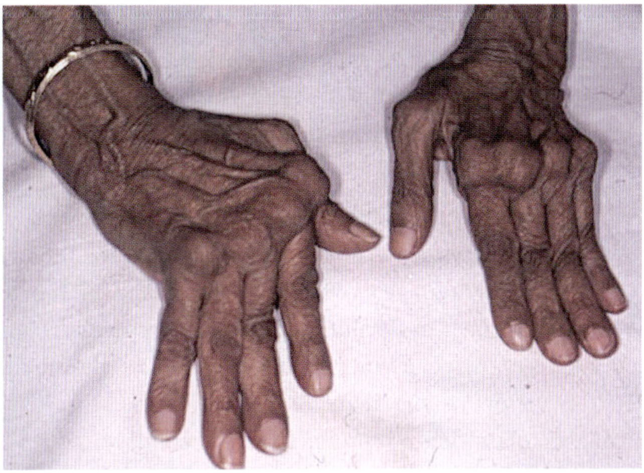

Fig. 18.1: Swan neck deformity in rheumatic arthritis

CLASSIFICATION

Rheumatoid arthritis is classified on the basis of number of joints involved (Table 18.1).[5] A scoring system is proposed for the diagnosing of the disease.

Patients receive the highest point level for each domain: 6 points is defined as definite RA, though those with lower scores may obtain more points with time and subsequently be defined as having RA.

Dry eye is the most common ocular involvement in RA. It is usually seen in patients with long-standing disease. About one third of patients suffer from keratoconjunctivits sicca (KCS) and in 10% it is combined with a dry mouth (Sjögren's syndrome). The severity of symptoms may not correlate with arthritis. Symptoms range from dry eyes, burning, gritty sensation and mucoid discharge.[6-9]

TABLE 18.1: 2010 ACR/EULAR classification criteria for rheumatoid arthritis[5]

Joint involvement	Serology	Duration	Acute phase reactants
1. 1 Large joint (0 points)	Negative RF and CCP (0 points)	Less than 6 weeks (0 points)	Abnormal ESR or CRP (1 point)
2. 2–10 Large joints (1 point)	Low titer positive CCP or RF (2 points)	6 or more weeks (1 point)	
3. 1–3 small joints (2 points)	High titer CCP or RF (3 points)		
4. 4–10 small joints (3 points)			
5. More than 10 joints (with at least one small joint) (5 points)			
Total possible points			
5	**3**	**1**	**1**

Sjögren's syndrome[9] is a condition of aqueous tear deficiency associated with dry mouth. Sjögren's syndrome is most commonly seen in women (95%). It can occur at all ages, with peak incidence in the fourth and fifth decades. The lacrimal and salivary glands are progressively infiltrated by activated T cells, which cause acinar and ductular cell destruction leading to decreased secretion of the tears or saliva.

The syndrome is classified as primary and secondary:

- Primary Sjögren's syndrome occurs in patients without a defined connective tissue disease
- Secondary Sjögren's syndrome occurs in patients with well-known connective tissue diseases like rheumatoid arthritis, systemic lupus erythematosus, polyarteritis, Wegener's granulomatosis, scleroderma, polymyositis, dermatomyositis, etc.

Episcleritis can be seen in 5% of patients of RA, usually correlating with the activity of RA. It may be nodular or diffuse, causing an ache and some discomfort, without affecting visual acuity. RA is the most common systemic association of scleritis. About 17–33% of all patients with scleritis have RA and 0.2–6.3% of patients with RA have scleritis. Patients with scleritis associated with RA more commonly have bilateral scleritis than patients with scleritis due to other collagen vascular disease. It correlates with long-standing disease, and with active inflammation. [10] Scleromalacia perforans is a very rare type of scleritis that occurs due to obliterative endarteritis. It is seen exclusively in patients with long-standing rheumatoid arthritis. It is clinically silent and pain-free, and is becoming extremely rare with improved treatments for rheumatoid arthritis.[10] Uveitis is rare in rheumatoid arthritis and involvement of the retinal vessels is very unusual.

Corneal involvement in RA occurs most often with scleritis, though it can be an isolated finding also. Sclerosing keratitis, acute stromal keratitis, peripheral ulcerative keratitis, and keratolysis occur in up to 50% of patients with scleritis. Peripheral ulcerative keratitis is most often associated with necrotizing scleritis. It is most probably due to immune complex deposition in the limbal vessels which results in immune-mediated vasculitis.[10] Various ocular manifestations of rheumatoid arthritis are summarized in Figure 18.2.

Laboratory findings usually include a raised ESR and CRP, anemia, thrombocytosis, and leucocytosis. Rheumatoid factor is an autoantibody directed against the Fc region of IgG. Rheumatoid factor and IgG join to form immune complexes that contribute to the disease process. Various immunoassays are available for detection of rheumatoid factor. The classic Rose-Waaler test is hemagglutination test for rheumatoid factor in the serum, which depends on the ability of rheumatoid factor to agglutinate sheep erythrocytes coated with anti-sheep immunoglobulin.[1] Latex agglutination test, in which latex particles coated with human IgG aggregate in the presence of IgM rheumatoid factor are also widely available. These tests identify only the IgM isotype of rheumatoid factor. Enzyme-linked immunosorbent assay (ELISA) can measure IgG, IgA, and IgM rheumatoid factors. It is important to mention here that some forms of rheumatoid arthritis like oligoarticular rheumatoid arthritis may be associated with a negative test for IgM rheumatoid factor but a positive test for IgG rheumatoid factor.[2]

Treatment of systemic rheumatoid arthritis involves the use of multiple

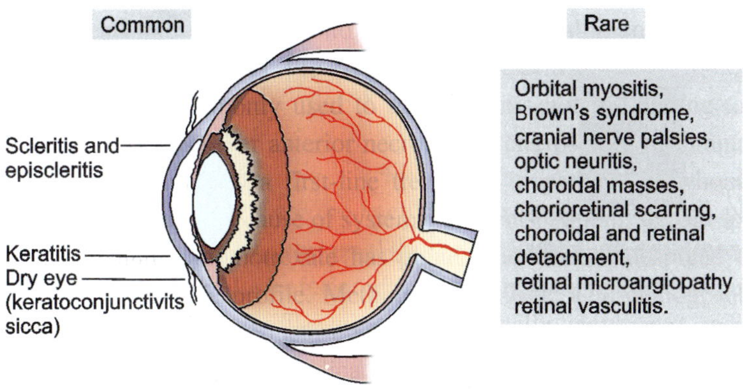

Fig. 18.2: Ocular involvement in rheumatoid arthritis

agents that affect the immune system and they can be divided into: nonsteroidal anti-inflammatory drugs (NSAIDs), corticosteroids, and disease-modifying antirheumatic drugs (DMARDs). NSAIDs improve the quality of life for patients with rheumatoid arthritis by reducing pain and inflammation; however, they have no role in prevention of joint damage, disability and organ involvement. Corticosteroids rapidly reduce inflammation, but they are not as effective as the DMARDs. DMARDs have been found to prevent bone and cartilage damage and improve quality of life for patients with RA by reducing the signs and symptoms of the disease.[1,2] DMARDs used in the treatment of RA include methotrexate, sulfasalazine, hydroxy-chloroquine, leunomide, penicillamine, azathioprine, cyclophosphamide, ciclosporin, tacrolimus, mycophenolate mofetil, and minocycline.

Treatment of ocular manifestations of rheumatoid arthritis is based on individual patient's symptoms and findings. Treatment for KCS always should include vigorous attention to the lid margins for meibomian glands and blepharitis. Allergic conditions and environmental changes triggering acute condition requires concurrent systemic and topical medications, and associated abnormalities should be identified and addressed.[11] Initial treatment of dry eye in rheumatoid arthritis remains ocular surface lubrication with artificial tear substitutes and lubricating ointments. In eyes not responsive to topical lubrication alone, additional modalities of management can be considered. Topical cyclosporine twice daily can result in decreased lacrimal gland lymphocytic infiltration and increased tear production.[12,13] Topical application of sterile autologous serum prepared in saline has been used with success.[14,15] Punctal occlusion is a technique used to maintain and prevent tear drainage from the ocular surface. If Schirmer values are consistently 3 mm or less, punctal occlusion can be considered.[16]

Peripheral ulcerative keratitis and other corneal involvement can be managed effectively with oral corticosteroid and topical cyclosporine.[17,18] It is very important to rule out infectious etiologies in such cases as treatment with immunosuppressives could lead to exacerbation.

Episcleritis in patients with rheumatoid arthritis are generally treated with topical and systemic nonsteroidal anti-inflammatory drug (NSAID). In severe episcleral inflammations topical steroid can be used.[10]

Unlike episcleritis, scleritis in patients with rheumatoid arthritis always requires systemic immunosuppressive therapy and topical steroids can be used as an adjunctive therapy. These patients should be monitored carefully and closely as they are at higher risk of developing necrotizing scleritis and chances of potentially lethal systemic vasculitis are more in them.[10] Various immunosuppressants have been tried for treatment of scleritis and these include antimetabolites (methotrexate, azathioprine, and mycophenolate mofetil), alkylating agents (chlorambucil and cyclophosphamide), and T-cell inhibitors (cyclosporine and tacrolimus). Newer biological agents like TNF-á inhibitors (infliximab or adalimumab), rituximab are reported to be used for the treatment of scleritis in patients with rheumatoid arthritis.[19,20]

Systemic Lupus Erythematosus

Systemic lupus erythematosus (SLE) is a chronic multisystem autoimmune disorder with heterogenous presentation. SLE is characterized by autoantibodies including double stranded DNA (dsDNA), anti-Smith, anti Ro and anti-La antibodies. The pathogenic significance of these antibodies is still unclear but some like dsDNA are very specific for SLE. Women, mostly in the childbearing years are nine times more commonly affected than men.

Skin is one of the frequently involved organs in SLE. In fact skin serves as the best window for the clinicians in diagnosis and assessment of disease activity. Malar rash on the bridge of the nose and cheeks is the most common skin lesion seen in SLE (Fig. 18.3). One should also look for Raynaud's phenomenon, acral cyanosis, periungual erythema and maculopapular rashes of the trunk or extremity. Alopecia, associated with inflammatory involvement of scalp can be seen in SLE. Photosensitivity,

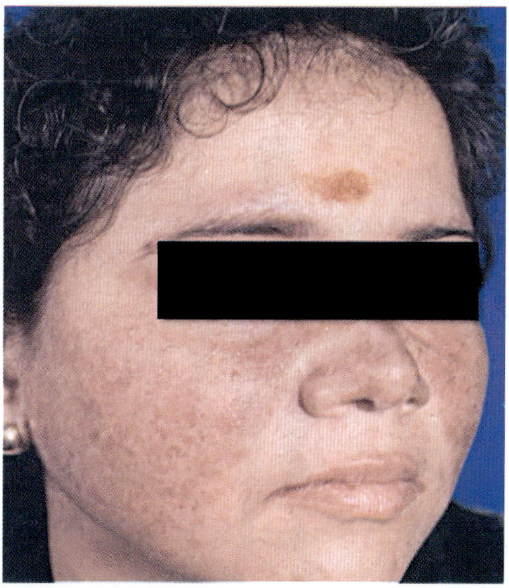

Fig. 18.3: Malar rash or butterfly rash seen in SLE

when the skin is exposed to UV light, is another important feature in SLE. The arthropathy seen in SLE, also known as *Jaccoud's arthropathy*, involves the same distribution as rheumatoid arthritis, including the metacarpophalangeal joints, wrists and metatarsophalangeal joints. This arthropathy is generally nonerosive in nature.[1,2] Systemic manifestations of SLE are presented in Figure 18.4.

Scleritis is seen in 5% patients of SLE. Sometimes, scleritis can be the initial presentation of SLE. Anterior uveitis is very rare in SLE and can be seen in association with severe scleritis. The cornea appears hazy because of corneal folds caused by hypotension in the eye secondary to severe ischemia.[22,23] Episcleritis and dry eye are also seen in association with SLE.

Optic nerve is involved in 1% patients with SLE. Optic neuropathy in SLE occurs due to vasculitis, with subsequent ischemia. Clinical manifestations of optic neuropathy in SLE include papillitis, retrobulbar neuritis, acute ischemic optic neuropathy associated with chronic progressive visual loss.[22] Retinal involvements in SLE or Lupus retinopathy may occur in the form of cotton-wool spots with or without retinal hemorrhages, and additional microvascular changes, including microaneurysms and capillary telangiectasia. Vasculitis in SLE is occlusive in nature and results due to deposition of immune complexes. The hallmark of occlusive vasculopathy is the cytoid body, which is the descriptive term used in SLE for cotton-wool spot. Retinal hemorrhages and occlusions of branch or central retinal arteries

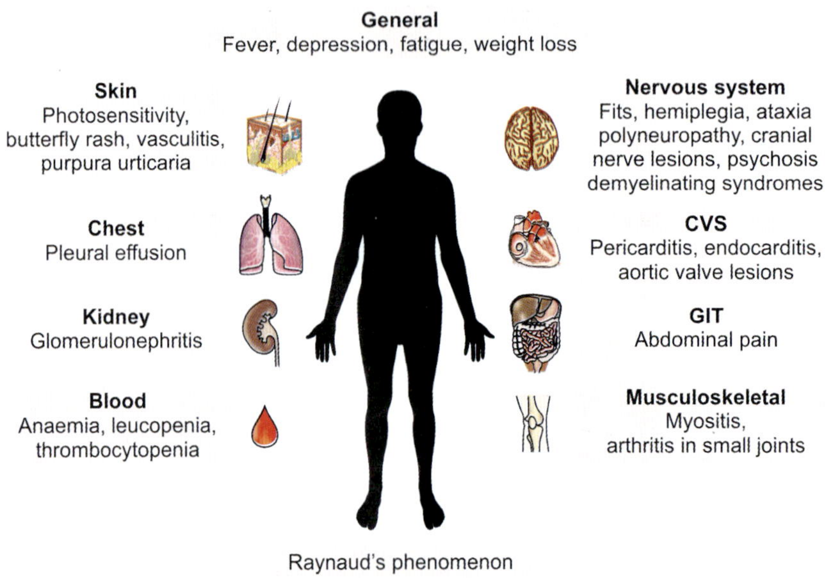

Fig. 18.4: Systemic manifestations of SLE are represented diagramatically

may occur. Occlusions of branch retinal veins are usually secondary to hypertension. Lupus choroidopathy is less common than lupus retinopathy. Lupus choroidopathy is usually associated with systemic vascular disease, such as hypertension due to lupus nephritis. Serous detachment of the retina and choroidal infarcts are salient features of Lupus choroidopathy.[1,22,23] Presence of anticardiolipin antibodies may be a marker for the development of retinal vascular occlusion. FFA should be ordered if retinal involvement is suspected in SLE. FFA helps to identify the areas of ischemia, shunt vessels and neovascularization.

Three groups of drugs are mainly used for the treatment of SLE: nonsteroidal anti-inflammatory drugs (NSAIDs), corticosteroids and immunosuppressive agents. Nonspecific manifestations of the disease, such as fever, arthralgia, arthritis and serositis are treated with NSAIDs and antimalarials (chloroquine or hydroxychloroquine). However, antimalarials can cause sight threatening macular disease, leading to decreased vision, abnormal color vision and visual field defects. Systemic corticosteroids are used orally (prednisolone 1–2 mg/kg/d) and intravenously (methylprednisolone 1–2 gm/d for 3 to 6 days) to treat major organ involvement and sight threatening conditions.[1,2,22] Patients unresponsive to systemic steroid often require immunosuppressive therapy. Various immunosuppressive drugs have been tried to treat the sight threatening conditions and complications of SLE and they include azathioprine, cyclophosphamide, chlorambucil, nitrogen mustard, methotrexate, and cyclosporine. It should be kept in mind that proper control of the systemic disease may lead to resolution of ocular manifestations in SLE as ocular involvement in SLE are generally associated with active systemic disease. Antiphospholipid antibodies are associated with the vasoocculusive ocular disease due to formation of microthrombi. Anticoagulation is required in such cases for prevention of thrombosis. Plasmapheresis is often required for the severe acute SLE flares, which involves removal of the plasma, the portion of blood containing antibodies.

Wegener's Granulomatosis

Wegener's granulomatosis (WG) is a granulomatous vasculitis typically involving small- to medium-sized vessels. It is characterized by formation of necrotizing granulomas within blood vessels. There is no specific gender or age predilection.[1,2] More recently WG has been renamed as granulomatosis with polyangitis (GPA).

The classic Wegener triad involves necrotizing granulomas of the respiratory tract, systemic vasculitis, and focal necrotizing glomerulonephritis

(Fig 18.5). However, more often the upper and lower respiratory tracts are affected first with progression to a generalized vasculitis if left untreated. Organs most often affected in WG, in decreasing order, are the upper respiratory tract, lung, kidney, skin, and orbit and eye.

The American Rheumatology Association has published following criteria for the classification and diagnosis of Wegener's Granulomatosis (WG).[24]

A patient shall be said to have Wegener's granulomatosis if at least 2 of these 4 features are present. The presence of any 2 or more features yields a sensitivity of 88.2% and a specificity of 92.0%.

1. Nasal or oral inflammation: Development of painful or painless oral ulcers or purulent or bloody nasal discharge.
2. Abnormal chest radiograph: Chest radiograph showing the presence of nodules, fixed infiltrates, or cavities.
3. Urinary sediment: Microhematuria (>5 red blood cells per high power field) or red cell casts in urine sediment.
4. Granulomatous inflammation on biopsy: Histologic changes showing granulomatous inflammation within the wall of an artery or in the perivascular or extravascular area (artery or arteriole).

Ocular manifestations develop in about 50% of patients with WG/GPA[25]. In 10–15% of patients ocular involvement may be the initial presentation

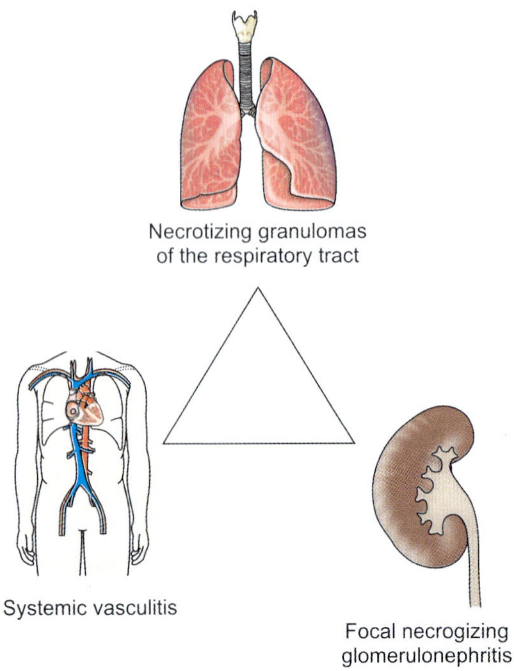

Fig. 18.5: Showing classical Wegener's triad

of the disease. The orbit is most often involved, usually with resultant proptosis. This is the only systemic inflammatory disease that may present with proptosis,[25] which is due to infiltration of the orbit with granulomatous tissue. Orbital inflammation or cellulitis can occur from extensive sinus involvement or secondary to purulent sinusitis and in such cases; bony erosion of the ethmoid and nasal bones is common. Orbital involvement often results in compressive optic neuropathy and ophthalmoplegia.[25]

Scleritis is common in patients with WG/GPA and sometimes it can be presenting manifestation. Scleritis in Wegener granulomatosis is severe and can lead to permanent blindness. Scleritis, which is of necrotizing variety, often associated with peripheral corneal changes and indicates severe systemic involvement and the need for more aggressive immunosuppressive therapy.[10]

The antineutrophil cytoplasmic antibody (ANCA) test has been very helpful in the diagnosis of WG/GPA. Cytoplasmic antineutrophi cytoplasmic antibody (cANCA) that react to proteinase 3 (PR£), is specific for WG/GPA. The sensitivity of cANCAs has been reported as high as 85–96% in patients with widespread Wegener's granulomatosis.[1,2]

With the advent of newer immunosuppressive therapies, patients with WG now have a low mortality rate (13%) and decreased morbidity. Unfortunately, most cases of limited WG eventually progress to renal involvement despite therapy.

The current treatment of choice for Wegener's granulomatosis is oral cyclophosphamide, 2 mg/kg per day along with oral prednisone, 1 mg/kg per day. Corticosteroids can be tapered after a few months as the acute phase of inflammation subsides. Cyclophosphamide therapy is generally continued for a year after remission is achieved. The drug is thus slowly tapered and doses are titrated to prevent leukopenia and neutropenia. Cyclophosphamide is well absorbed orally and completely metabolized within 24 hours by the liver to metabolites which are excreted in the urine. One of these metabolites, acrolein, is known to be responsible for causing hemorrhagic cystitis and bladder cancer. Therefore, it is essential to encourage the patients to drink copious amounts of fluid to reduce the chances of these complications. In severe and nonresponsive cases, infusion of 500 mg of cyclophosphamide (given over 1 to 2 hours) is often required.[1,2,25]

Scleroderma or Systemic Sclerosis

Scleroderma or systemic sclerosis (SS) is a chronic multi-system disorder of unknown etiology. Women are affected three times more often than men and common between 30 and 50 years of age. Black patients are affected twice as frequently as white patients.[1,2]

Systemic involvement of SS can be best defined with the help of following ABCDCREST criteria[2] (Fig 18.6):

- Autoantibodies to various body proteins
- Basilar pulmonary fibrosis detected by chest radiograph as linear shadows or "honeycomb" reticular appearance.
- Contracture of the joints defined as permanent limitation of joint motion. The prayer sign is detected when a patient opposed the palmar surfaces of both hands with extended wrists. The sign is positive when the patient is unable to oppose the palms.
- Dermal thickening
- Calcinosis cutis, most often located on the fingers, is intra- and/or subcutaneous deposits of hydroxyapatite that can ulcerate the skin
- Raynaud's phenomenon is a sudden pallor of an acral structure (e.g. fingers, whole hand, toes, and tip of nose, earlobe, or tongue). Raynaud's phenomenon is observed in 90–98% of SS patients

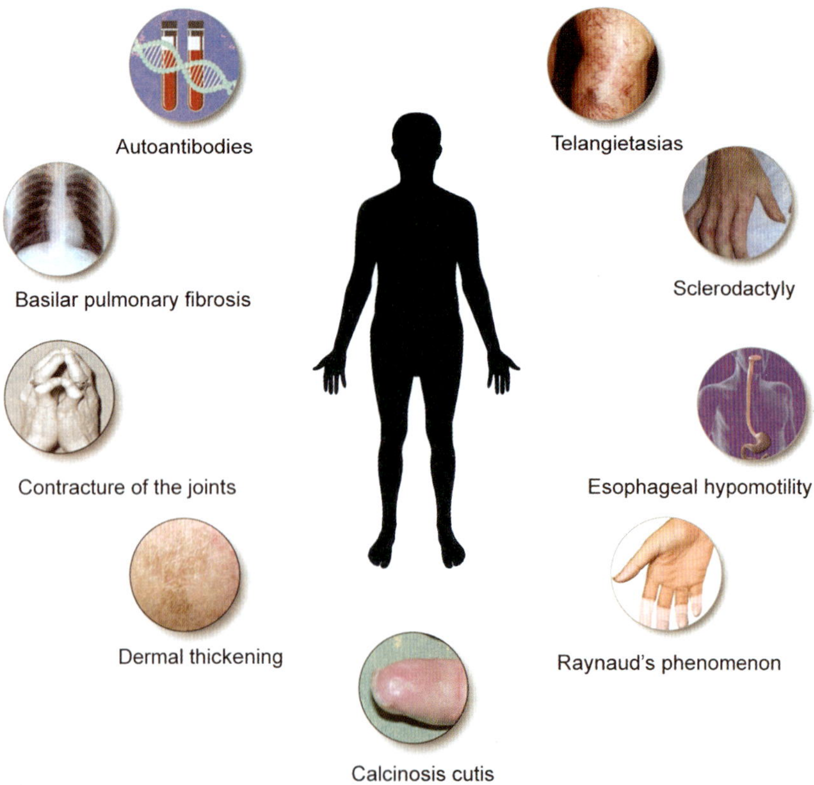

Fig. 18.6: Showing systemic involvement in systemic sclerosis (ABCDCREST Criteria)

- Esophageal distal hypomotility
- Sclerodactyly is symmetric thickening and tightening of the skin on the digits
- Telangiectasias are seen in digits, face, lips, and tongue.

The American Rheumatology Association's criteria for the classification of systemic sclerosis is based on the presence of major and minor features:[1]The patient should fulfil the major criterion or two features of the three minor criteria. (97% sensitive and 98% specific for systemic sclerosis)

Major criteria

- Proximal diffuse (truncal) sclerosis (skin tightness, thickening, non-pitting indurations).

Minor criteria

- Sclerodactyly (only fingers and/or toes)
- Digital pitting scars or loss of substance of the digital finger pads (pulp loss)
- Bilateral basilar pulmonary fibrosis.

Lid stiffness or "woody" texture of the eyelids is seen in 29–65% of patients.[26] Telangiectasia is seen in 17–21% of SS patients and it can be found on either upper or lower lids. It is very small, rarely exceeds 1 mm in diameter, and is best observed with biomicroscopic examination.

The most common ocular manifestation of SS is keratoconjunctivitis sicca, which has been identified to occur in 37–79% of patients.[26,27] Secondary Sjogren syndrome is frequently seen in these patients (Keratoconjunctivitis sicca in association with xerostomia or dry mouth). Corneal involvement in SS is rare; however, filamentous keratitis, exposure keratitis secondary to lid changes and peripheral ulcerative keratitis have all been reported. Retinopathy in SS is similar to that seen in the other systemic vasculitides, with cotton-wool spots, exudates, neuroretinal edema, intraretinal hemorrhages and lipid degeneration. However, retinal involvements were mainly reported in advanced case of scleroderma (with renal involvement and hypertension) and were indistinguishable from hypertensive retinopathy *per se*. And hypertension itself due to renal involvement is a finding affecting 50% of SS patients.[26,27]

There is no disease specific therapy is available for SS as no single drug has been found to treat all of the manifestations of scleroderma. Thus management of SS is based on the symptoms and disease manifestations of each individual patient and is often organ-specific. Various agents used in the treatment of SS include corticosteroids, topical vitamin D3 or calcipotreine ointment, oral antimalarials for morphea, D-penicillamine for skin lesions, and limiting visceral involvement. Keratoconjunctivitis sicca is managed with topical lubricants. As the other ocular manifestations are rare, treatment and management must be dealt with on an individual case basis.

Polyarteritis Nodosa

Polyarteritis nodosa (PAN) is a necrotizing vasculitis of medium-sized arteries. Inflammation in this disorder is mediated by circulating immune complexes. Essentially, all organs can be affected. Men are almost twice as affected as women, usually in the fourth to sixth decades.[1-3]

This disease has almost similar ophthalmic manifestations as seen in systemic lupus erythematosus. However, necrotizing scleritis with peripheral corneal ulceration is relatively more common in PAN patients.[28] Episcleritis is also common in patients with PAN and can be one of the earliest manifestations of the disease.[29] The retinopathy seen in PAN is usually secondary to accelerated hypertension and therefore, characterized by arteriovenous nipping, cotton-wool spots, and flame-shaped hemorrhages. However, cotton-wool spots and arterial occlusion is unusual. Optic nerve involvement is rare.

Corticosteroids and cytotoxic agents remain the cornerstones of treatment in patients with PAN. Approximately, 50% patients with PAN achieve remissions or cures with high doses of corticosteroids alone.[28] Cyclophosphamide is indicated in patients who are refractory to corticosteroids or having serious involvement of major organs.

Ankylosing Spondylitis and the Seronegative Arthropathies

Seronegative spondyloarthropathies are a group of disorders characterized by sacroilitis, oligoarthritis affecting large joints of lower limbs, enthesitis and dactylitis. In these arthopathies tests for rheumatoid factor are usually negative.

Seronegative spondyloarthropathies may be associated with following disorders:
- Ankylosing spondylitis
- Reiter's syndrome, now called as "reactive arthritis"
- Psoriatic arthritis
- Arthritis associated with inflammatory bowel disease (Crohn's, Whipple's, or idiopathic).

ANKYLOSING SPONDYLITIS

Ankylosing spondylitis (AS) is an HLA-B27-associated chronic inflammatory disease of unknown etiology. The term ankylosing spondylitis is derived from the Greek words ankylos ("bent") and spondylos ("vertebral disk"). It affects mainly the sacroiliac joints and the axial skeleton, but peripheral

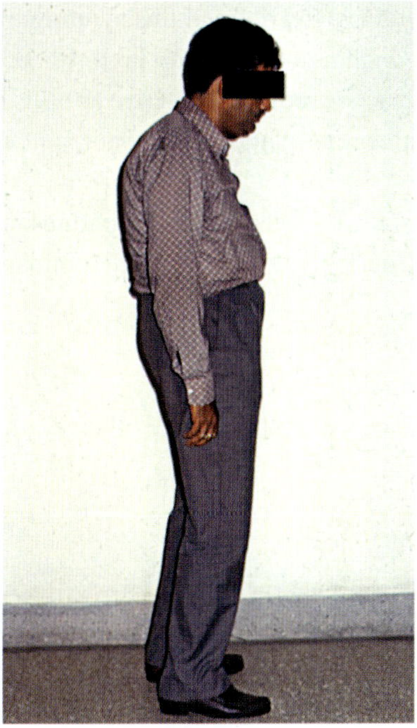

Fig. 18.7: Showing spinal deformity in seronegative spondyloarthropathy

joint involvement may also be seen. The disease is also characterized by extraskeletal manifestations, which includes acute anterior uveitis, aortic incompetence, cardiac conduction defects, and fibrosis of the upper lobes of the lungs, neurologic involvement, or renal (secondary) amyloidosis.

It occurs in 0.2% of the general population and 2% of the HLA B27-positive population.[30-32] Males predominate with a male: female ratio ranging from 2.5:1 to 5:1. It typically begins in young adulthood, but symptoms may start in adolescence or earlier.

Symptoms of spondyloarthropathies usually start with inflammatory back pain. The insidious onset of low back pain and/or buttock pain that persists for more than 3 months, awakens the patient from sleep, is accompanied by early morning stiffness and is typically improved by exercise. If inflammation is not adequately treated, leads to persistent stiffness and progressive loss of spinal mobility (Fig. 18.7).

REITER'S SYNDROME

Reiter's syndrome was first described as a clinical triad of arthritis, nongonoccocal urethritis, and conjunctivitis by Hans Reiter in 1916. Conjunctivitis occurs in one-third of patients with Reiter's disease but there is no increased incidence in the other groups. In 1981 the American

Rheumatism Association (ARA) defined this syndrome as peripheral arthritis lasting longer than 1 month associated with urethritis or cervicitis or diarrhea. Reiter syndrome is a "reactive arthritis. Reactive arthritis differs from infectious arthritis in that the infectious pathogens cannot be cultured from the joint fluid or synovium.[30]

Following characteristics of spondyloarthropathies are reported.[30-33]

- Typical pattern of peripheral arthritis: predominantly of lower limb—asymmetrical
- Tendency to radiographic sacroiliitis
- Absence of rheumatoid factor
- Absence of subcutaneous nodules and other extra-articular features of rheumatoid arthritis
- Overlapping extra-articular features characteristic of the group (e.g., anterior uveitis)
- Significant familial aggregation
- Association with HLA-B27.

European Spondyloarthropathy Study Group (ESSG) has suggested following criteria for the classification of spondyloarthropathies: [1,30]

- Inflammatory spinal pain or synovitis (asymmetric, predominantly in lower limbs) and any one of the features:
- Positive family history
- Psoriasis
- Inflammatory bowel disease
- Alternate buttock pain
- Enthesopathy

It has a sensitivity rate of 77% and specificity of 89%. Adding sacroiliitis, sensitivity becomes 86% and specificity 87%.

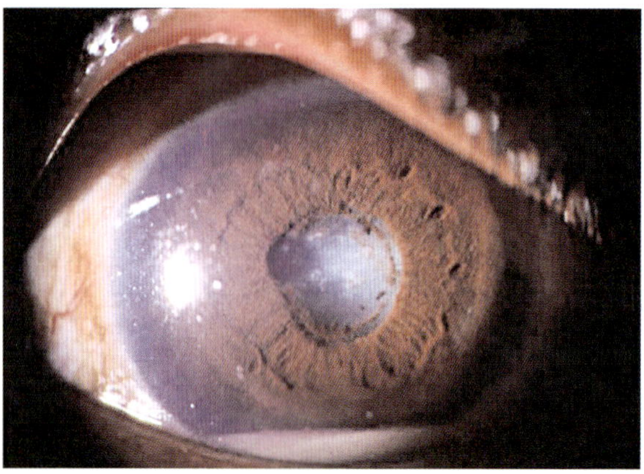

Fig. 18.8: Anterior uveitis with hypopyon in a patient with spondyloarthopathy HLA B27 positive

Acute anterior uveitis with hypopyon (Fig. 18.8) is the most important ocular disease in patients with spondyloarthropathies. It is seen in 25% of patients with ankylosing spondylitis and in 10–15% of patients with other causes of seronegative arthropathy. The clinical symptoms and signs are similar, regardless of the accompanying disease. Attacks are usually unilateral but both eyes become affected during the course of the disease. Acute anterior uveitis is typically abrupt in onset and associated with significant circumcorneal congestion (ciliary flush) and symptoms of pain, photophobia, and watering. Slit-lamp examination reveals a sticky, fibrinoid aqueous in the anterior chamber and posterior synechiae are common. Very few cases (approximately 10% cases) involve the posterior segment secondarily, leading to vision threatening complications, such as cystoid macular edema, vitritis, papillitis, or pars planitis. During acute phase, IOP is usually lowered due to ciliary body shutdown. Increased IOP is due to iris bombé or synechial angle closure, which is a well-recognized complication of the HLA-B27-associated anterior uveitis. It has been observed that patients who are HLA-B27 positive tend to be younger at the time of the first attack,[30,31] and have more severe acute ocular inflammation, which persists for a longer duration.

JUVENILE IDIOPATHIC ARTHRITIS

Juvenile idiopathic arthritis (JIA) was formerly known as juvenile rheumatoid arthritis in the United States and referred to as juvenile chronic arthritis in Europe. It is a group of idiopathic arthritides with an onset before 16 years of age (Fig.18.9) that persists for at least 6 weeks. JIA is the most common cause of arthritis and chronic anterior uveitis in children. The most frequent extra-articular manifestation of JIA is asymptomatic chronic anterior uveitis. Although prognosis of uveitis has shown improvement due to advances in monitoring and treatment, JIA still remains one of the major causes of visual impairment in children with uveitis. Uveitis associated with juvenile idiopathic arthritis has an insidious onset and is usually asymptomatic before the development of sight threatening complications. If juvenile idiopathic

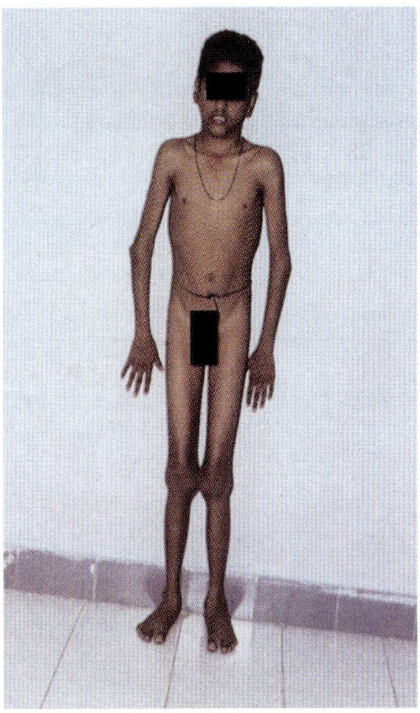

Fig. 18.9: General profile of a child with juvenile ideopathic arthritis

TABLE 18.2: International League of Association of Rheumatology classification of JIA

Arthritis	Definition	Salient features	Uveitis
Systemic arthritis	Arthritis in 1 or more joints accompanied or preceded by fever and accompanied by 1 or more of the following:· • Evanescent (no fixed) erythematous rash· • Generalized lymph node enlargement· • Hepatomegaly and/or splenomegaly· • Serositis	Systemic arthritis is the least common subtype of JIA. Affects girls and boys of any age with equal frequency. The early course is dominated by features including fever, rash, and hepatosplenomegaly. Uveitis is rare in children with this subtype of JIA.	Rare
Oligoarthritis	Arthritis affecting 1–4 joints during the first 6 months of the disease.	Occurs predominantly in young girls.The peak age of onset is 2 to 4 years. The knee is the most commonly affected joint. Rheumatoid factor (RF) is almost always negative.	Most important extra-articular manifestation
Polyarthritis, (rheumatoid factor-negative)	Arthritis affecting 5 or more joints during the first 6 months of the disease; RF is negative.	It is more common in girls. Mean age at onset is older than in children with oligoarthritis. Antinuclear antibody (ANA) is often present whereas RF is absent.	Occurs in approximately 10% of patients
Polyarthritis, (rheumatoid factor-positive)	Arthritis affecting 5 or more joints during the first 6 months of the disease; 2 or more tests for RF, at least 3 months apart during the first 6 months of disease, are positive.	Onset in older children. It shows symmetrical involvement of small joints, especially of hands and feet and large joints.	Very rare
Psoriatic arthritis	Arthritis and psoriasis, or arthritis and at least 2 of the following:· • Dactylitis· • Nail pitting or onycholysis· • Psoriasis in a first-degree relative.		Uveitis occurs in 10% to 20% of patients. Uveitis is reported to be more resistant to therapy than that of oligoarthritis.

Contd...

TABLE 18.2: Contd...

Arthritis	Definition	Salient features	Uveitis
Enthesitis-related arthritis	Arthritis and/or enthesitis (tenderness at the insertion of a tendon, ligament, fascia, or capsule to bone) with at least 2 of the following:· • The presence of or a history of sacroiliac joint tenderness and/ or inflammatory lumbosacral pain· • The presence of HLA-B27 antigen· • Onset of arthritis in a male over 6 years of age· • Acute symptomatic anterior uveitis· • History of ankylosing spondylitis, enthesitis-related arthritis (ERA), sacroiliitis with inflammatory bowel disease, Reiter's syndrome, or acute anterior uveitis in a first-degree relative.	Typically in older boys, most often affects the hip joints. Most patients are HLA-B27 positive and will eventually develop lumbosacral spine disease and sacroiliitis It is more common in older adolescents and adults than in younger children.	Uveitis occurs in 10% to 15% of patients
Undifferentiated or other forms of arthritis	Arthritis that fulfills criteria in no category or in 2 or more of the above categories.	Children in this category account for 5–15% of JIA patients.	NA

arthritis is more severe and widespread, the less likely the child develops uveitis.

The International League of Associations for Rheumatology recently revised the JIA classification system. The classification of JIA defined by the International League of Associations for Rheumatology is tabulated in Table 18.2.

JIA is more common in girls than boys, with a ratio of 3:2. The girls are likely to have 5 times more prolonged course of the disease than boys. They carry a distinctly higher risk of developing uveitis than boys. Risk factors for developing JIA uveitis include ANA positivity and early age at onset of arthritis (<6 years).[34-36]

JIA-associated uveitis is typically a nongranulomatous, asymptomatic anterior uveitis with a chronic course. The condition is bilateral; in majority of cases both eyes are involved either simultaneously or within few months of each other. Keratic precipitates are from small to medium in size; sometimes mutton fat keratic precipitates are also seen. In severe cases, cells can be seen in the anterior vitreous and the inflammation may involve the posterior parts of the eye, sometimes resulting in cystoid macular edema.

Generally, uveitis is diagnosed after the onset of arthritis. As it is primarily a joint disease, most of the patients remain under care of a pediatric rheumatologist. However, it is essential that all of the arthritis patients should be evaluated by an ophthalmologist for any evidence of uveitis. Similarly, all children with uveitis should be examined by a pediatric rheumatologist. Reported risk factors for ocular involvement in patients with JIA include female sex, oligoarticular arthritis, onset of arthritis at young age, ANA seropositivity, and RF seronegativity.

JIA-associated uveitis may result in severe visual impairment due to complications like cataract, glaucoma, hypotony, maculopathy, and amblyopia. Chronic uveitis can cause damage to ocular tissue. Long-standing intraocular inflammation, such as is seen in JIA may cause band keratopathy, where an accumulation of calcium is seen at the level of Bowman's membrane in the cornea, usually confined to the interpalpebral zone.

Although the inflammation in JIA-associated uveitis is primarily anterior in nature, chronic active inflammation can result in permanent structural alterations also in the posterior parts of the eye. Predictive factors for poor visual outcome include increased severity of uveitis at initial examination, onset of uveitis before or at the time of arthritis diagnosis, short duration between onset of arthritis and ocular involvement, and male sex.

JIA is a diagnosis of exclusion, there is no particular specific laboratory test to diagnose this condition. Evaluation of such patient includes a detailed history and general examination, with particular attention to the musculoskeletal system including joints, muscles, enthuses and soft tissues. Frequent periodic examinations are recommended (Table 18.3).

Treatment

Early diagnosis followed by prompt treatment is critical if one is to preserve vision in children with JIA uveitis. The goal of treatment is to achieve complete quiescence of inflammation in order to prevent sight threatening complications.

Topical corticosteroids are usually the first line of therapy. The dose of topical steroid should be titrated based upon the cellular reaction in the anterior chamber. Ultimate aim is to use as little topical steroid as possible to maintain quiescence of the inflammation. If a child requires more frequent topical steroids, one can consider adding systemic therapy.

TABLE 18.3: Showing periodic examinations of JIA patients

Frequency of screening	Eyes	Clinical conditions Joints
Every 6 weeks	High risk for the development of asymptomatic uveitis and of complications	Oligoarthritis, RF-negative polyarthritis, early onset psoriatic arthritis
Every 3 months	High risk for the development of asymptomatic uveitis and of complications that did not develop uveitis after a 2-year follow-up	Oligoarthritis/RF-negative polyarthritis/early onset psoriatic arthritis
	Low risk of asymptomatic uveitis should be continued until 7 years after diagnosis	Systemic arthritis /RF-positive polyarthritis
Every 6 months	Typical symptomatic uveitis	Enthesitis related arthritis/late onset psoriatic arthritis
	Others that did not develop uveitis until 7 years after arthritis	

Short-acting mydriatics and cycloplegics are of paramount importance, to keep the pupil mobile and prevent formation of posterior synechiae. However, it should be kept in mind that constant cycloplegia may result in amblyopia and synechiae in dilated position can develop, if the pupil is not moving. Periocular depot corticosteroid injections are sometime helpful in reducing ocular inflammation in cases unresponsive to topical corticosteroids. The periocular corticosteroid injections should be used with caution because of the steroid induced glaucoma.

Methotrexate is the most commonly used first-line agent when long-term systemic immunosuppression or adjunctive therapy is required. Due to their overwhelming side effects on growth and bone formation, many clinicians avoid oral prednisone and start oral methotrexate when systemic therapy is required. It should be kept in mind that methotrexate usually takes 4 to 8 weeks to produce a desired immunosuppressive effect. Methotrexate is usually given orally, however it can be administered intramuscularly or subcutaneously. The most common side effects are gastrointestinal, including nausea, vomiting, diarrhea, dyspepsia. Other side effects include hepatotoxicity and bone marrow suppression, both of which are usually reversible with dose reduction. Liver enzymes and complete blood counts are monitored every 4–6 weeks. Folic acid supplementation is recommended to reduce risk of bone marrow suppression. Dosage of methotrexate is 0.1–0.5 mg/kg/week; low dose therapy is started at a dose of 7.5 mg/week and it can be increased to 25 mg/week, generally given orally once a week.

Azathioprine and cyclosporine are often used in the treatment of JIA. Azathioprine is a purine analog that is rapidly converted to 6-mercaptopurine in the liver. The major adverse effect of azathioprine is bone marrow suppression; however, this affect is generally dose related and reversible. Cyclosporine is an amino acid peptide that selectively inhibits T cells. The most common and serious side effect of cyclosporine is nephrotoxicity, which is seen almost universally at high doses of 10 mg/kg. Lower doses of 3–5 mg/kg are generally used to treat uveitis, and are associated with a lower risk of nephrotoxicity. Toxicity is usually reversible with discontinuation of the medication.

GIANT-CELL ARTERITIS

Giant-cell arteritis (GCA) is a necrotizing vasculitis which involves large and medium-sized vessels. Patients are generally older than 60 years of age. Giant-cell arteritis forms a clinical spectrum with polymyalgia rheumatica, which is characterized by arthralgia and myalgia of the shoulder and pelvic girdle.

Approximately 25% of patients of giant cell arteritis develop ocular disease and the majority experience sudden loss of vision in one eye, with a dense, inferior, altitudinal field defect. It is an ophthalmic emergency and an important cause of preventable blindness in elderly people. The cause of the blindness is ischemic optic neuropathy (infarction of the optic nerve), and occlusion of the central retinal artery in a minority of cases. The American College of Rheumatology suggested criteria of diagnosis of GCA[1,3] (Table 18.4).

Rare neuro-ophthalmological complications of giant-cell arteritis are oculomotor palsies, Horner's syndrome, cortical blindness, internuclear ophthalmoplegia and visual hallucinations.

When GCA is strongly suspected in some patient and there is no associated history of visual loss, oral corticosteroid should be administered and the patient should be referred for a temporal artery biopsy. Temporal artery biopsy has almost zero mortality and very low morbidity and it is the only test that can confirm the diagnosis of GCA. Unilateral temporal artery

TABLE 18.4: American College of Rheumatology criteria for diagnosis of giant-cell arteritis

1. Age over 50 years
2. New onset of headache
3. Scalp tenderness or decreased temporal artery pulse
4. Erythrocyte-sedimentation rate greater than 50 mm/h
5. Positive temporal-artery biopsy.

biopsy is about 90% sensitive and bilateral biopsies are about 95% sensitive.

Patients with suspected GCA who have experienced transient visual loss for a few hours should be admitted and given high-dose intravenous methylprednisolone for 3–5 days as soon as possible. Visual loss of more than 24 hour's duration is almost always permanent. It has been shown in various retrospective studies that the addition of low-dose aspirin (80–100 mg/day) reduces by five folds the risk of blindness or stroke in GCA.[3]

References

1. Imboden JB, Hellmann DB, Stone JH: Current Rheumatology Diagnosis and Treatment, Second Edition, McGraw-Hill Companies Inc; 2007
2. Isenberg DA, Maddison PJ, Woo P, Glass D, Breedveld FC: Oxford Textbook of Rheumatology. 3rd Edition, Oxford University Press; 2004.
3. Firestein GS, Budd RC, Harris ED Jr., et al, Kelley's Textbook of Rheumatology. 8th ed. Philadelphia, Saunders Elsevier; 2008
4. Gabriel SE. The epidemiology of rheumatoid arthritis. *Rheum Dis Clin North Am*. 2001;27:269.
5. Aletaha D, Neogi T, Silman AJ, Funovits J, Felson DT, Bingham CO, III et al. 2010 Rheumatoid arthritis classification criteria: an American College of Rheumatology/ European League Against Rheumatism collaborative initiative. *Ann Rheum Dis.* 2010;69(9):1580-8.
6. Fuerst DJ, Tanzer DJ, Smith RE. Rheumatoid diseases. *Int Ophthalmol Clin*. 1998;38:47-80.
7. Harper SL, Foster CS. The ocular manifestations of rheumatoid disease. *Int Ophthalmol Clin*. 1998;38:1-19.
8. Whitcher JP Jr, Gritz DC, Daniels TE. The dry eye: a diagnostic dilemma. *Int Ophthalmol Clin*. 1998;38:23-37.
9. Friedlaender MH. Ocular manifestations of Sjögren's syndrome: keratoconjunctivitis sicca. *Rheum Dis Clin North Am*. 1992;18:591-608.
10. Pavesio CE, Meier FM. Systemic disorders associated with episcleritis and scleritis. *Curr Opin Ophthalmol*. 2001;12(6):471-8.
11. Calonge M: The treatment of dry eye. Surv Ophthalmol 2001; 45(Suppl 2)): S227-S239.
12. Stevenson D, Tauber J, Reis BL: Efficacy and safety of cyclosporin a ophthalmic emulsion in the treatment of moderate-to-severe dry eye disease: A dose-ranging, randomized trial. The Cyclosporin A Phase 2 Study Group. *Ophthalmology.* 2000;107:967-74.
13. Sall K, Stevenson OD, Mundorf TK, et al: Two multicenter, randomized studies of the efficacy and safety of cyclosporine ophthalmic emulsion in moderate to severe dry eye disease. CsA Phase 3 Study Group. *Ophthalmology*. 2000;107: 631-639.
14. Tananuvat N, Daniell M, Sullivan LJ, et al: Controlled study of the use of autologous serum in dry eye patients. *Cornea*. 2001;20:802-6.
15. Noble BA, Loh RS, MacLennan S, et al: Comparison of autologous serum eye drops with conventional therapy in a randomised controlled crossover trial for ocular surface disease. *Br J Ophthalmol.* 2004;88:647-652.
16. Murube J, Murube E: Treatment of dry eye by blocking the lacrimal canaliculi. *Surv Ophthalmol.* 1996;40:463-480.

17. Liegner JT, Yee RW, Wild JH: Topical cyclosporine therapy for ulcerative keratitis associated with rheumatoid arthritis. *Am J Ophthalmol.* 1990;109:610-12.
18. Holland EJ, Olsen TW, Ketcham JM, et al: Topical cyclosporin A in the treatment of anterior segment inflammatory disease. *Cornea*. 1993;12:413-9.
19. Rachitskaya A, Mandelcorn ED, Albini TA.: An update on the cause and treatment of scleritis. *Curr Opin Ophthalmol*. 2010;21(6):463-7.
20. Thomas AA, Narsing AR, Ronald ES. The Diagnosis and Management of Anterior Scleritis. *Int Ophthalmol Clin*. 2005;45(2):191-204.
21. American College of Rheumatology Ad Hoc Committee on Systemic Lupus Erythematosus Guidelines. Guidelines for referral and management of systemic lupus erythematosus in adults. *Arthritis Rheum*. 1999;42:1785.
22. Arevalo JF, Lowder CY, Muci-Mendoza R. Ocular manifestations of systemic lupus erythematosus. *Curr Opin Ophthalmol*. 2002;13(6):404-10.
23. Davies JB, Rao PK. Ocular manifestations of systemic lupus erythematosus. *Curr Opin Ophthalmol*. 2008;19(6):512-8.
24. Leavitt RY, Fauci AS, Bloch DA, Michel BA, Hunder GG, Arend WP, et al. The American College of Rheumatology 1990 criteria for the classification of Wegener's granulomatosis. *Arthritis Rheum*. 1990;33:1101-07.
25. Harman LE, Margo CE. Wegener's granulomatosis. *Survey of Ophthalmology.* 1998;42:458-80
26. Tailor R, Gupta A, Herrick A, Kwartz J. Ocular manifestations of scleroderma. *Surv Ophthalmol*. 2009 Mar-Apr;54(2):292-304.
27. West RH, Barnett AJ. Ocular involvement in scleroderma. *Br J Ophthalmol.* 1979;63(12):845-847.
28. Akova YA, Jabbur NS, Foster CS: Ocular presentation of polyarteritis nodosa: clinical course and management with steroid and cytotoxic therapy. *Ophthal-mology.* 1993,100:1775-81.
29. Yamamoto S, Takeuchi S: Episcleritis as the primary clinical manifestation in a patient with polyarteritis nodosa. *Jpn J Ophthalmol.* 2000,44:151-3.
30. Ali A, Samson CM. Seronegative spondyloarthropathies and the eye. *Curr Opin Ophthalmol*. 2007;18(6):476-80.
31. Wakefield D, Montanaro A, McCluskey P. Acute anterior uveitis and HLA-B27. *Surv Ophthalmol*. 1991;36:223-32.
32. Brewerton DA, Caffrey M, Nicholls A. Acute anterior uveitis and HLA-B27. *Lancet.* 1973;2:994-6.
33. Chang JH, McCluskey PJ, Wakefield D. Acute anterior uveitis and HLA-B27. *Surv Ophthalmol*. 2005;50:364-88.
34. Foster CS. Diagnosis and treatment of juvenile idiopathic arthritis-associated uveitis *Curr Opin Ophthalmol*. 2003,14:395-398
35. Holland GN, Denove CS, YU F. Chronic Anterior Uveitis in Children: Clinical Characteristics and Complications. *Am J Ophthalmol*. 2009;147:667-78.
36. Kotaniemi K, Savolainen A, Karma A, Aho K. Recent advances in uveitis of juvenile idiopathic arthritis. *Surv Ophthalmol*. 2003;48(5):489-502.

19

chapter

Paramdeep Singh
Rupinderjeet Kaur

An Update on Imaging in Neuro-ophthalmology

ABSTRACT

Advancements in imaging techniques such as, computed tomography, and magnetic resonance imaging in the last century have revolutionized the early diagnosis, prognosis, and treatment of many neuro-ophthalmological disorders. The relatively recent techniques comprise magnetic resonance (MR) spectroscopy, magnetic resonance angiography, computed tomography angiography, single photon emission computed tomography, positron emission tomography and functional MR imaging. A timely prescription of an appropriate imaging technique and the appropriate sequence can increase the diagnostic yield. The basic principles and applications of neuroimaging in neuro-ophthalmology are described.

Introduction

Imaging techniques for visualizing pathology of the brain and orbit continue to advance and develop. Revolutionary advancements in the speed of data acquisition and resolution of CT scanning and MRI have provided essential tools for assessment of the brain and orbit. The relatively new techniques such as magnetic resonance (MR) spectroscopy, computed tomography (CT) angiography, positron emission tomography (PET), and functional MR imaging have guided to early anatomical and functional diagnosis and treatment of many neurovisual disorders. This chapter provides a brief review of the most frequently used imaging techniques of value to ophthalmologists (e.g., CT and MRI, digital subtraction angiography [DSA]) and also reviews the recent literature on newer modalities for imaging. It will also update clinicians regarding special MR imaging sequences and discusses functional imaging. Ophthalmologists should be familiar with these neuroimaging techniques as well as with the typical or characteristic images of the pathological conditions.

Indications for Neuroimaging in Ophthalmology

The most frequent indications[1] for an ophthalmologist to request a neuroimaging study are:

1. Visual acuity or visual field loss (e.g. amaurosis fugax, optic neuropathy, scotoma, and hemianopsia)
2. Anisocoria or ptosis (e.g. Horner's syndrome, third nerve palsy)
3. Proptosis (e.g. thyroid eye disease, orbital tumor or orbital pseudotumor)
4. Diplopia or ophthalmoplegia (e.g. ocular motor cranial neuropathy, supranuclear and internuclear ophthalmoplegia)
5. Oscillopsia (e.g. nystagmus)
6. Ophthalmoscopic abnormalities (e.g. papilledema).

Imaging Techniques

Following imaging techniques will be briefly discussed:

1. Computed tomography (CT)
2. Magnetic resonance imaging (MRI), including MR spectroscopy
3. Digital subtraction angiography
4. CT and MR angiography
5. Functional imaging techniques (fMRI, PET and SPECT).

COMPUTED TOMOGRAPHY

Basic Principles

The CT imaging involves the rapid rotation of a large X-ray tube around the patient and is based on attenuation of ionizing radiation (X-rays) by different tissues possessing different densities. The resultant transmitted radiation is measured by multi detectors housed in a gantry, and the data collected by the detectors is analyzed by a computer. Newer CT scanners can obtain continuous data in a helical fashion. Helical CT allows the X-ray tube and the detectors to continually rotate around the patient. The advantages of helical CT over conventional CT are: (i) shorter scan times, (ii) less motion artifacts and radiation exposure, and (iii) better sensitivity for detecting a foreign body.

The Hounsfield unit (HU) is a quantitative scale for describing radiodensity. This scale allocates water as an attenuation value of zero. Denser tissues attenuate the X-ray beam, and less dense tissues allow the beam to pass through to the detectors. Consequently, dense tissues like bone appear brighter (positive Hounsfield units) on CT and less dense tissues such as air appear darker (negative Hounsfield units).

Orbital and cranial CT scans are commonly advised. They are simple to perform, relatively economical and can be acquired rapidly. An orbital CT is different from a head CT, since it is angled in a different way and uses thinner slices. It is often imperative to obtain at least two views of the orbit on imaging. The most frequently performed views are axial and coronal (Figs 19.1 and 19.2). The contrast material for CT scanning is iodinated. Contrast allergy and renal failure are contraindications to iodinated contrast for CT.[2]

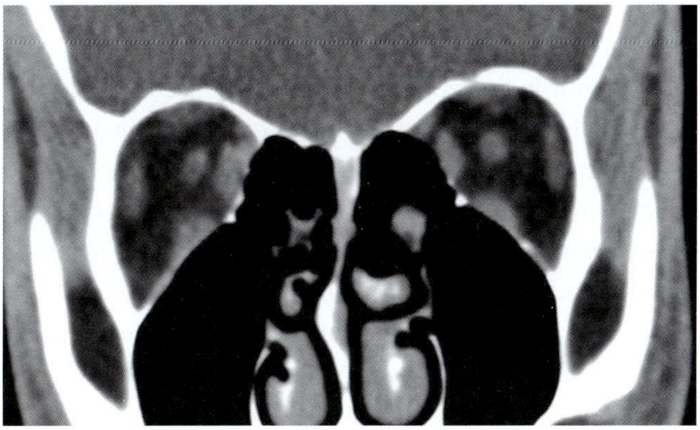

Fig. 19.1: Coronal CT scan of the orbit at the mid orbit level showing normal optic nerves and extraocular muscles

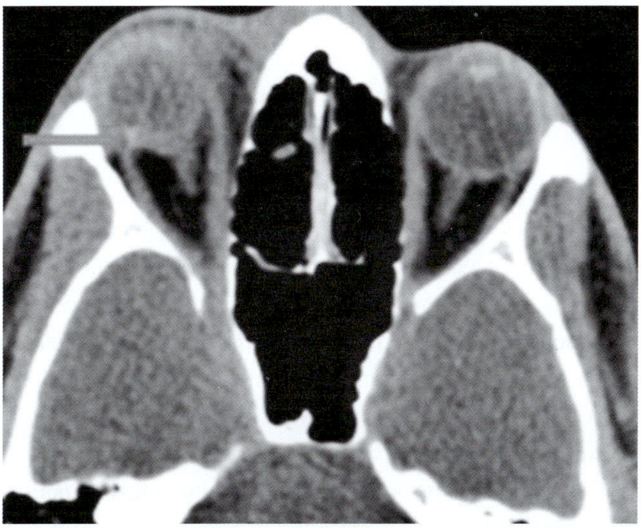

Fig. 19.2: Axial CT scan of the orbit showing hyperdense foreign body (arrow) and thickened coats of right eyeball

Clinical Indications

The clinical indications[3] for CT scanning for neuro-ophthalmologists and orbital surgeons include:

1. Orbital disorders, such as thyroid, trauma, infection, and tumor
2. Sinus and lacrimal disorders
3. Calcification
4. Acute intracranial bleeds
5. Contraindications to MR imaging
6. Osseous abnormalities, such as erosion, hyperostosis, fractures, and calcifications.

In emergency setting, a C T scan may be requested by an ophthalmologist for severe acute headache, an acute bitemporal hemianopsia or diplopia (e.g. pituitary apoplexy), or acute papilledema.

Enhancement with iodinated contrast agents is used to detect intracranial extension of orbital tumors and to evaluate optic chiasmal lesions. CT has the advantage over MR imaging of requiring less time period, being less costly, and being valid in patients in whom MR imaging is contraindicated or in whom it cannot be done. CT is superior to MRI in the assessment of bony structures and the presence of blood; therefore, it is excellent in trauma. Other advantages of CT include detection of calcification, orbital tumors, or even optic disk drusen.

The disadvantages of CT scanning include ionizing radiation exposure, reactions to iodinated contrast agents, and dental or osseous artifacts. MR imaging more sensitive than CT for the detection of soft tissue pathology such as brain, and is the investigation of choice for almost all neuro-ophthalmic disorders. Although the common availability of CT scan and the fast scan time make it more valuable than MR for patients requiring imaging in an emergency setting, a MR scan can still be needed later for further assessment of the pathology.[4-9]

MAGNETIC RESONANCE IMAGING

Basic Principles

Magnetic resonance imaging (MRI) is the technically most complex imaging modality in radiodiagnosis but it also has the largest diagnostic potential. In the simplest terms, MRI is a technique that produces images by means of magnetic fields and radio waves. MR imaging is based on the ability of a small number of protons within the body to absorb and emit radio wave energy when the body is placed within a strong magnetic field. The soft tissue contrast provided by MRI is significantly superior to any other imaging procedure. Differences in the density of protons available to contribute to the MR signal discriminate one tissue from another. Different tissues absorb and release radio wave energy at different, detectable, and characteristic rates.

Examples of MRI Pulse Sequences

T1- and T2-weighted images

Various pulse-sequence techniques are used in MRI, but the most archetypal are T1- and T2-weighted images. What do T1 and T2 mean? T1 measures the ability of protons in a tissue to exchange energy with the surrounding environment, or how fast the tissue can become magnetized? T2 measures how quickly it loses its magnetization. Fat appears relatively bright and water relatively dark on T1-weighted images, whereas the reverse is true on T2-weighted images (Figs 19.3 and 19.4). As a common rule, T1-weighted images are good for viewing anatomy, and T2-weighted images are superior for detecting pathology.

T1 orbital sequence with fat suppression

Fat-suppression techniques are used in MR imaging to identify the presence of fat or to suppress signal from fat (Fig. 19.5) to augment recognition of the pathology (tumor invasion into fat or edema in fat). Gadolinium is administered to improve detection of pathology. This sequence is helpful to make a diagnosis of optic nerve sheath meningiomas and optic neuritis, which take up gadolinium and look bright. These pathologies are not concealed

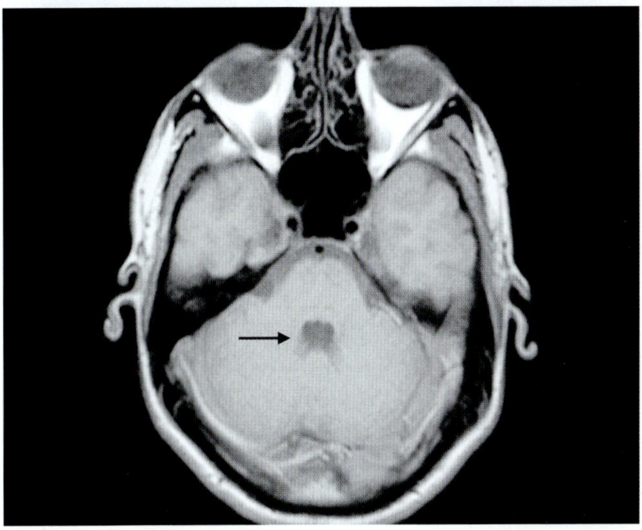

Fig. 19.3: T1-weighted MR image showing dark CSF in 4th ventricle (arrow) and bright orbital fat

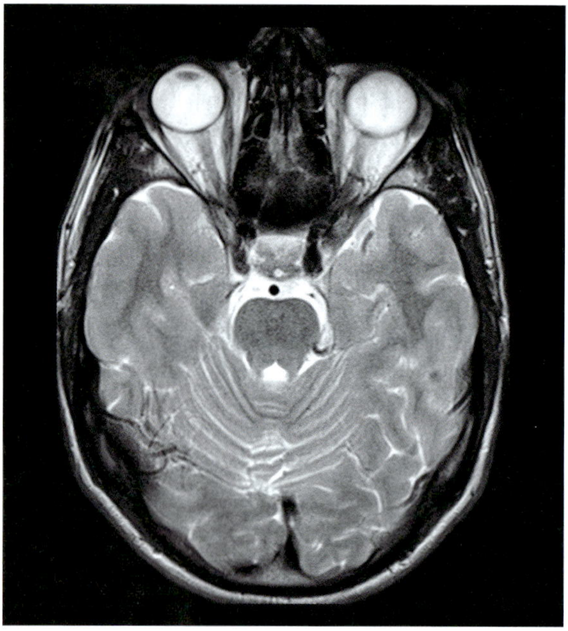

Fig. 19.4: T2-weighted image showing bright CSF in 4th ventricle and bright orbital fat

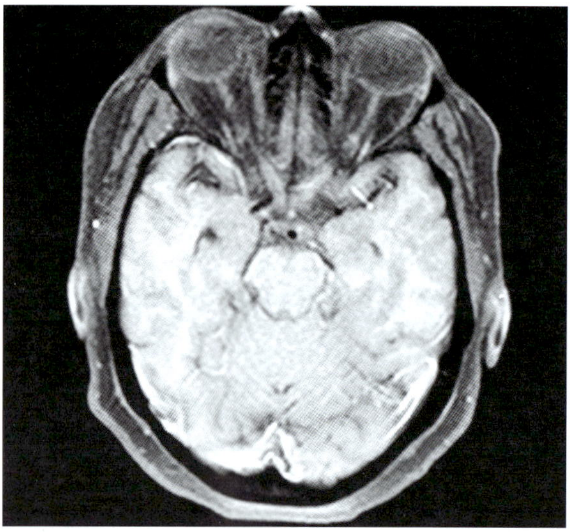

Fig. 19.5: T1 orbital sequence with fat suppression showing dark orbital fat (due to fat suppression) as well as dark CSF in 4th ventricle

by orbital fat once fat suppression is used.

T2-weighted sequence with fat suppression

T2-weighted sequence with fat suppression sequence is helpful for accurately imaging the anatomy of the optic nerve and the CSF-space surrounding the optic nerve (perioptic space).

Fluid-attenuated inversion recovery

Fluid-attenuated inversion recovery (FLAIR) sequence suppresses the bright signal from fluid in T2-weighted images (Fig. 19.6). Therefore, the CSF looks dark which allows the bright MS plaques to be better visualized (particularly when located close to the ventricular system) and let not concealed them by bright-appearing CSF.

Diffusion-weighted sequence

Diffusion-weighted sequence (DWI) is used to identify the acute cerebral infarctions (Fig. 19.7) within the first hours of stroke. The most valuable application of DWI for the neuro-ophthalmologist, is the capability to detect hyperacute ischemic lesions (bright on DWI) producing a homonymous hemianopia or cortical visual impairment.

Gradient echo sequences

Gradient echo sequences (GRE) can show hemorrhage on MR scans (Fig. 19.8) in patients with underlying vascular malformations, intracerebral hemorrhage, or traumatic brain injury.

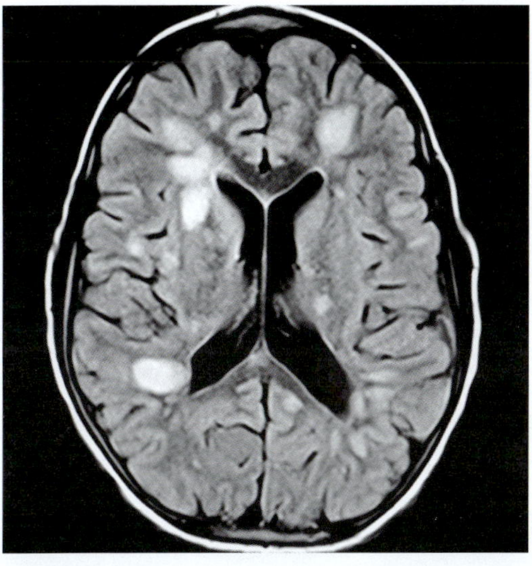

Fig. 19.6: Axial FLAIR image at the level of the lateral ventricles showing multiple periventricular white matter hyperintense lesions, suggestive of multiple sclerosis

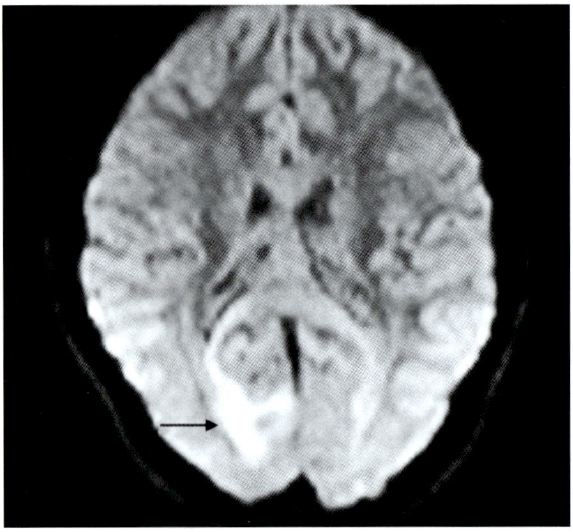

Fig. 19.7: Axial diffusion-weighted image showing hyperintense area of diffusion restriction (arrow) in right occipital lobe

Contrast material for MR imaging improves recognition of primary pathology by demonstrating areas of breakdown of the blood-brain barrier. In comparison to the iodinated contrast for CT, the contrast used for MRI is a paramagnetic substance called gadolinium. Gadolinium does not produce cross-reactions in patients with allergies to iodinated contrast.[10-13]

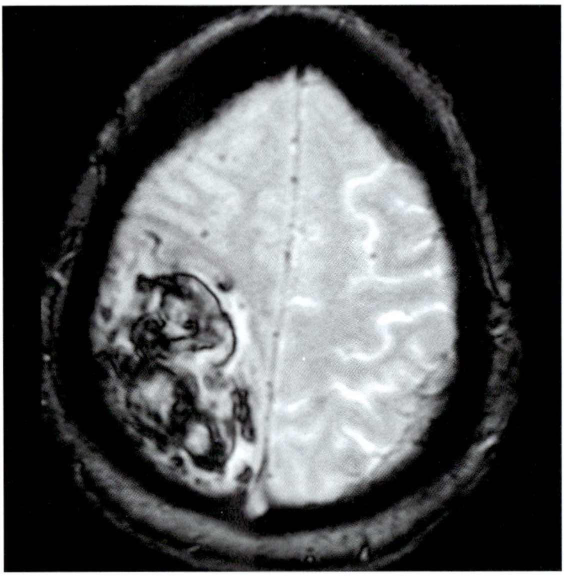

Fig. 19.8: Axial GRE image showing area of hemorrhage (blooming) in right high parietal region

APPEARANCE OF VARIOUS TISSUES AND BODY FLUIDS ON MRI

Appearance of different tissues and body fluids on MRI is shown in Table 19.1.[14]

Advantages of MRI

There are many advantages of MRI over the other cross-sectional imaging modalities. It does not use ionizing radiation. It can generate images through an entire section of the body, and the image quality is not affected by the presence of bone or air in the imaging plane. MR imaging provides a superior soft tissue contrast as compared to other imaging modalities and is able to create images in multiple planes, including sagittal, coronal and axial. It also enables visualization of vascular structures with or without the administration of contrast material.

Disadvantages of MRI

As compared with the other imaging modalities, MRI is relatively costly and not commonly available. Some patients cannot undergo MRI examination, for instance those who are having cardiac pacemakers or other electrical devices in which the magnet would create currents, patients with certain ferromagnetic foreign objects, for example, cerebral aneurysm clips and highly claustrophobic patients.

TABLE 19.1: Appearance of tissues and body fluids on MRI

Tissue/body fluid	Examples	T1W signal	T2W signal
• Gas	Air in lung, gas in bowel	Absent	Absent
• Mineral-rich tissue	Cortical bone, calculi	Absent	Absent
• Collagenous tissue	Ligaments, tendons, fibro-cartilage, scar tissue	Low	Low
• Fat	Adipose tissue, fatty bone marrow	High to high	Intermediate
• High bound water tissue	Liver, pancreas, adrenal, muscle, hyaline cartilage	Low	Low to intermediate
• High free water tissue	Kidney, testes, prostate, seminal vesicles, ovary, thyroid, spleen, penis, simple cysts, bladder, gallbladder, edema, urine, bile, CSF	Low	High
• Proteinaceous fluid	Complicated cysts, abscess, synovial fluid, nucleus pulposis	Intermediate	High

MR SPECTROSCOPY

MR spectroscopy (MRS) is a noninvasive technique capable of measuring chemicals within the body. It distinguishes various metabolites on the basis of their slightly different chemical shifts or resonance frequencies. The metabolic information received is displayed as a graph (Fig. 19.9). The magnetic resonance spectroscopy is used in neuro-ophthalmology in distinguishing ischemic, neoplastic, demyelinating, inflammatory, and mitochondrial disorders affecting the visual pathway as well as side effects of radiation therapy. [10-13]

ANGIOGRAPHY

Digital Subtraction Angiography

Digital subtraction angiography (DSA) uses X-rays and iodine-based intra-arterial contrast material delivered through a catheter. DSA subtracts the other structures like bone. A picture of just blood vessels is generated, unobscured by unnecessary bone and other tissue. DSA remains the gold standard for imaging the extracranial and intracranial vasculature and particularly for detecting cerebral aneurysms. Nowadays, many DSA studies have been replaced by less invasive techniques, such as three-dimensional CT angiography (3D CTA) and MR angiography.

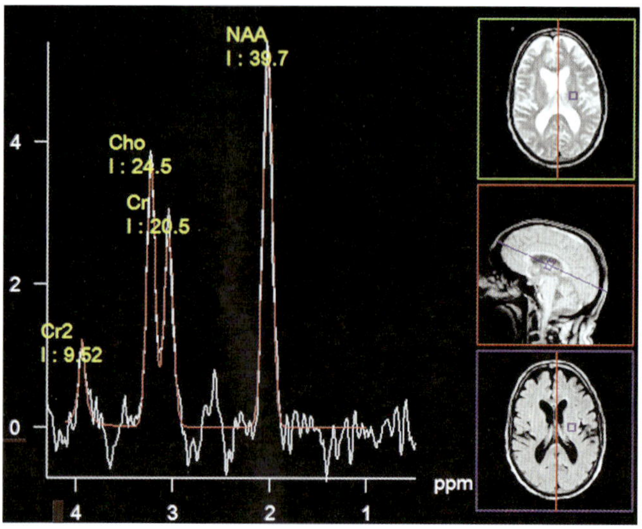

Fig. 19.9: Magnetic resonance spectroscopy (MRS). This normal MRS graph shows the magnetic resonance spectra for choline, creatinine, and N-acetyl-aspartate peaks

CT Angiography

CT angiography (CTA) also involves the use of X-rays and iodine-based contrast material; the contrast is injected into the antecubital vein. Intravenous bolus of contrast material is followed by high-speed spiral CT scanning during which patient is moved through the scanner during one breath hold.

The data are extracted, and by post-processing three-dimensional displays (Figs 19.10A and B) are generated. There are two main types of three-dimensional displays: shaded surface display (SSD) and maximum intensity projection (MIP). The SSD shows surface anatomy with color, in a three-dimensional view. The MIP shows only the blood vessel, without color. The advantages of CT angiography over MR angiography are a shorter examination time, a superior image resolution, harmless in patients with aneurysm clips and pacemakers, and less claustrophobia issues. CT angiography can also outline surgical anatomy finer than MR angiography, and the data are obtained faster and safer than with DSA.

MR Angiography

Main advantage of MR angiography (Fig. 19.11) is that it does not use ionizing radiation or iodinated contrast material. Three types of procedures are used: (i) three-dimensional time of flight (3D TOF), (ii) two-dimensional time of flight (2D TOF), and (iii) gadolinium MR angiography. The first two methods need no gadolinium. However, these are dependent on directional blood flow to generate the image. Gadolinium MR angiography does not depend on directional flow to generate the image. [15-24]

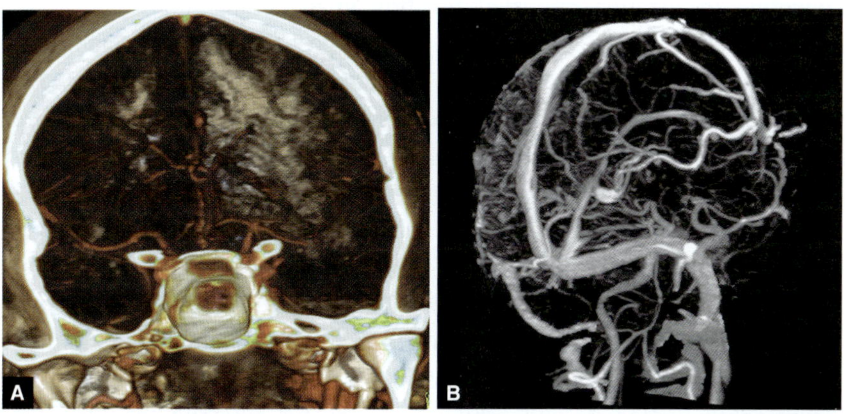

Figs 19.10A and B: Three-dimensional computed tomography angiograms of the brain. Note the simultaneous demonstration of the surrounding osseous landmarks in Figure A

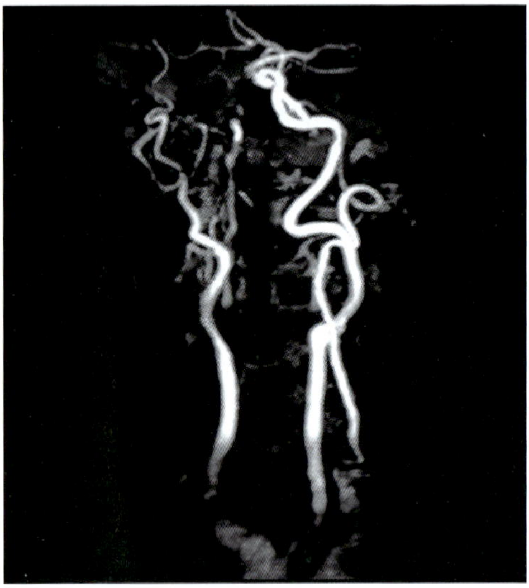

Fig. 19.11: Maximum intensity projection (MIP) of 2D time of flight (TOF) angiogram showing extra-cranial neck vessels

FUNCTIONAL MAGNETIC RESONANCE IMAGING

Functional MR imaging is based on changes in T2 signal because of deoxyhemoglobin. This signal change is termed the blood oxygenation level dependent (BOLD) mechanism. A local increase in neuronal activity leads to increased cerebral blood flow and a decrease in deoxyhemoglobin. The functional magnetic resonance (MR) imaging techniques have been used for presurgical mapping of brain function and have provided new information regarding localization of visual function in the brain.[25]

Other functional imaging studies include positron emission tomography (PET) and single photon emission computed tomography (SPECT). PET and SPECT imaging (Fig.19.12) are done with systemically administered isotopes that release protons to image biological processes that measure regional cerebral blood flow (CBF) and glucose consumption and therefore, indirectly, metabolism of tissues. Patients undergoing functional imaging might show hypometabolism ("cold") or hypermetabolism ("hot") in areas where structural imaging procedures (CT or MR imaging) were normal.

PET is presently used by vision neuroscientists to understand the anatomical correlates of visual function. PET imaging is also used by the neuro-ophthalmologists and orbital surgeons for studying the functional correlates of human diseases such as cancers and metastatic disease.

Positron emission tomography can also be useful in the study of visual pathways involved in amblyopia and also the oculomotor repair during the

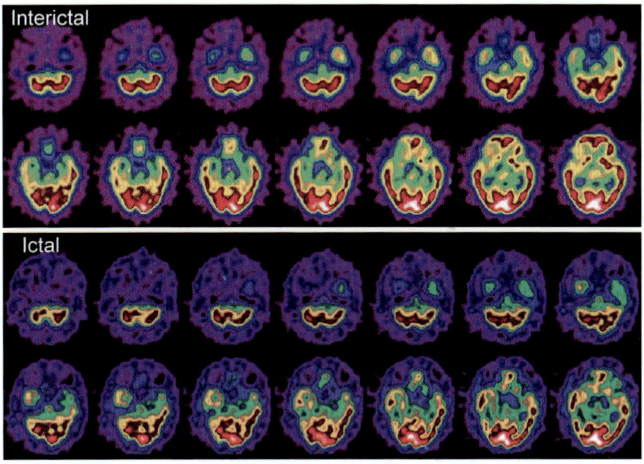

Fig. 19.12: Images of SPECT scan in a patient presenting with epilepsy and visual disturbances showing hypoperfusion in right temporal region in both interictal and ictal phases

period just after a stroke. PET has also proved to be a successful tool for understanding the effects of pharmaceutical agents, such as neuroprotectants, as well as new and evolving drugs for dementia, Alzheimer's disease, and optic neuropathies.[26-30]

Conclusion

Recent advances in imaging techniques for brain and orbit have improved the diagnostic yield. A well-timed communication with the radiologist can optimize the prescription and interpretation of imaging in ophthalmology.

References

1. Lee AG, Brazis PW, Garrity JA, White M. Imaging for neuro-ophthalmic and orbital disease. *Am J Ophthalmol.* 2004;138:852-62.
2. Lee AG, Johnson MC, Policeni BA, Smoker WR. Imaging for neuro-ophthalmic and orbital disease - a review. *Clin Experiment Ophthalmol.* 2009;37:30-53.
3. Bose S. Neuroimaging in neuroophthalmology. *Neurosurg Focus.* 2007;23:E9.
4. Fuchs T, Kachelriess M, Kalender WA. Technical advances in multi-slice spiral CT. *Eur J Radiol.* 2000;36:69-73.
5. Kalender WA, Seissler W, Klotz E, Vock P. Spiral volumetric CT with single-breath-hold technique, continuous transport, and continuous scanner rotation. *Radiology.* 1990;176:181-3.
6. Flohr TG, Schaller S, Stierstorfer K, Bruder H, Ohnesorge BM, Schoepf UJ. Multi-detector row CT systems and image-reconstruction techniques. *Radiology.* 2005;235:756-73.
7. Zagoria RJ. Iodinated contrast agents in neuroradiology. *Neuroimaging Clin N Am.* 1994;4:1-8.

8. Lee AG, Hayman LA, Ross AW. Neuroimaging contrast agents in ophthalmology. *Surv Ophthalmol*. 2000;45:237-53.
9. Morcos SK, Thomsen HS. Adverse reactions to iodinated contrast media. *Eur Radiol*. 2001;11:1267-75.
10. Grossman CB. Physical principles of computed tomography and magnetic resonance imaging. In: Grayson TH, editor. Magnetic resonance imaging and computed tomography of the head and spine. Baltimore: Williams & Wilkins; 1990. pp. 8-21.
11. Grossman CB. Clinical MR application. In: Grayson TH, editor. Magnetic resonance imaging and computed tomography of the head and spine. Baltimore: Williams & Wilkins; 1990. pp. 41-2.
12. Grossman CB. The Sella region. In: Grayson TH, editor. Magnetic resonance imaging and computed tomography of the head and spine. Baltimore: Williams & Wilkins; 1990. pp. 254- 68.
13. Grossman CB. Clinical computed tomography application. In: Grayson TH, editor. Magnetic resonance imaging and computed tomography of the head and spine. Baltimore: Williams &Wilkins; 1990. pp. 22-37.
14. Mitchell DG, Burk DL Jr, Vinitski S, Rifkin MD. The biophysical basis of tissue contrast in extracranial MR imaging. *Am J Roentgenol*. 1987;149:831-7.
15. Jacobson DM, Trobe JD. The emerging role of magnetic resonance angiography in the management of patients with third cranial nerve palsy. *Am J Ophthalmol*. 1999;128:94-6.
16. Horikoshi T, Fukamachi A, Nishi H, Fukasawa I. Detection of intracranial aneurysms by three-dimensional time-of-flight magnetic resonance angiography. *Neuroradiology*. 1994;36:203-7.
17. Anderson GB, Ashforth R, Steinke DE, Ferdinandy R, Findlay JM. CT angiography for the detection and characterization of carotid artery bifurcation disease. Stroke 2000;31:2168-74.
18. Prokop M, Debatin JF. MRI contrast media—new developments and trends: CTA vs. MRA. Eur Radiol 1997;7(Suppl 5):29-306.
19. Hamed LM, Silbiger J, Silbiger M, Quisling R, Fanous M, Arrington J, et al. Magnetic resonance angiography of vascular lesions causing neuro-ophthalmic deficits. *Surv Ophthalmol*. 1993;37:425-34.
20. Kaufman DI. Magnetic resonance angiography, computed tomographic angiography, conventional angiography—when to use and why: Recent advances in brain angiography and the impact on neuroophthalmology. In: Neuro-ophthalmology subspecialty day course book. New Orleans7 AAO; 2001. pp. 47-52.
21. Kassell NF, Torner JC. Size of intracranial aneurysms. *Neurosurgery*. 1983;12:291.
22. Tampieri D, Leblanc R, Oleszek J, Pokrupa R, Melancon D. Three-dimensional computed tomographic angiography of cerebral aneurysms. *Neurosurgery*. 1995;36:749-55.
23. Hope JK, Wilson JL, Thomson FJ. Three-dimensional CT angiography in the detection and characterization of intracranial berry aneurysms. *Am J Neuroradiol*. 1996;17:439-45.
24. Jager HR, Grieve JP. Advances in non-invasive imaging of intracranial vascular disease. *Ann R Coll Surg Engl*. 2000;82:1-5.
25. Thulborn KR: A BOLD move for fMRI. *Nat Med*. 1998;4:155-6.
26. van den Hoff J: Principles of quantitative positron emission tomography. *Amino Acids*. 2005;29:341-53.

27. Mizoguchi S, Suzuki Y, Kiyosawa M, Mochizuki M, Ishii K: Differential activation of cerebral blood flow by stimulating amblyopic and fellow eye. *Graefes Arch Clin Exp Ophthalmol.* 2005;243:576-82.
28. Moll AC, Hoekstra OS, Imhof SM, Coans EF, Schouten-van Meeteren Ay, van der Valk P, et al: Fluorine-18 fluorodeoxyglucose positron emission tomography (PET) to detect vital retinoblastoma in the eye: preliminary experience. *Ophthalmic Genet.* 2004;25:31-35.
29. Pickard JD, Hutchinson PJ, Coles JP, Steiner LA, Johnston AJ, Fryer TD, et al: Imaging of cerebral blood flow and metabolism in brain injury in the ICU. *Acta Neurochir Suppl.* 2005;95:459-64.
30. Freudenberg LS, Schueler AO, Beyer T, Antoch G, Kuhl H, Bornfeld N, et al: Whole-body fluorine-18 fluordeoxyglucose positron emission tomography/computed tomography (FDGPET/ CT) in staging of advanced uveal melanoma. *Surv Ophthalmol.* 2004;49:537-40.

20

chapter

Shubhra Goel
Ashwin Mohan
Rashmin Gandhi

Giant Cell Arteritis

ABSTRACT

Giant cell arteritis (GCA) is a systemic, sight threatening, medical emergency affecting the large and medium sized vessles and is known to cause blindness. Visual manifestation like transient or complete sudden visual loss is a common mode of presentation. Temporal artery biopsy (TAB) is one of the gold standard for the confirmation of diagnosis. Corticosteroids remain the mainstay of treatment.

Introduction

Giant cell arteritis (GCA) is a systemic, sight threatening, medical emergency known to cause blindness.[1] Visual manifestations like transient or complete sudden visual loss is a common mode of presentation requiring a high index of suspicion. Many newer modalities of investigation like magnetic resonance imaging (MRI), ultrasonography (USG), and fundus fluorescein angiography have been used in aiding diagnosis. Temporal artery biopsy (TAB) remains the gold standard for the confirmation of diagnosis. Corticosteroids remain the mainstay of treatment, although other treatment modalities include methotrexate, aspirin and infliximab.

Historical Perspective

As early as the 10th century, Ali-ibn-Isa of Baghdad described the association of blindness with temporal arteritis[2]. Since then temporal arteritis has been referred to by various names[3], such as giant cell arteritis, Horton's disease, thrombotic arteritis of the aged, cranial arteritis, granulomatous arteritis, and senile arteritis. The first complete description of this disease was given by to Hutchinson in 1890.[4] Later it was reported that the temporal artery biopsy specimens were positive for arteritis in many patients having symptoms of polymyalgia rheumatica[4] and it is suggested that the two may represent the same pathology with different clinical manifestations.

Epidemiology

The incidence of giant cell arteritis shows variability in different studies. The worldwide annual incidence rate of GCA ranges from 1.28 to 29.1 per 100,000 among persons aged 50 years or more.[5] Highest rates are found in th white individuals of northern European descent (e.g. about 30/1000,000 in Norway) and lowest rates are found in African, Asian and Arab populations (e.g. 1.47/100,000 in Japan).[6] The incidence increases with age, with a mean age at presentation of 71 years.[7] In Europe, GCA is the most common form of systemic vasculitis.[1] GCA has rarely been reported in India and there are only sporadic case reports documenting its occurrence. Singh et al[8] have recently reported only 21 patients over a period of 15 years from Mumbai. The disease is more common (2–4 times) in women than men.

Etiology

The etiology of GCA is not known. Genetic, infectious and autoimmune mechanisms are implicated in the etiology. Familial aggregation has been reported in patients with HLA-DR4 suggesting a genetic linkage or hereditary predisposition in patients with giant cell arteritis. Some studies using DNA detection technique implicated *Chlamydia Pneumoniae, Mycoplasma pneumona* and parvovirus B19 for the destrctive arterial lesion.

Two different immunopathogenetic mechanisms underlie the clinical manifestations of GCA. One is a systemic inflammatory reaction that results from the over activation of the innate acute phase response and the other is a maladaptive, antigen specific immune response that directs an attack on the arterial walls and is responsible for the focal ischemic complications of GCA. The innate response is the basis for systemic inflammatory syndrome of GCA while the antigen-specific response mediates the arteritis (Flowchart 20.1). The acute phase response involves a cascade of chemical signals driven in large part by IL-6, which derives from circulating monocytes, neutrophils and macrophages.[9]

A complete understanding of the immunological events that lead to arterial wall inflammation and destruction is not fully established. It is accepted

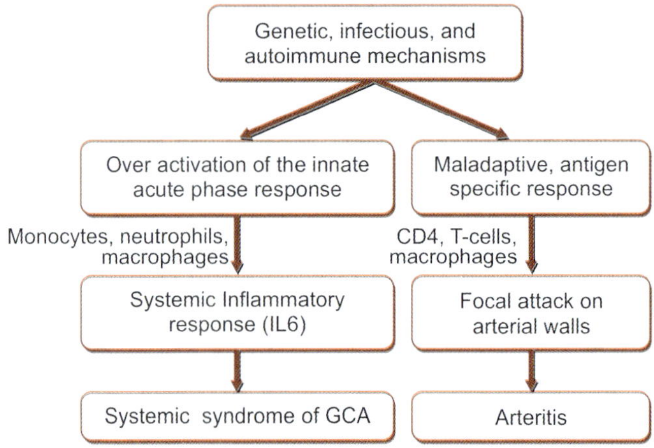

Flowchart 20.1: Immunopathogensis of GCA

that the arteritis of GCA is an adaptive, antigen driven T-cell mediated process; the inflammatory infiltrate is composed mainly of CD4, T-cells and macrophages.[9]

Activation of T-cells, differentiation of macrophages and intimal hyperplasia and vascular occlusion are the main events leading to ischemia in GCA. A definite initiating event for the activation of T-cells is not known. A microbial event has been a popular but still unsubstantiated hypotesis for the activation of T-cells. Another hypothesis states that the triggering element may be an endogenous element in the arterial wall. Once activated, advential T-cells undergo rapid clonal proliferation and recruit macrophages and stimulate giant cell formation. Reactive oxygen metabolites that induce lipid peroxidation for the smooth muscle cell membranes as well as metallo-proteinase enzymes that break down and digest the internal elastic lamina are produced by the macrophages. Once the internal elastic lamina is damaged, migration of smooth muscle cells and their proliferation, under the influence of PDGF cause intimal hyperplasia and vessel occlusion (Flowchart 20.2). Neoagiogenesis driven by VEGF accompanies this event. Thus T-cell differentiation is the chief event in determining the extent and course of the vascular inflammation.[9]

Pathology

Histopathology of the biopsied vessel may present different pictures in the early and late cases of GCA:

Early cases: Infiltration of lymphocytes are found in the internal and external adventitia associated with the thickening of the wall of the arteries.

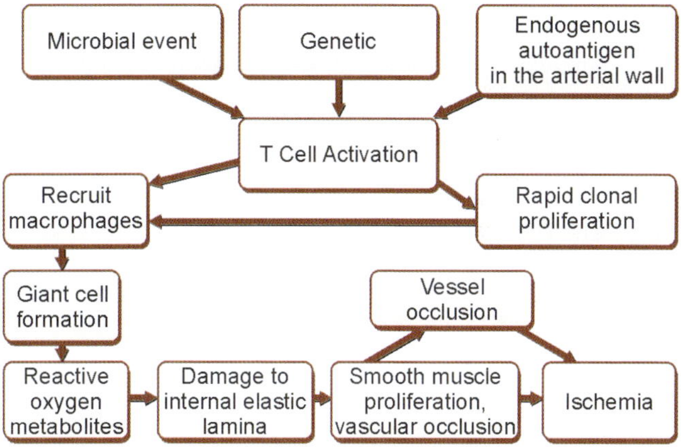

Flowchart 20.2: Immunopathogensis of GCA

Late cases: All layers of the artery are affected—panarteritis (Fig. 20.1). There is a widespread destruction of some portions of arterial wall. The arterial walls are infiltrated with multinucleated histiocytes, foreign giant cells, T-helper cell lymphocytes, and some plasma cells and fibroblasts. The lumen of the vessel may be occluded due to thrombus formation or sub-intimal edema and cellular proliferation.[10] Fragmentation and disintegration of the internal elastic lamina due to digestion by matrix metalloproteinases[11] and patchy degeneration of the smooth muscle cells is found. The vessel walls are characterized by skip lesions.

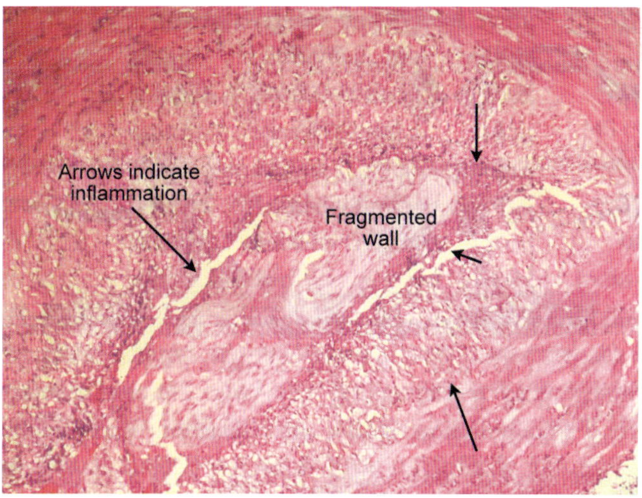

Fig. 20.1: Microphotograph showing the inflammation of the arterial wall with fragmentation and disruption of the internal elastic lamina. (H and E, 20x)

The American College of Rheumatologists have laid down the histological criteria for the diagnosis of GCA which include segmental cellular infiltrates of the vessel wall with predominantly T-helper and suppressor lymphocytes, plasma cells, and macrophages.[12]

Clinical Features

The American College of Rheumatologists (ACR) have defined following five diagnostic criteria for GCA:[13]

1. Age at onset of 50 years or older.
2. Onset of a new headache.
3. Temporal artery tenderness or reduced pulsation.
4. Raised ESR (50 mm/hr by the Westergren method).
5. Histological evidence of necrotizing arteritis in the temporal artery with predominantly mononuclear cell infiltration or granulomatous inflammation usually with multinucleate giant cells.

At least three out of five of the above features should be present for definitive diagnosis of GCA. The presence of three or more features yields a sensitivity of 93.5% and a specificity of 91.2% [1] (Table 20.1).

The onset of giant cell arteritis may be sudden or gradual. It is usually characterized by both systemic and ophthalmic features.

Patient characteristically presents with headaches, anorexia, weight loss, fatigue, malaise, sweating, depression, and arthralgia. Scalp tenderness, aching, stiffness, lower back pain, pain in neck, shoulder and hip are common. Headache of new-onset, characteristically temporal and lancinating in quality is attributed to the stimulation of sensory fibers within inflamed extracranial arteries. It is the most common symptom occurring in up to 90% of patients and tends to be located over the temporal or occipital areas. Fever and respiratory symptom (dry cough) are also common. Other features include enlargement of lymph nodes (50%), glossitis, Raynauld phenomenon,

TABLE 20.1: ACR criteria
• Age at onset of 50 years or older
• Onset of a new headache
• Temporal artery tenderness or reduced pulsation
• Raised ESR (50 mm/hr by the Westergren method)
• Histological evidence of necrotising arteritis in the temporal artery with predominantly mononuclear cell infiltration or granulomatous inflammation usually with multinucleate giant cells
• Any 3 out of 5 should be positive

nonpulsatile prominent temporal arteries, subclavian bruits, and diminished pulse.

In a recent review by Alexandra Villa-Forte[14], four main phenotypes of the disease spectrum have been defined:

1. Cranial arteritis is characterized by headache, visual loss, scalp and temporal tenderness and jaw claudication. Jaw claudication with pain on chewing has been associated with a high number of positive biopsies.[15]
2. Polymyalgia rheumatica is marked by aching of the shoulder and hip girdle with morning stiffness.
3. Nonspecific systemic inflammatory response consists of fever, malaise, night sweats along with very high ESR and C-reactive protein.
4. Large vessel vasculitis causes thoracic aortic aneurysm.

Broadly speaking, two kinds of vessels are affected in GCA. The cranial vessels are affected most frequently followed by large vessel vasculitis also now as extracranial GCA.

In cranial vasculitis, focal inflammation limited to the branches of the carotid arteries occurs most commonly. Scalp necrosis occurs very rarely only if all four vessels supplying the scalp are affected. Internal and external carotid arteries and central retinal arteries are affected less frequently. Intracranial cerebral vasculature is spared in GCA because cerebral arteries lack internal elastic lamina.

In large vessel vasculitis, the inflammation is more aggressive and is limited to or dominated by involvement of the subclavian and axillary arteries and the aorta often and is termed *extracranial large-vessel GCA.*[9]

Ocular Features

The true incidence of ocular involvement in GCA is not known. It is reported that the incidence ranges between 14 and 70%.[1] Transient visual loss, transient repeated episodes of blurred vision, and sudden partial and complete loss of vision are common symptoms. The most common and serious ophthalmic presentation is permanent visual loss (81.2%) in one or both eyes[17] and the common cause for this visual loss in GCA is due to anterior arteritic ischemic optic neuropathy (AAION) resulting from occlusive inflammation in the posterior ciliary arteries causing infarction of the optic nerve head.[18,19] A high percentage of patients with early GCA, can initially present with AAION[16] (Figs 20.2 and 20.3). The optic neuropathy may present with the edema of the optic nerve head, splinter hemorrhages and chalky white optic disk. Amaurosis fugax is commonly caused by transient ischemia of the optic nerve head and can signify impending blindness.[19,21]

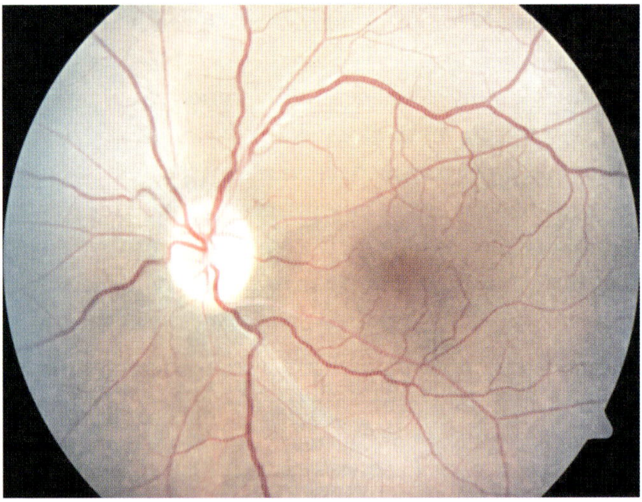

Fig. 20.2: Hyperemia of the optic nerve head can be seen along with blurring of the disk margins

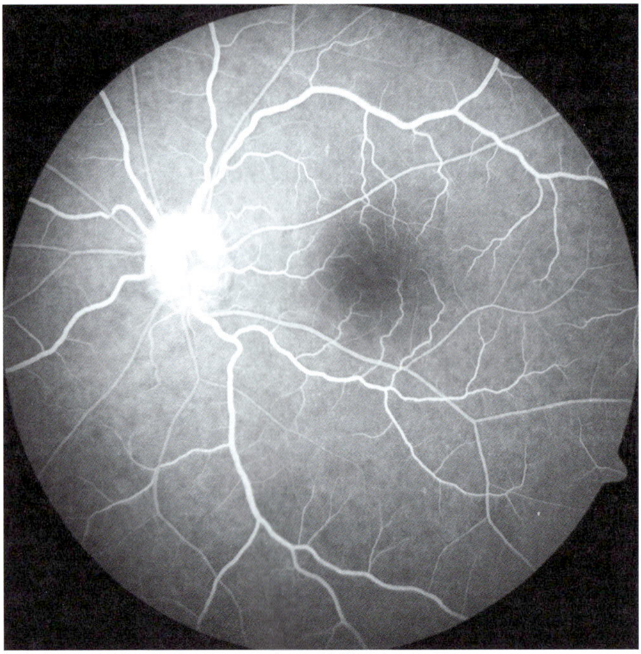

Fig. 20.3: FFA of the same patient showing hyperfluorescence in the superonasal quadrant

In patients presenting with acute visual loss without obvious signs of GCA, it is often confusing to differentiate between posterior arteritic ischemic optic neuropathy (PAION), nonarteritc ischemic optic neuropathy (NAION) and AAION. Some of the salient features which can be useful to differentiate between these are:

1. A normal appearing disc with visual loss and RAPD is suggestive of a PAION.
2. In contrast to NAION, AAION is characterized by more severe visual loss, chalky white optic disc and a positive temporal artery biopsy.

As mentioned earlier, the occlusion of posterior ciliary arteries is most commonly implicated, but involvement of the central or branch retinal arteries and the cilioretinal artery is not uncommon. These will result in filing defects in angiographic studies. Posterior ischemic (retrobulbar) optic neuropathy, central retinal artery occlusion, branch retinal artery occlusion, cilioretinal occlusion and choroidal ischemia can, hence, occur in GCA.

The neuro-ophthalmic manifestations of giant cell arteritis include diplopia, ptosis, nystagmus, pupillary abnormalities and internuclear ophthalmoplegia. Diplopia and ocular motor imbalance occurs in 2–15% of GCA patients due to ischemia of the extraocular muscles, ocular motor nerves or brainstem. On treatment, this diplopia and motor imbalance usually reverts back to normal.[19,20] The characteristic visual AION, an altitudinal defect, usually inferior is commonly found on perimetry. Inferior sectorial field defect and central scotoma are not uncommon.

Differential Diagnosis

The differential diagnosis includes autoimmune vasculitis like polyarteritis nodosa, Wegener's granulomatosis, rheumatoid arthritis and systemic lupus erythematous (SLE). Infection, malignancy and amyloidosis can also present like GCA. At times, trigeminal neuralgia and sinus/dental infections, and optic neuritis can be confused with GCA.[1] GCA can be differentiated based on the histopathology, location of findings and organ involvement (Tables 20.2 and 20.3).

TABLE 20.2: Red flags
• Transient or sudden visual loss
• Recent onset headaches with weight loss
• Associated fatigue, malaise, night sweats and muscle aches

TABLE 20.3: Differential diagnosis

Disease	Feature
NAION	Optic neuropathy
Polyarteritis nodosa	Autoimmune vasculitis
Wegener's granulomatosis	Autoimmune vasculitis
Rheumatoid arthritis	Autoimmune vasculitis
Systemic lupus erythematosus	Autoimmune vasculitis
Malignancy	Vasculitis & vision loss
Amyloidosis	Infiltration and vasculitis
Trigeminal neuralgia	Pain

Diagnosis

Temporal artery biopsy (TAB) is considered as the gold standard for the diagnosis of GCA, and must be performed as soon as a patient is suspected of having GCA or AAION.[16] We know that GCA is characterized by granulomas and skip-lesions; hence, a chance of obtaining a false-negative result do exists. It is generally agreed that an adequate biopsy specimen should have a minimum length of 2 cm.[22] This helps reduce the chance of getting a false negative biopsy. This is a relatively safe surgical procedure, although a chance of hematoma, infection, facial nerve damage and scalp necrosis exists. Treatment must be started as soon as GCA is suspected clinically without waiting for the biopsy to be taken, as the sensitivity is not significantly affected with 2 weeks of starting therapy.[23]

After marking, a sharp dissection is carried out through the subdermal fibrofatty tissue to reach the superficial temporalis fascia. Following the blunt dissection of the superficial temporalis fascia care is taken to locate the branch of the frontal branch of the facial nerve traversing the superficial temporal artery within the superficial temporalis fascia. Superficial temporal artery is separated with blunt dissection underneath it. The artery is ligated inferiorly and superiorly with 4-0 silk. The artery is then dissected and tributaries are cauterized with the radiofrequency cautery. Artery of more than 2 cm is harvested. It is important to palpate the biopsied artery to check for hard lumps or ropiness—suggestive of GCA. Hemostasis is achieved before closure. Wound is sutured in layers (Fig. 20.4).

Fundus fluorescein angiography typically shows filling defects affecting the choroid, which may be patchy or generalized, and peripapillary or peripheral.[26] It is mainly due to inflammatory occlusion of the posterior ciliary arterial supply.

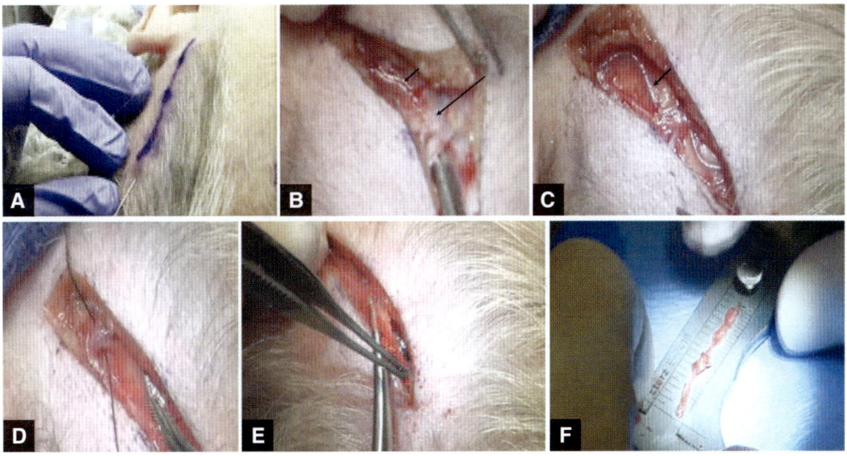

Figs 20.4A to F: Steps of temporal artery biopsy (TAB)

A. Marking of the proposed area for TAB with local infiltration without adrenaline.
B. Separation through the subdermal fibrofatty layer and locating frontal branch of facial nerve (small arrow) at the superficial temporlais fascia (big arrow).
C. Locating the superficial temporalis artery (small arrow) piercing superficial temporalis fascia.
D. Ligation of artery with 4-0 mersilk.
E. Separation of artery from the underlying deep temporalis fascia plane
F. 30 mm of temporal artery harvested

Courtesy: Dr John G Rose, Dean hospital, Madison, Wisconsin, USA

Ultrasonography can also be used as a non invasive diagnostic tool. Schmidt et al detected a hypoechoic halo (halo sign) around the perfused lumen of the temporal artery in 73% of patients with GCA.[27] Sonography is not intended to be a replacement for a temporal artery biopsy in the diagnostic evaluation of GCA. It does, however, play an important role in the evaluation of patients with GCA, some of which includes: providing non-histological evidence of arterial wall inflammation in the extracranial arteries; guiding the biopsy site or finding alternative sites other than the temporal arteries; evaluating the axillary arteries for the presence of large-vessel involvement; and assessing disease activity following treatment.[28]

In a recent study of 64 patients who underwent contrast-enhanced high-resolution MRI, sensitivity and specificity for detecting temporal artery inflammation were 80.6% and 97%, respectively, compared against a positive diagnosis using ACR clinical criteria or histopathological findings.[29]

An elevated ESR strongly supports a clinical suspicion of GCA but a normal ESR does not rule out a diagnosis of GCA. According to the American College of Rheumatology, an ESR by Westergren method is elevated if it is >50 mm D hr. About 85% of patients have an ESR >50 mm D hr and almost all patients have an ESR greater than 20 mm D hr.[24] ESR is highly elevated.

C-reactive proteins (CRP) level is elevated and reflects underlying inflammatory process. CRP greater than 2.45 mg/dl and elevated platelet count show a positive correlation with the temporal artery biopsy. Its advantages over the ESR are faster responsiveness to inflammation (within 4–6 hr), insensitivity to age, gender and hematological factors, and notably higher sensitivity and specificity for GCA in the appropriate clinical setting. The disadvantages of CRP include the higher cost of testing compared to ESR and perhaps a relative unfamiliarity with the test amongst clinicians.[9]

Both ESR and C-reactive proteins are the most sensitive and reliable parameters to monitor GCA and to regulate steroid therapy.[25]

Enzymes alkaline phosphatase and asparate aminotransferase are usually raised. Many patients with GCA present normochromic, normocytic anemia with raised prothromxbin time.

Complications

GCA can lead to permanent blindness in about 60% of patients. Systemic complications of the disease include peripheral neuritis, myopathy, neurologic syndromes, neuropsychiatic syndromes, aortic aneurysm, and regurgitation. Approximately 50% of the patients die suddenly as a result of cerebrovascular accidents.

Treatment

As noted earlier, the natural history of GCA is spontaneous remission. However, the disease activity may smoulder on for months or years before extinguishing. The need for treatment stems from the high rate of morbidity related to ischemic complications caused by GCA, particularly blindness. Treatment of GCA is aimed at controlling and arresting the inflammatory process in order to prevent an ischemic complication such as visual loss, neurological dysfunction or other organ infarction.[9] Thus corticosteroids are the mainstay of treatment. Other drugs like methotrexate, infliximab and aspirin which have immunomodulatory effects have also been tried as second line of management.

CORTICOSTEROIDS

In a retrospective study, corticosteroids have been shown to prevent progression of visual loss.[32] The initial dosing is usually maintained for 4 weeks and then decreased slowly. The duration of therapy varies; most patients remain on therapy for at least 1 year, and some cannot stop it completely without recurrence of symptoms.[14] The following schedule is recommended for corticosteroid therapy:[9]

a. In patients without visual or neurological manifestations who have only rheumatic and systemic symptoms, treatment with oral prednisolone is used and is generally 40–60 mg daily or 1 mg/kg/day.
b. In patients with acute visual or neurological symptoms or signs, higher doses are generally recommendedan equivalent of prednisone 80 mg daily more daily or 1–2 mg/kg/day. Pulse methylprednisolone study conducted by Mazlumzadeh et al shows an equal risk for adverse effects from glucocorticoids.[33]
c. Maintenance: High-dose daily oral prednisone is maintained for at least 4-6 weeks until systemic symptoms have subsided and markers of disease activity (ESR and/ or CRP) have normalized.[9]
d. Tapering and duration: Steroid tapering is a slow process and highly individualized with constant monitoring of symptoms and serum markers.[9] In the study by Hayreh et al[25] after 2 years, more than 92% of patients (with and without visual loss at presentation) were still on steroids, emphasizing the long duration of treatment.

IMMUNOSUPPRESSIVE AGENTS

Given the concern about glucocorticoid toxicity, several studies have evaluated alternative strategies, especially treatment with immunosuppressive drugs. The common side effects of steroid treatment include diabetes, hypertension, secondary infections, osteoporosis and bone fracture, myopathy and psychiatric changes, such as anxiety, depression, confusion and occasionally psychosis.[9] However, no study has confirmed that other medications are effective in the treatment of giant cell arteritis[18]. The following strategies have been attempted.

Methotrexate (MTX)

Two studies performed by Spiera et al[34] and Jover et al[35] showed neither a significant difference in the prednisolone requirement with and without methotrexate, nor a the difference in the adverse effects. In patients with severe adverse reactions to steroids or steroid-refractive disease, MTX is considered a viable second-line alternative.[36]

Infliximab

Infliximab is a tumor necrosis factor-alpha inhibitor. The study by Hoffman et al[37] shows no difference in the relapse rate, but a higher rate of infections, therefore, it drug is not recommended in the treatment of GCA. A recent randomized, prospective placebo-controlled multi-center trial of infliximab as adjunctive treatment in 44 patients with GCA showed no significant benefit.[38]

Aspirin

Daily low-dose aspirin therapy has been shown in several studies to be effective in preventing the ischemic complications of giant cell arteritis, including stroke and visual loss. It is currently recommended that all patients with giant cell arteritis, without a major contraindication, should take aspirin 81 mg daily[14]. A retrospective review of 143 patients with GCA who received either antiplatelet or anticoagulant therapy found a lower incidence of ischemic events with such treatment.[38]

In the light of the treatment trials it may be recommended that the treatment of GCA suspects should be started with prednisolone 1 mg/kg/day and the dose to be increased if the visual loss or optic disc findings are more severe. ESR and CRP levels should guide the tapering of steroids. Methotrexate and pulse methylprednisolone have not shown to have any advantage over prednisolone. Infliximab is ineffective but aspirin 81mg daily has been shown to be beneficial.

Conclusion

Giant cell arteritis is a rare autoimmune disease that can lead to blindness if left undiagnosed and untreated. The important signs of the disease should be known to clinicians especially to help them to detect early cases with high index of suspicion. Appropriate diagnostic tests may confirm the diagnosis. A prompt initiation of treatment may be vision saving.

References

1. Rahman and Rahman. Giant cell (temporal) arteritis: an overview and update. *Surv Ophthalmol.* 2005;50(5):415-28
2. Wood CA: A memorandum book of a tenth century oculist, a translation of Tadkivate Ali Ibn Isa. Chicago: Northwestern University Press. 1936;225-226
3. Hunder. The early history of giant cell arteritis and polymyalgia rheumatica: first descriptions to 1970. *Mayo Clin Proc.* 2006;81(8):1071-83
4. Hutchinson J. Diseases of the arteries. *Arch Surg (London).* 1889-90;1:323.
5. Ramstead CL, Patel AD: Giant cell arteritis in a neuro-ophthalmology clinic in Saskatoon 1998-2003. *Can J Ophthalmol.* 2007:42;295-8.

6. Miller NR: Epidemiology of Giant Cell Arteritis in Arab Population: a 22 year study. *Br J Ophthalmol.* 2007:91;705-6.
7. Nordborg C, Johansson H, Petursdottir V, et al: The epidemiology of biopsy-positive giant cell arteritis: special reference to changes in the age of the population. Rheumatology (Oxford) 2003:42;549-552
8. Singh S et al: Giant cell arteritis in Mumbai. *J Assoc Physicians India.* 2010:58;372-4.
9. Kawasaki A, Purvin V. Giant cell arteritis: an updated review. *Acta Ophthalmologica.* 2009;87(1):13-32.
10. Weyand CM, Goronzy JJ: Pathogenic mechanisms in giant cell arteritis. *Cleve Clin J Med.* 69(Suppl 2) 2002:SII ;28-32
11. Rittner HL, Hafner V, Klimiuk PA, et al: Aldose reductase functions as a detoxification system for lipid peroxidation products in vasculitis. *J Clin Invest.* 1999;103: 1007-13
12. Albert DM, Searl SS, Craft JL: Histologic and ultrastructural characteristics of temporal arteritis. The value of the temporal artery biopsy. *Ophthalmology.* 1982;89: 1111-1126
13. Hunder GG, Bloch DA, Michel BA, et al: The American College of Rheumatology 1990 criteria for the classification of giant cell arteritis. *Arthritis Rheum.* 1990;33:1122-8
14. Villa-Forte. Giant cell arteritis: Suspect it, treat it promptly. *Cleve Clin J Med.* 2011;78(4):265-70
15. Huston KA, Hunder GG, Lie JT, et al: Temporal arteritis: A 25-year epidemiologic, clinical, and pathologic study. *Ann Intern Med.* 1978;88:162
16. Hayreh SS, Podhajsky PA, Zimmerman B: Occult giant cell arteritis: ocular manifestations. *Am J Ophthalmol.* 1998;125:521-6
17. Font C, Cid MC, Coll-Vinent B, et al: Clinical features in patients with permanent visual loss due to biopsy-proven giant cell arteritis. *Br J Rheumatol.* 1997;36: 251-4
18. Hayreh SS, et al: Acute ischemic disorders of the optic nerve: Pathogenesis, clinical manifestations and manage- ment. Ophthalmol Clin North Am 1996:9; 407-42
19. Hayreh SS, Podhajsky PA, Zimmerman B: Ocular manifestations of giant cell arteritis. *Am J Ophthalmol.* 1998;125:509-20
20. Hayreh SS: Ophthalmic features of giant cell arteritis. *Baillieres Clin Rheumatol.* 1991;5:431-59
21. Hayreh SS: Factors influencing blood flow in the optic nerve head. *J Glaucoma.* 1997;6:412-25
22. Carroll SC, Gaskin BJ & Danesh-Meyer HV: Giant cell arteritis. *Clin Exp Ophthalmol.* 2006:34;159-173
23. Achkar AA, Lie JT, Hunder GG, et al: How does previous corticosteroid treatment affect the biopsy findings in giant cell (temporal) arteritis? *Ann Intern Med.* 1994:120;987-92
24. Schmidt WA: Current diagnosis and treatment of temporal arteritis. *Curr Treat Options Cardiovasc Med.* 2006:8;145-151
25. Hayreh SS, Zimmerman B: Management of giant cell arteritis. Our 27-year clinical study: new light on old controversies. *Ophthalmologica.* 2007:217;239-59
26. Mack HG, O'Day J, Currie JN: Delayed choroidal perfusion in giant cell arteritis. *J Clin Neuroophthalmol.* 1991;11:221-7
27. Schmidt WA: Doppler ultrasonography in the diagnosis of giant cell arteritis. *Clin Exp Rheumatol.* 2000:18;540-2

28. Schmidt WA: Technology insight: the role of color and power Doppler ultraso- nography in theumatology. *Nat Clin Pract Rheumatol.* 2007:3;35-42.
29. Bley TA, Uhl M, Carew J, Markl M, Schmidt D, Peter HH, Langer M & Wie-ben O: Diagnostic value of high-resolution MR imaging in giant cell arteritis. *Am J Neuroradiol.* 2007:28;1722-27.
30. Bhatti MT, Tabandeh H: Giant cell arteritis: diagnosis and management. *Curr Opin Ophthalmol.* 2001:12;393-9.
31. Mizen TR, et al: Giant cell arteritis: diagnostic and therapeutic considerations. *Ophthal Clin North Am.* 1991:4;547-56.
32. Birkhead NC, Wagener HP, Shick RM. Treatment of temporal arteritis with adrenal corticosteroids; results in fifty-five cases in which lesion was proved at biopsy. *J Am Med Assoc.* 1957:163;821-7.
33. Mazlumzadeh M, Hunder GG, Easley KA, et al. Treatment of giant cell arteritis using induction therapy with high-dose glucocorticoids: a double-blind, placebo-controlled, randomized prospective clinical trial. *Arthritis Rheum.* 2006:54; 3310-3318.
34. Spiera RF, Mitnick HJ, Kupersmith M, et al. A prospective, double- blind, randomized, placebo controlled trial of methotrexate in the treatment of giant cell arteritis (GCA). *Clin Exp Rheumatol.* 2001:19;495-501.
35. Jover JA, Hernández-García C, Morado IC, Vargas E, Bañares A, Fernández-Gutiérrez B. Combined treatment of giant-cell arteritis with methotrexate and prednisone. a randomized, double-blind, placebo-controlled trial. *Ann Intern Med.* 2001:134;106-114.
36. Hall JK & Balcer L: Giant cell arteritis. *Curr Treat Options Neurol.* 2004:6; 45-53.
37. Hoffman GS, Cid MC, Rendt-Zagar KE, et al. Infliximab-GCA Study Group. Infliximab for maintenance of glucocorticosteroid-induced remission of giant cell arteritis: a randomized trial. *Ann Intern Med.* 2007:146;621-630.
38. Lee MS, Smith SD, Galor A, Hoffman GS. Antiplatelet and anticoagulant therapy in patients with giant cell arteritis. *Arthritis Rheum.* 2006:54; 3306-9.

21

chapter

Karobi Lahiri Coutinho

Radiation Retinopathy

ABSTRACT

Radiation retinopathy follows exposure to radiation in high doses and over a prolonged period. It causes progressive occlusive vasculopathy and manifests as microaneurysm, neovascualarization, exudates, hemorrhages, and macular edema. Anti-VEGF, steroids, and laser have been tried in the management of radiation retinopathy with variable results.

Introduction

Radiation retinopathy is a predictable complication following exposure to any source of radiation. It was first described in 1933 by Stallard following treatment of retinoblastoma. Radiation retinopathy is a slowly progressive occlusive vasculopathy characterized by radiation induced endothelial damage. It appears clinically as microaneurysms, telangiectases, neovascularization, retinal hemorrhage, hard exudates, cotton-wool spots and macular edema.

Etiology

Exposure to any radiation source including external beam and plaque brachytherapy specifically, external beam radiation as treatment for nasopharyngeal, paranasal sinus or orbital tumors, where there is limited protection for the eye, often can lead to clinically significant radiation retinopathy.[1] Plaque brachytherapy in the treatment of intraocular tumors can also cause severe damage to the immediate retina and choroid. Radiation retinopathy is seen following radiation for ocular tumors like retinoblastoma, choroid melanoma, angioma, head and neck cancers, optic nerve sheath meningioma, Hodgkin's lymphoma and ill defined choroidal neovascular membranes (CNVMs). Head and neck irradiation can cause ophthalmic complications like cataracts, optic neuropathy and radiation retinopathy.

Radiation Therapy

RADIATION TIMING AND MODALITY

The optimum timing of therapy (before, during, or after visual changes) and the optimum radiation strategy — lateral port external beam, fractionated conformal, fractionated stereotactic, intensity-modulated radiation therapy (IMRT)—remain evolving concepts.

EFFECTS OF RADIATION TREATMENT

Most systemic side effects are transient and self-limited. They include nausea, vomiting, focal alopecia, swelling, pain, and mild erythematous skin changes. Ocular side effects are less frequent and often delayed; they include radiation retinopathy, optic neuropathy, cataract formation, and dry eye. Cranial nerve dysfunction, pituitary dysfunction, brain necrosis, hearing loss, and new tumor induction can develop after decades.

Recent advances in achieving greater precision for delivering higher isodose levels to smaller volumes of tissue (thereby reducing the dosage to uninvolved tissue) should theoretically reduce side effects to the surrounding tissues.

The duration of follow-up in published cases that detail new techniques is more limited, and the future side effect incidence rate should be determined with a longitudinal follow-up.

Risk Factors

Higher total radiation dose has been shown to increase the risk of radiation retinopathy. The fractionation, field design, type and rate of administration of radiation should also be accounted for. While there are no definite thresholds, estimates for external beam radiation range from 15 to 60 Gy. The incidence of retinopathy increases steadily at doses greater than 45 Gy.[2] Radiation retinopathy has been reported in doses as low as 11 Gy but infrequent below 45 Gy dose. The risk of induction of retinopathy increases with dose used from 25 to 35 Gy. The external beam irradiation is more likely to induce changes.

Hyperfractionation has been associated with a decreased incidence of radiation retinopathy.[3] Patients who receive less than 25 Gy in fractions of 2 Gy or less are unlikely to develop significant retinopathy.

With local or external beam irradiation patients develop retinopathy 6 months to 3 years after treatment.

With plaque brachytherapy, the risk of radiation retinopathy is related to total radiation dose. In the treatment of uveal melanoma, therapeutic apical doses range from 80 to 100 Gy. Factors that affect total radiation dose such as tumor height and location also increase the risk of retinopathy. Tumor thickness greater than 4 mm has been associated with a greater risk for radiation maculopathy.[4] A decreased distance to the fovea has also been associated with decreased time to maculopathy.[5] Increased fraction size correlated with increase in retinal complications.

Comorbidities

Comorbidities such as diabetes, hypertension, autoimmune disorders, concurrent chemotherapy and pregnancy are associated with an increased risk of radiation retinopathy.[6] Risk factors for developing proliferative radiation retinopathy include younger age, preexisting diabetes mellitus and shorter tumor distance from the optic disc.[7] Patients with preexisting vascular diseases such as collagen vascular disease, hypertension, or previous chemotherapy have also been reported to develop radiation retinopathy at even lower doses of radiation.

Pathogenesis

Radiation can cause both acute and chronic effects on retina:

Acute changes occur within 6 hours of radiation and show nuclear pyknosis among rods, and edema in the outer retinal layers.

Chronic changes occur due to endothelial cell injury owing to retinal ischemia resulting in necrosis of the nerve tissue, and fibrovascular proliferation. Exposure of radiation is thought to cause preferential loss of vascular endothelial cells with relative sparing of the pericytes.[8] It is hypothesized that differential sensitivity between endothelial cells and pericytes is the result of direct exposure of the endothelial cells to high ambient oxygen and iron found in the blood which generates free radicals and leads to cell membrane damage.[9] This damage leads to occlusion of capillary beds and microaneurysm formation. The retinal ischemia from areas of retinal nonperfusion ultimately leads to macular edema, neovascularization, vitreous hemorrhage and tractional retinal detachment.

Diagnosis

HISTORY

Patients will have a history of radiation exposure or radiotherapy few months to years ago. Intelligent patients often remember the nature of the disease and mode of therapy. They may give history of malignant melanoma for which radiation therapy, brachytherapy or cobalt plaque therapy was instituted.[10-14] It has been reported that radiation retinopathy can develop anywhere from 1 month to 15 years. However, it most commonly occurs between 6 months and 3 years.[6] Attempts have been made to attenuate the ill effects of radiotherapy by vitreous substitution[15] or by injecting periocular triamcinolone.[16]

PHYSICAL EXAMINATION

Evaluation for radiation retinopathy includes a complete ophthalmologic examination including a dilated funduscopy to look for pathologic features of retinopathy described below.

SYMPTOMS

Patients with early or mild retinopathy may be asymptomatic but advanced disease can present with decreased vision or floaters. Sudden loss of vision after radiation is not rare. Chronic blurring of vision, distorted vision and defective color vision are common.

SIGNS

Dilated funduscopic examination (Fig. 21.1) may reveals the following features:

- Retinal microaneurysms
- Retinal hemorrhages
- Retinal telangiectatic vessels
- Retinal hard exudates
- Macular edema
- Cotton-wool spots
- Retinal neovascularization
- Vitreous hemorrhage
- Tractional retinal detachment
- Capillary dilation
- Capillary closure
- Perivascular sheathing
- RPE atrophy
- Central retinal artery or vein occlusion

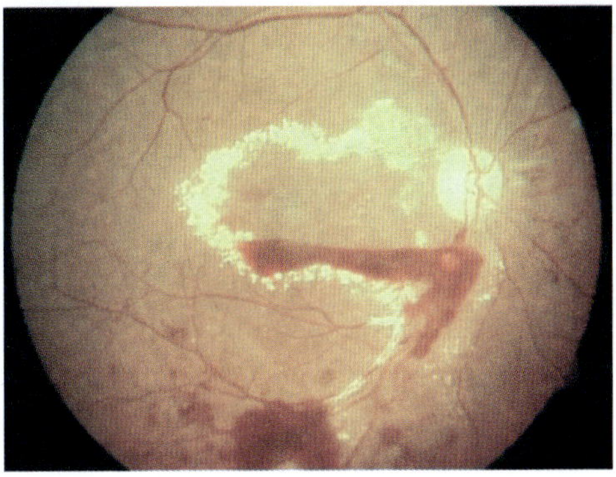

Fig. 21.1: Radiation Retinopathy

Optic disk edema, neovascularization of the iris, neovascularization of the angle, neovascular glaucoma and cataract are associated features of the radiation retinopathy.

Visual impairment ranges from mild to severe and is secondary to macular ischemia or edema. The most severe change is a progressive development of capillary nonperfusion (CPN) areas in periphery and posterior pole. These features are similar to changes in diabetic retinopathy with exception that microaneurysms are less frequent in radiation retinopathy. RPE atrophy due to vaso-obliteration is seen in radiation retinopathy.

In proliferative retinopathy, ischemia is seen in area that receives highest dose of radiation as compared to nasal location and diabetic retinopathy. Latency by radiation exposure and clinical manifestations of vascular changes may range either from 3 weeks to 7 years or 6 months to 3 years.

Macular changes include hard exudates, cystoid and noncystoid edema, and serous detachment that can lead to significant visual loss.

Optic neuropathy occurs in the acute phase which is marked by disk edema, intraretinal hemorrhages, hard exudates, and presence of subretinal fluid (SRF). The optic nerve appears progressively pale and atrophic with variable visual acuity during a few weeks or months.

BIOMICROSCOPY

Biomicroscopic examination may show conjunctival hemorrhage, conjunctival scars, signs of dry eye, symblepharon, corneal aberrations, corneal opacification, anterior uveitis, and cataract.

FINGER CLASSIFICATION

Radiation retinopathy is classified according to Finger in to 4 stages:

- Stage 1: It is located outside the macula and visual acuity is good.
- Stage 2: It is located at the macula and has guarded prognosis.
- Stage 3: It presents some vision loss and carries a severe risk of neo-vascularization, macular edema, and retinal ischemia.
- Stage 4: Any of the above combination with vitreous hemorrhage and retinal ischemia can affect vitreous, macula and extra macular area (> or = to 5 DA).

DIAGNOSTIC PROCEDURES

Fundus fluorescein angiogram can be helpful in highlighting the microvascular features of radiation retinopathy.

Indocyanine green angiography can reveal precapillary arteriolar occlusion and areas of choroidal hypoperfusion.

Optical coherence tomography (OCT) can be helpful in evaluating macular edema. A study by Horgan et al found that OCT was able to detect evidence of macular edema approximately 5 months earlier than clinically detectable radiation maculopathy.[17]

Differential Diagnosis

Following conditions should be considered in the differential diagnosis of radiation retinopathy:

- Diabetic retinopathy
- Branch retinal vein occlusion
- Central retinal vein occlusion
- Hypertensive retinopathy
- Coats' disease
- Perifoveal telangiectasia.

Management

MEDICAL

Anti-VEPF Therapy

Vascular endothelial growth factor (VEGF) is a secreted protein that promotes vascular leakage and angiogenesis.[18] Bevacizumab is a humanized monoclonal antibody to VEGF. Several studies have examined the use of intravitreal bevacizumab (1.25 mg in 0.05 ml) in the treatment of radiation retinopathy and maculopathy;[18-21] and demnstrated an improvement in macular edema following intravitreal bevacizumab though a sustained decrease often required multiple injections. However, visual acuity was not found to improve significantly in most of the studies. Anti-VEGF agents can decrease edema, hemorrhages, exudates, microaneurysms and may improvement of visual acuity with decrease of macular edema.

Finger et al[19] reported on a series of 21 patients in which intravitreal bevacizumab (1.25 mg/0.05 mL) was injected every 6–12 weeks. At a mean follow-up of 7.8 months, 18 patients (86%) had improvement or stabilization of visual acuity, and three (14%) improved by two or more lines of vision. The authors also reported improvement in vascular leakage as determined by fluorescein angiography. Another report by the same group[20] investigated the usc of ranibizumab for radiation retinopathy in five patients. A mean of 8.2 injections of ranibizumab (0.5 mg) was given over a mean follow-up of 8 months. Visual acuity improved by a mean of six letters, with four patients showing a modest improvement on average of 9.5 letters, and one patient losing seven letters. A decrease in vascular leakage and macular edema was seen, and CMT thickness decreased from 416 µm to 270 µm, a 35% reduction. Adverse effects were minimal, including subconjunctival hemorrhage at the injection site and transient post-injection IOP elevations. These studies show that periodic dosing, such as is used in treatment of AMD, may be beneficial in sustaining a treatment effect.

At Bascom Palmer Eye Institute, a study[21] was performed on a series of patients who were given 5,496 intravitreal bevacizumab injections for radiation retinopathy. Based on the observations, it was concluded that early identification of radiation retinopathy (using OCT), followed by early treatment, results in stability and often improvement. It was also observed that combined therapy with triamcinolone and bevacizumab, in the radiation-induced macular edema, possibly has a synergistic effect. Contrary to earlier reports, a limited usefulness of anti-VEGF agents in radiation retinopathy was found on a longer follow-up. These preliminary reports and observations, therefore, warrant further studies to define the precise role of these agents in the management of radiation retinopathy.

Triamcinolone Acetonide Therapy

Triamcinolone acetonide is thought to downregulate various cytokines and regulate capillary permeability. It is used to treat macular edema secondary to various retinal pathologies and has similarly been used to treat radiation maculopathy. While the data is limited, some studies suggest that intravitreal triamcinolone acetonide (4 mg/0.1 ml) does transiently reduce macular edema and improve visual acuity.[22,23] Further studies are needed to determine whether these results are sustainable and whether the benefit of frequent injections outweigh the known risks of glaucoma, cataract and endophthalmitis.

LASER

Grid Macular Laser Photocoagulation

Grid macular laser photocoagulation has been used to treat radiation maculopathy with variable success. Studies by Kinyoun et al[24] and Hykin et al[25] demonstrated a beneficial effect of photocoagulation in visual acuity. However, the effect was not sustained with longer follow-up in the study conducted by Hykin et al.

Sector Scatter and Panretinal Laser Photocoagulation

Sector scatter and panretinal laser photocoagulation have also been used to treat nonproliferative and proliferative radiation retinopathy. In a study by Finger et al., patients received sector scatter laser photocoagulation at the first sign of retinopathy, proliferative or nonproliferative.[26] Retinopathy regressed in 64% of their treated patients. Similarly, in a study by Bianciotto et al. panretinal photocoagulation was found to cause regression of neovascularization in 66% of eyes with proliferative radiation retinopathy.[7] There are also case reports of successful treatment of radiation retinopathy using hyperbaric oxygen[27] and oral pentoxifylline.[28]

SURGERY

Advanced proliferative radiation retinopathy complicated by vitreous hemorrhage and/or tractional retinal detachment may require pars plana vitrectomy.

Conclusion

Radiation is a time-honored treatment for intraocular tumors. The resultant radiation retinopathy is a well known formidable complication, which has no effective treatment. The retinopathy with macular edema must be detected early. Currently, intravitreal triamcinolone, repetitive treatment with anti-VEGF drugs, a combined therapy and laser photocoagulation are recommended to reduce macular edema and improve visual acuity. However, these modalities particularly anti-VEGF and corticosteroids, warrant further evaluation. Preventive PRP or avastin injection is helpful in prevention of neovascularization of retina, vitreous hemorrhage and neovascular glaucoma.

To date there is no prevention of radiation retinopathy except to fractionate the doses and decrease the total cumulative dose of radiation.

References

1. Yanoff M, Duker JS, Augsburger JJ. *Ophthalmology*. 2nd ed. St. Louis, MO: Mosby; 2004.
2. Parsons JT, Bova FJ, Fitzgerald CR, Mendenhall WM, Million RR. Radiation retinopathy after external-beam irradiation: analysis of time-dose factors. *Int J Radiat Oncol Biol Phys*. Nov 15 1994;30(4):765-73.
3. Monroe AT, Bhandare N, Morris CG, Mendenhall WM. Preventing radiation retinopathy with hyperfractionation. *Int J Radiat Oncol Biol Phys*. Mar 1 2005;61(3):856-64.
4. Stack R, Elder M, Abdelaal A, Hidajat R, Clemett R. New Zealand experience of I125 brachytherapy for choroidal melanoma. *Clin Experiment Ophthalmol*. Oct 2005;33(5):490-94.
5. Puusaari I, Heikkonen J, Kivela T. Ocular complications after iodine brachytherapy for large uveal melanomas. *Ophthalmology*. Sep 2004;111(9):1768-77.
6. Durkin SR, Roos D, Higgs B, Casson RJ, Selva D. Ophthalmic and adnexal complications of radiotherapy. *Acta Ophthalmol Scand*. May 2007;85(3): 240-50.
7. Bianciotto C, Shields CL, Pirondini C, Mashayekhi A, Furuta M, Shields JA. Proliferative radiation retinopathy after plaque radiotherapy for uveal melanoma. *Ophthalmology*. May;117(5):1005-12.
8. Archer DB, Amoaku WM, Gardiner TA. Radiation retinopathy—clinical, histopathological, ultrastructural and experimental correlations. *Eye*. 1991;5 (Pt 2):239-51.
9. Archer DB, Gardiner TA. Ionizing radiation and the retina. *Curr Opin Ophthalmol*. Jun 1994;5(3):59-65.
10. Damato B, Patel I, Campbell IR, Mayles HM, Errington RD. Visual acuity after Ruthenium (106) brachytherapy of choroidal melanomas. *Int J Radiat Oncol Biol Phys*. Oct 1 2005;63(2):392-400.
11. Puusaari I, Heikkonen J, Kivela T. Effect of radiation dose on ocular complications after iodine brachytherapy for large uveal melanoma: empirical data and simulation of collimating plaques. *Invest Ophthalmol Vis Sci*. Oct 2004;45(10):3425-34.
12. Char DH, Lonn LI, Margolis LW. Complications of cobalt plaque therapy of choroidal malanomas. *Am J Ophthalmol*. Oct 1977;84(4):536-41.
13. Stallard HB. Radiotherapy for malignant melanoma of the choroid. *Br J Ophthalmol*. Mar 1966;50(3):147-55.
14. Horgan N, Shields CL, Mashayekhi A, Teixeira LF, Materin MA, Shields JA. Early macular morphological changes following plaque radiotherapy for uveal melanoma. *Retina*. Feb 2008;28(2):263-73.
15. Oliver SC, Leu MY, DeMarco JJ, Chow PE, Lee SP, McCannel TA. Attenuation of iodine 125 radiation with vitreous substitutes in the treatment of uveal melanoma. *Arch Ophthalmol*. Jul;128(7):888-93.

16. Horgan N, Shields CL, Mashayekhi A, et al. Periocular triamcinolone for prevention of macular edema after plaque radiotherapy of uveal melanoma: a randomized controlled trial. *Ophthalmology*. Jul 2009;116(7):1383-90.
17. Mason JO, 3rd, Albert MA, Jr., Persaud TO, Vail RS. Intravitreal bevacizumab treatment for radiation macular edema after plaque radiotherapy for choroidal melanoma. *Retina*. Sep 2007;27(7):903-7.
18. Finger PT, Chin K. Anti-vascular endothelial growth factor bevacizumab (avastin) for radiation retinopathy. *Arch Ophthalmol*. Jun 2007;125(6):751-6.
19. Finger PT. Radiation retinopathy is treatable with anti-vascular endothelial growth factor bevacizumab (Avastin). *Int J Radiat Oncol Biol Phys*. Mar 15 2008;70(4):974-7.
20. Gupta A, Muecke JS. Treatment of radiation maculopathy with intravitreal injection of bevacizumab (Avastin). *Retina*. Jul-Aug 2008;28(7):964-8.
21. Cavalcante LL, Cavalcante ML, Murray TG, et al. Intravitreal injection analysis at the Bascom Palmer Eye Institute: evaluation of clinical indications for the treatment and incidence rates of endophthalmitis. *Clin Ophthalmol*. 2010;4:519-24.
22. Shields CL, Demirci H, Dai V, et al. Intravitreal triamcinolone acetonide for radiation maculopathy after plaque radiotherapy for choroidal melanoma. *Retina*. Oct-Nov 2005;25(7):868-74.
23. Sutter FK, Gillies MC. Intravitreal triamcinolone for radiation-induced macular edema. *Arch Ophthalmol*. Oct 2003;121(10):1491-3.
24. Kinyoun JL, Zamber RW, Lawrence BS, Barlow WE, Arnold AM. Photocoagulation treatment for clinically significant radiation macular oedema. *Br J Ophthalmol*. Feb 1995;79(2):144-9.
25. Hykin PG, Shields CL, Shields JA, Arevalo JF. The efficacy of focal laser therapy in radiation-induced macular edema. *Ophthalmology*. Aug 1998;105(8):1425-9.
26. Finger PT, Kurli M. Laser photocoagulation for radiation retinopathy after ophthalmic plaque radiation therapy. *Br J Ophthalmol*. Jun 2005;89(6):730-8.
27. Gall N, Leiba H, Handzel R, Pe'er J. Severe radiation retinopathy and optic neuropathy after brachytherapy for choroidal melanoma, treated by hyperbaric oxygen. *Eye*. Jul 2007;21(7):1010-12.
28. Gupta P, Meisenberg B, Amin P, Pomeranz HD. Radiation retinopathy: the role of pentoxifylline. *Retina*. 2001;21(5):545-7.

Index

Page numbers followed by *f* refer to figure and *t* refer to table

C

D